"As a long-time adult patient, and parent of a son also diagnosed, I am so happy to have this supportive resource. It is an important contribution to the awareness of the complexities of living with and managing a disease that is little known, even in medical circles. This invaluable compendium of information will be helpful not only to families, patients, and caregivers, but also the medical community, schools and resource people."
—Jean Shepherd, retired Deaf Educator

Living Well with Mitochondrial Disease

A Handbook for Patients, Parents, and Families

Cristy Balcells, R.N., M.S.N.

"This is the book I wish I had been given when my daughter was diagnosed with mitochondrial disease and the resource I've been looking for every since. Balcells's unique perspective as both a Mito parent and a medical practitioner results in advice that is personal and practical, compassionate and comprehensive, accessible and expert. After reading the book I understand so much more about my daughter's illness and feel better equipped to serve as her advocate. Balcells defines the ideal 'Mito Survival Kit'; the only thing she left out was this book!"
—Jessica Fein, mother of a six-year-old daughter with mitochondrial disease

"Parents of children with mitochondrial disease face a two-fold challenge—supporting their families and navigating a complex medical care system. What better person to 'sherpa' parents through this process than a mother of a child with mitochondrial disease, a nurse, and a foundation leader. Cristy is all three. As a CEO of a pharmaceutical company developing drugs for mitochondrial disease, I have experienced first-hand the challenges families and care providers face in creating a unified standard of care, and family and physician resources. This is a long overdue body of work that needs to become a living document to guide care, and serve as a benchmark for best practices."
—Guy Miller, MD, CEO & Founder of Edison Pharma

Woodbine House 2012

D1131865

© 2012 Cristy Balcells

Publisher & Author's Disclaimer: The purpose of this book is education and support. The information contained in this book is not intended as a substitute for consultation with your (or your child's) health-care providers. Although the author, editor, and publisher made every attempt to ensure that the information in this book was up to date and accurate at the time of publication, recommended treatments and drug therapies may change as new medical or scientific information becomes available. Additionally, the author, editor, and publisher are not responsible for errors or omissions or for consequences from application of this book. Any practice described in this book should be applied by the reader in close consultation with a qualified physician.

Library of Congress Cataloging-in-Publication Data

Balcells, Cristy, 1974-
 Living well with mitochondrial disease : a handbook for patients, parents, and families / Cristy Balcells. -- 1st ed.
     p. cm.
 Includes bibliographical references and index.
 ISBN 978-1-60613-014-8
 1. Mitochondrial pathology. I. Title.
 RB147.5.B35 2012
 616.042--dc23
                                                                    2011046335

Printed in the United States of America

First edition
10 9 8 7 6 5 4 3 2

For Eva

Table of Contents

Introduction &
Chapter Outline

Who Can Use this Book:

If you, your child, or someone in your life has been given a diagnosis of mito-chondrial disease, consider this book a personal gift from a friend. Like an atlas you might receive before embarking on a world tour, this book is the roadmap for your journey. While we don't know where this diagnosis will take us, we know that a pocket companion can be a compass when we are lost. This book is also your refreshment along the way, giving you positive encouragement and practical information to help you move forward. *Living Well with Mitochondrial Disease* will help you not only un-derstand what it means to you or a loved one to have mitochondrial disease, but also change how you live by teaching you to manage symptoms, understand and imple-ment recommended treatments, and overcome emotional challenges inherent to this complex diagnosis.

Mitochondria affect all of us by making the energy for our bodies to work and play. There are many people in a community that can benefit from knowing how to live with and understand mitochondrial disease. In particular, this guide will be espe-cially useful for those who are directly affected by mitochondrial disease, including:

- parents of children with a mitochondrial disorder, including complex defects, mtDNA mutations, Mito-Autism, PDCD, POLG mutations, and abnormal mitochondria (such as depletions or deletions);

- adult patients diagnosed with mitochondrial disorders, including those above as well as other types, such as MELAS and MERFF;
- anyone—patient or caregiver—facing a suspected or potential mitochondrial disease diagnosis;
- spouses of adult patients;
- teens learning about and living with mitochondrial disease;
- parents of children with autism (including ASD, Aspergers Syndrome, PDD, PDD-NOS) who also have "unexplained" medical issues;
- mothers who are also symptomatic or have some symptoms but don't have a true mitochondrial disease diagnosis;
- fathers of children with mitochondrial disease, and men with family history of mitochondrial disease; and
- family members, including siblings, grandparents, aunts, and uncles supporting a child or loved one dealing with the diagnosis.

In the same vein, think of all of the people who play a role in the everyday lives of those who are directly affected by Mito. This book is also very useful for:

- home health nurses, patient care aides, babysitters, and caregivers helping a person with suspected or diagnosed mitochondrial disease;
- therapists, including physical therapists, occupational therapists, speech therapists, and developmental specialists;
- school nurses, teachers, individual aides, and special education directors educating a child with mitochondrial disease;
- family advocates and individuals involved in legislation and policy-making for genetic diseases; and
- friends interested in helping a family struggling with the disease.

Finally, it should be noted that there are many individuals among us who are walking around with a misdiagnosis. Many of these children and adults may actually have mitochondrial disease that, due to the complexity of the diagnosis, has not been accurately identified. Consequently, this book is also useful for:

- adults with chronic fatigue syndrome, multiple sclerosis, muscular dystrophy, early-onset Alzheimer's disease, or Parkinson's;
- adult patients, teens, spouses, and parents of children with a history of "unexplained," "unrelated" health problems that are getting worse with time;
- parents of children who are "failure to thrive," developmentally delayed, very weak or tired, intolerant of heat and exercise, and who do not have a definitive diagnosis;
- spouses of adults who suffered from strokes at a young age, deteriorating memory, and muscle weakness, all of which cannot be explained; and
- anyone who suffers from unexplained fatigue, muscle weakness, exercise intolerance, and has unexplained "health issues," such as severe constipation, migraine headaches, frequent nausea and vomiting, dizziness, vision or hearing loss, and pain.

How to Use this Book:

If you are confused or a little panicked by the diagnosis (or possible diagnosis) of mitochondrial disease, you are not alone! I have a few suggestions for you on how to approach the chapters in this book.

1. Go straight to the chapters most relevant to you. Are you or your child suffering from so many confusing and upsetting symptoms that you can barely make it through the day? Go straight to the chapters on symptom management (Chapter 5) and treatment (Chapter 4). On the other hand, perhaps you are the type of person who really needs to understand the big picture of what you are facing in order to be able to process it and move forward. You will benefit from the chapters that explain the biochemistry of mitochondrial disease (Chapters 1 and 10). Facing a muscle biopsy, or decision about diagnosis, in the immediate future? Get all the facts in the chapter on the journey to a diagnosis (Chapter 2). Fill your heart and your head with the information that you need to know, based on where you are in this process, first.

2. Once you feel more empowered by answering your most pertinent questions, step back and begin again at the beginning. Take time to read each chapter, as each is filled with patient stories, real examples, and practical tips and advice on top of the information consolidated by topic.

3. Use the glossary at the back of the book. The glossary is extremely comprehensive, and was written with careful attention to define medical terms in "plain English." When you come across an unfamiliar word, take a second and go to the glossary.

4. Use this book as a reference. Keep it handy so that when new symptoms or issues arise, you can look them up. Share specific chapters with teachers, nurses, and clinicians as appropriate.

5. Take the examples and analogies in this book and use them to teach the people around you about mitochondrial disease, and what living with Mito means. Use the numerous examples of how mitochondria act as energy sources like batteries to help doctors, nurses, friends, therapists, teachers, legislators, and family learn about your life with Mito.

6. Prepare yourself for important appointments. If you can speak the same language as the doctors making decisions about your health, or as your child's teacher and principal, you are so much better equipped to be able to move forward. Use this book as a crash-course or as a refresher before these meetings, just as you would prep by reviewing material before a test.

7. Remember to use this book as a pick-me-up as well as a resource guide. *Living Well with Mitochondrial Disease* was not written with the intention of being an impersonal textbook. Instead, this book was

written tenderly, knowing that there are dark moments on the path when you or someone you care about has mitochondrial disease. This book should not only explain different aspects of the disease, it should also help you mentally and emotionally refocus and recharge. When you need a pep talk, inspiration, and ideas about what you can do to start feeling better, go to this book.

What This Book Covers—Chapter Outline

Chapter 1: What is Mitochondrial Disease?

There exists a connection between mitochondria and virtually everything about life as we know and understand it. This chapter provides the basic answers to the questions we all have about mitochondrial disease, including what are the hallmark symptoms, who does it affect, what causes it, and why is it so hard to diagnose. Further, this chapter revisits high school biology to explain what our mitochondria do, i.e., what really happens from the time we eat our breakfast until it is converted into usable energy. Technical and confusing concepts of energy metabolism, including genetic inheritance patterns, oxidative phosphorylation, and the electron transport chain are explained in terms that make sense to lay readers. The mitochondria have long been understood to be the "powerhouses of the cell" but scientists are still uncovering the relationship between mitochondrial function, aging, and disease.

Chapter 2: The Journey to Diagnosis and Understanding the Causes

Misdiagnosis is very common with Mito. In fact, because the symptoms can affect so many body systems and be so perplexing, adult patients are often stereotyped as hypochondriacs and parents of children with Mito are often unfortunately scrutinized as child abusers. Diagnosis of mitochondrial disease is highly complex and involves a range of invasive and upsetting tests including MRI, multiple blood tests, and biopsies of the skin and muscle. Many readers may be waiting for a diagnosis or for test results, investigating a possible Mito diagnosis for themselves, their child, or their loved one, or have been assigned a "suspected" diagnosis based on their symptoms. Recommendations of the most efficient and effective methods in order to solidify a diagnosis are offered in detail. This chapter also examines various diagnostic techniques, and takes a detailed look at each test and what the findings may mean. It provides clear information on the existing classifications of mitochondrial disease and what they mean. Descriptive explanations of where and how mitochondrial defects occur help readers understand the "big picture" surrounding a diagnosis of mitochondrial disease.

Chapter 3: Accepting the Diagnosis and Learning to Live WELL with Mito

For adults, children, and caregivers, there is a natural tendency to be overwhelmed, frenetic even, when trying to understand volumes of complex test results while watching symptoms fluctuate out of control. This chapter puts you back on solid ground by providing practical tips that can be put to use right away and helps patients and families find their footing when they get lost. Patient stories in sidebars help demonstrate the spectrum of mitochondrial disease and show that "quality of life" is defined many different ways.

Chapter 4: Approaches to Treatment, Including Vitamins, Supplements, and Therapies

Pharmacists and physicians call the slurry of vitamins, amino acid supplements, and medical foods that are a recommended daily regimen for mitochondrial disease patients a "Mito cocktail." The ingredients of the Mito cocktail vary depending on where the defect in the energy metabolism mechanism occurs (if it can be identified), and dosing is typically 1,000 to 10,000 times more than the recommended daily allowance for a healthy person. Dosing is very important, and each compound has unique properties that a patient should understand, especially when taking the supplements in hopes of slowing disease progression and stabilizing symptoms. Recommendations regarding therapeutic levels, how to take the Mito cocktail, tips for better absorption, possible side effects, how to have insurance cover the expense, and where to get the Mito cocktail, including helpful pharmacies and companies, are described in this chapter.

Chapter 5: Managing and Preventing Symptoms

Different expressions and related symptoms of each mitochondrial diagnosis are described at length in this chapter. The premise of "symptom management" is introduced, and teaches parents, patients, and caregivers the process of learning to recognize and identify symptoms. Home health teaching and advice helps patients and parents learn to watch blood pressure, heart rate, thirst, fatigue level, and fine motor coordination as part of a daily approach to maintaining an optimum baseline. Advice on energy management approaches during periods of illness or stress is outlined in detail, along with an explanation of how common colds, heat, infections, and stress affect the adult or child with mitochondrial disease differently than healthy individuals. This chapter also outlines important information regarding pre-op/post-op surgical protocol and a protocol for dehydration.

Chapter 6: Children & Teens with Mitochondrial Disease

This chapter gives parents the hope they need to face a devastating and complex medical diagnosis and survive in a medical community that is still learning about Mito, and that does not know how to serve their children. Stories and examples of real children and families help illustrate the various symptoms most common for children. Parents who struggle with finding "normal" for their child will appreciate the practical advice for approaching everything from feeding and keeping your baby well hydrated, to early intervention therapies, to school obstacles and IEPs, puberty, and well-meaning comments, such as "You must be such a wonderful mother/father to have a child like that." Parents who have learned to guide their family with a loving heart and hope offer their stories as well as inspiration and insight into how a devastating diagnosis can actually be a blessing for your family.

Chapter 7: Adults with Mitochondrial Disease

Mito was once described as a pediatric condition, and many physicians are still slow to recognize the onset of adult mitochondrial disease. Adult patients are forced to be their own advocates, making difficult choices about keeping their jobs and caring for their families, finding insurance coverage and medical support, and keeping an optimistic attitude. Adult patients face some distinct challenges as well as some misconceptions. Patient vignettes and quotes add a degree of richness to this chapter and directly address the adult patient's biggest complaint, "*I am all alone.*"

Chapter 8: Autism and Mitochondrial Disease: Special Challenges and the Diagnosis Debate

In the landmark 2008 case of Hannah Poling, the United States government conceded that nine-year-old Hannah's autism-mitochondrial disease was triggered by the administration of multiple vaccines at her two-year-old checkup, and that the physiologic stress of the vaccines triggered her behavioral symptoms. Suddenly, thousands of parents of children with autism began to question if mitochondrial disease could be the root cause of their child's autism. Subsequent clinical research studies, cohort studies, case studies, and expert opinions have brought further debate, along with an estimate that between 6-20 percent of children with autism also have a mitochondrial disease (which may or may not have been diagnosed yet).

This chapter outlines the history of the autism-mitochondrial disease connection, details the similarities as well as distinct differences between the two diagnoses independent of each other, addresses the vaccine debate, compares the DAN! Protocol with supplements commonly used to treat Mito, and includes personal stories from parents of children with this dual-diagnosis.

Chapter 9: Your Mito "Survival Kit"

"But you don't look sick!" is what parents of affected children and adult patients often hear. Many adults and children with Mito defy every medical norm, and are subject to frequent life-threatening hospitalizations that make having a "normal" life impossible. How can parents and patients be advocates for themselves without falling into the abyss of depression and frustration? "Looking normal" is a constant challenge that parents and adult patients alike share as they try to navigate their world with a "low battery," life-threatening symptoms, and no energy. This chapter will teach you to pack and plan ahead for daily obstacles, organize and keep up-to-date medical records, use a multi-disciplinary approach to treatment, make difficult decisions about things like moving and palliative care and hospice options, keep your perspective, and be an active participant in the Mito community.

Chapter 10: Mitochondrial Biochemistry

A more in-depth look at the science behind mitochondrial function, energy production, and the mitochondrial disease process is offered. The structure and function of the mitochondria are explored in detail in order to help the reader understand every reaction that occurs within the cell in order to make energy. Important components of energy metabolism are defined, including ATP, ADP, CoQ10, glucose, the electron transport chain complexes, and oxidative phosphorylation. Along with the biochemistry of mitochondrial function, the potential for mitochondrial defects, mitochondrial dysfunction, and ideas related to aging and slowing disease processes are described.

Note: In an effort to make the information in this book more readable, gender is alternated by chapter. Also, the names of people in the case studies have been changed to protect their identities.

Author's Note

When my daughter Eva was born, my other children were only two and four years old. My husband was finishing his fellowship in cardiology, I had just finished graduate school in nursing and public health, and we were beginning a new business. Initially, I thought that Eva was just a very sleepy newborn. She napped a lot, and often fell asleep while I was nursing her. I had a lot of experience helping new moms learn about breastfeeding and infant development from my background as a maternal-child health nurse, so I felt confident in my ability to nurture and nourish Eva.

Unfortunately, Eva stopped gaining weight completely by the time she was three months old. She seemed exhausted all of the time. She was still so small, only eleven pounds at three months. By the time she was six months old, she was still only responding to her environment like a newborn. I knew something was wrong, but no one except my husband believed me. Her pediatrician sent us to have a gastroenterology consult because she was so constipated and could barely eat two tiny spoonfuls of rice cereal without gagging and going to sleep. At that appointment, the GI doctor told me that if I gave her formula and tried harder, she would gain weight and catch up on her milestones. She sent me away with a sample of Enfamil®.

Six weeks later, Eva still hadn't gained weight and continued to be very, very weak. She could barely hold her head up at seven months of age, when she should have been vigorously crawling. I remember taking her outside to the park with our other children and becoming frantic as I watched her get more and more overheated despite lying still in a shaded stroller. That was the first time I realized that I had never seen her sweat, and I knew that something was really wrong. Eva's health issues would not be solved by eating more or switching to formula!

We pushed the gastroenterologist to run lab tests. She ran basic metabolic profiles, which didn't tell us much except that Eva's blood levels were abnormally acidotic. Eva was hospitalized. Even in the hospital, she still didn't get better. After struggling to determine the cause of Eva's abnormal tests, the pediatrician looked me straight in the eye and asked, "What are you giving her that is poisonous?" I was incredulous and simultaneously devastated. The best that our medical system had to offer my sick daughter was to automatically assume it must be my fault?

My husband and I began actively calling in favors with everyone we knew from our years of medical training. We became Eva's advocates, and were relentless in asking questions and seeing specialists with hopes of figuring out what we could do to help our baby. During Eva's first year, we lived with several misdiagnoses, including cerebral palsy and renal tubular acidosis.

We began physical therapy and sought early intervention services for Eva when a friend whose daughter had autism encouraged me to get help. Eva's therapists were my lifeline. They could push her in ways that I couldn't; they could envision her being able to crawl, walk, and talk one day…while I was too afraid to imagine anything at all.

We finally met with a metabolic specialist who suggested that Eva could have a mitochondrial disease. He urged us to go see a specialist and arrange for a muscle biopsy. Neither my husband nor I had ever heard of mitochondrial disease, despite our collective medical background. We were shocked and horrified when we began reading about mitochondrial disease. The medical literature was full of case studies of children who were dying horrific deaths, and there was very little information about management or treatment. There was an incredible amount of biochemistry to absorb, while still trying to care for Eva, help her grow, and make the most difficult decision of our lives about the muscle biopsy. We looked for support everywhere and found none. We needed help to understand all of the information as well as how to help Eva right now.

We put off the muscle biopsy for about a year. If our worst fears were realized— that Eva's diagnosis was fatal—we were uncertain how a definitive and invasive test could help her. Our family suffered terribly from grief. Even though Eva was with us, I felt I had lost her. I sobbed my way through therapy sessions and stayed up with her at night, holding her, afraid that she would stop breathing as had been described in the case studies published in the medical literature. My husband scoured the Internet and clinical trials for answers. Both of us put one foot in front of the other, going through the motions every day while carrying such a heavy burden in our hearts.

Meanwhile, our other children were growing and becoming more involved with and attached to Eva every day. Some special home health therapists and a new pediatrician gave me gentle guidance and support and helped me to see Eva's progress, albeit very small. I made two friends online whose little girls also had mitochondrial disease and were a lot like Eva. One lived in the US, the other in the UK. Despite the vast geographic differences, these two moms became my lifeline. I started to feel hopeful that we were not alone. I decided then that no one should ever have to face those years leading to the diagnosis without support.

At my middle daughter's third birthday party, my friend who was watching Eva inside brought her out to me. Eva was limp and listless in her arms. She had had a fever from an ear infection for a couple days, but our pediatrician had encouraged us to just give her Tylenol and ride it out.

We immediately rushed Eva to the hospital, where once again, everyone was perplexed. Without a definitive diagnosis of mitochondrial disease, and without a specialist to call who knew her, everyone was at a total loss. She decompensated so badly that our church began a prayer chain and the priest stayed on call with us. The medical staff was so focused on her labs and imaging studies (MRI, etc.) that no one really paid attention to her nutrition and fluid intake. She was not eating at all and was not even getting IV fluids for the first forty-eight hours of her hospitalization. I pleaded, desperate, with the doctors and nurses to give her fluids and nutrition through her veins. We were overwhelmed with relief when Eva began to respond to us again within hours after the fluids and TPN (total parenteral nutrition) had started. My husband and I knew, without speaking, that we also had to see the specialist and get a muscle biopsy for a definitive diagnosis. Without a diagnosis, how could we (or anyone else) help her?

The journey to get the diagnosis was grueling. We paid at least $10,000 out of pocket for the tests, and traveled out of state for the consult as well as the procedure. Even though we had been told to expect that Eva had a very serious form of mitochondrial disease, the actual definitive diagnosis was another brutal blow. Once again, we grieved for Eva and for all that we were afraid we had lost. We were so overwhelmed that we could barely have the objectivity to see that she was slightly improving before our very eyes every day. She was taking the slurry of supplements called the Mito cocktail. She was gaining weight and strength. She was making slow (very slow) progress toward the milestones she had missed. She responded to us, and to her brother and sister. She smiled a lot and had a gurgling, wheezy, emphysema kind of laugh that was distinctly hers. She made great strides with her ability to chew and swallow (thanks to speech therapy) and I began to give her a homemade diet of whole foods pureed to a consistency like velvety mashed potatoes.

One evening when my husband was reading more articles about Eva's diagnosis, I realized that Eva was unaware that she had a terrible prognosis. She didn't know that her life expectancy was just four years. I turned off the computer and pulled my husband away from the desk, telling him, "All Eva knows is that she loves us. She loves it when we read books to her, and blow kisses on her belly. She loves to be rocked and to be bounced to music. We have to be with her."

We made a decision together at that moment that we would, forever in the future, always be thinking about quality of life for Eva, not quantity of life. We started changing the way we made decisions, even about her medical care, by asking if it was best for Eva. As a family, we embodied the "don't sweat the small stuff" rule. We had to be very strong and let go of many other people's expectations in order to rebuild our family.

During that time, I found MitoAction.org. MitoAction had just been formed by a group of parents, patients, doctors, and nurses in Boston who had a vision that research for a cure was not the only support needed for the children, adults, and families with mitochondrial disease. They wanted "action" right now, to help provide support and advocacy that would make a difference to those affected immediately. At that time, MitoAction's website was a one-page brochure, and their outreach was limited to a walk in Boston once a year for about 100 families. But the Internet age was booming, and I was completely energized by the ideas and the mission of MitoAction. I knew with my background as a nurse and my husband's medical training that there was so much more that we could offer to families like ours.

I became very passionately involved with MitoAction, bringing all of my ideas from my background in public health to the table along with my sometimes horrific experiences as a "Mito mom." Eventually, I became the executive director of MitoAction. The growth of the organization has been incredible over the last five years, and actually parallels the incredible growth of my daughter. She has outlived her prognosis, and although she is still very disabled by her diagnosis, she has exceeded our expectations. When I see her pull herself up to stand and joyously stand on her own for a second or two, we are ecstatic. Rather than see her as "not being able to walk," we see that she CAN stand for a second, she CAN take a step and we see the possibilities for the future! As an advocate for so many parents and adult patients, I have felt very passionately for many years that I had a responsibility to every Mito patient and parent to write this book. We are building this community of hope together.

I'd like to dedicate this book to my family. To my daughter Eva, who has taught me that some blessings are disguised as tragedy; to my husband Eduardo, who put the pen in my hand and said "start writing" as many times as it took; and to Sophie and Diego for their innocent devotion and brilliant light that has helped me to refocus again and again.

Acknowledgements

There are countless people, both clinicians and patients, who should be thanked for their help with this book and for their contribution to the field of mitochondrial medicine. To that end, I would like to acknowledge all of the nurses, therapists, physicians, and healthcare providers who have dedicated their practices to the care of mitochondrial disease patients. As a mother, as a nurse, and as an advocate and voice for the Mito community—thank you. I wrote this book in order to help establish mitochondrial disease as a mainstream condition, deserving of a patient and family handbook and providing the opportunity for others to follow suit by sharing their expertise.

I would additionally like to acknowledge the many adult patients, parents, and family members who shared their personal stories with me for use in this publication. Their words convey the struggle and the triumph that we feel as patients and caregivers fighting for an under-recognized cause. Thank you for giving so freely of yourself in order to help me with this book and to help others who will benefit from hearing your story. To that end, I would like to thank MitoAction and all of the people who are part of the MitoAction community for supporting me and my vision to improve quality of life for all who are affected by Mito. I am hopeful that this book helps to serve that purpose.

A very special thanks goes to Dr. Katherine Sims and Nancy Slate of Massachusetts General Hospital and Harvard Medical School for their invaluable support and review of the most technically difficult chapters in this book. The endeavor of simplifying the complex biochemistry associated with energy metabolism simply would not have been possible without their support, patience, and attention to detail.

I would also like to thank all of the physicians who contributed to my and the Mito community's understanding of the physiology and management of mitochondrial disease by sharing their expertise as guest lecturers and authors of useful publications. These people are pioneers that should be recognized for their tireless dedication to the quest of knowledge and better patient care. Some of these physicians are acknowledged within the chapters herein, and I can only hope that I represent their wealth of knowledge and expertise appropriately and with the full respect that they deserve.

Dr. Mark Korson, thank you for your poignant snippets of advice and for your most thoughtful state of the union piece on mitochondrial medicine. Dr. Guy Miller, thank you for breaking down century-old barriers in order to offer promising therapeutic options for our children and loved ones who suffer from mitochondrial disease, and thank you for helping all of us to see the bigger picture through your written contribution following the chapter on treatment.

Kirsten Casale is an incredible advocate for parents struggling for appropriate educational goals for their children with Mito, and should be gratefully acknowledged for acting as an invaluable resource for me and helping provide the information necessary to put together the information in the chapters about children, education, and Mito adolescents.

Jane Adams is an incredibly talented and professional young woman who provided the illustrations used throughout the book. I hope that your work with this book leads to many more opportunities.

Thank you to Trudy Friar for assistance with the glossary and for supporting me from beginning to end.

I'd like to thank my agent Kate from Epstein Literary Agency for helping me to transform my passion and experience into an opportunity.

The team at Woodbine House, especially my editor Nancy Gray Paul, took such enthusiastic interest in this subject that they should be showered with gratitude by the entire mitochondrial disease patient community for taking the leap and publishing the first layperson's book on mitochondrial disease.

Finally, thank you to my husband, on whom I was forever leaning. His help with this book as well as his patience and support really cannot be adequately described or acknowledged.

—Cristy Balcells RN, MSN

1

What Is Mitochondrial Disease?

BENJAMIN

My name is Benjamin and I'm six years old. I was diagnosed with mitochondrial disease when I was two years old after lots of things in my body weren't working right. I am tired—really, really tired—most of the time and sometimes my legs hurt a lot. I go to school but sometimes I get sick and it takes me a really long time to get better. I have a tube in my stomach that helps me get enough food and water and a special formula that helps me grow. I can't see right sometimes because everything gets all blurry or I feel like the room is spinning around so I take rests a lot. My doctor says that my problems with my eyes, my tummy, and my muscles are because I have Mito. He says it's like my energy factories are broken…like my batteries are running low.

For most people, waking up in the morning, getting dressed, running off to school or to work, and keeping active throughout the day happens without much thought. Typically, children don't need to plan ahead if they want to be able to have the energy to play and learn, and adults don't need to pace themselves in the early morning in order to be able to think and speak coherently by the afternoon. In addition, for most people, everyday bodily functions happen as expected, again with little recognition. Food digests, eyes focus, voices sing and speak, muscles relax and contract to provide movement, and the sweat glands kick in to cool the skin when it's hot outside.

However, for people with mitochondrial disease, energy is a commodity. Their bodies' energy demands, even with minimal activity, are greater than the available supply. For them, a "typical day" is unpredictable. The tasks and activities that many people take for granted can be exhausting. For these adults and children, planning and conserving energy is crucial to avoid an energy crash. Something as inconsequential as hot weather or the common cold can be a huge energy drain. It takes a long time to generate enough energy to feel restored or "normal," and even then, the restorative energy supply goes quickly. Automatic body functions don't happen normally like they are supposed to, and may slow down or stop working altogether. It is like comparing the effectiveness of a turbine being operated by a hand crank versus a power grid.

Children and adults with mitochondrial disease face, at the most fundamental level, an energy shortage. However, sometimes this very basic problem takes years to recognize due to manifestation of multiple, confusing symptoms. Health problems such as seizures, failure to thrive, muscle pain and weakness, pervasive developmental delay, and gastroparesis (slow digestion) are just a few. Despite the wide spectrum of potential symptoms that can occur, the underlying issue for anyone with a mitochondrial disorder is a basic inability to keep up with his body's energy demand.

Imagine that you just moved into a house. In this house, one day the oven stops working. You focus on the oven and you consult an appliance repair service to investigate and try to fix the problem. Unfortunately, a few days later, the microwave blows up! Now what? You go back to the appliance repair shop, where you ultimately purchase a new microwave altogether. Then, to your disbelief, the following week the lights in all of the bedrooms won't turn on! This seems like an uncanny coincidence, but an electrician eventually finds a faulty fuse and replaces it, which temporarily fixes the problem. But, lo and behold, soon the refrigerator begins to have issues, freezing the food one hour and overheating it the next. You throw your hands up. How many service calls should one homeowner need to make?

What you don't know and eventually find out is that ALL of the problems in your house are related to an inadequate power unit that is unable to provide enough voltage to your home during peak hours, causing a drop in voltage and electrical energy. As a result, your appliances stopped working or were working sporadically and performing less effectively. The truth is that there was never anything wrong with the appliances or light fixtures per se; instead, the brownouts were caused by an underlying energy issue.

Why is Mitochondrial Disease Hard to Diagnose?

Children and adults with mitochondrial disease often show a myriad of symptoms that are fundamentally caused by a defect in their bodies' ability to effectively and appropriately produce energy. However, the symptoms may not have clear indicators that point to this energy metabolism issue, and a great deal of medical detective work often must occur before the diagnosis of mitochondrial disease is exposed. Like

Possible Symptoms That Result From Ineffective Energy Production

Our bodies' organs and systems need power to work properly. Just like the battery in a car, or a power plant in a community, the mitochondria are the power supply for living things. Mitochondria must work effectively in order for the energy demands of our body to be met. Any defect in the mitochondria can result in the production of less "power." It's a cause and effect relationship that has the greatest impact on organs and body systems that require the most power, such as those listed below.

Brain—Impaired mitochondrial function in the brain and central nervous system can lead to seizures, memory loss, cognitive delay or loss of skills, stroke-like episodes, difficulty with speech or problem solving (especially when tired), migraines, cortical blindness, pyramidal signs, extra pyramidal signs (that can look like cerebral palsy), hearing loss, vision loss, peripheral neuropathy, and pain.

Heart—Impaired mitochondrial function in the heart and cardiovascular system can lead to dizziness (especially when going from lying down to standing), impaired heart function, low blood pressure, and poor circulation (seen as purplish, mottled skin).

Gut—Impaired mitochondrial function in the organs necessary for digestion can lead to digestive problems, constipation, belly pain, nausea, reflux, lack of appetite, and difficulty gaining weight.

Muscles—Impaired mitochondrial function in the muscles can lead to muscle weakness, muscle cramps (especially in large muscles, like the legs), muscle pain, fatigue, exercise intolerance, and "heavy" legs and arms.

Eyes—Impaired mitochondrial function can affect the eyes and vision and may include vision loss, eye fatigue, blurry vision or vision loss that comes and goes, and droopy eyelids.

all of the appliances that stopped working in the house with inadequate power, many people find themselves living with symptoms for months or years before finally getting a diagnosis of mitochondrial disease. In other words, the symptoms get our attention first—seizures, lack of energy, failure to thrive, muscle pain and weakness, memory and concentration issues, heat intolerance, developmental delay, constipation, reflux, slow motility, nausea, difficulty recovering from fever, illness, or anesthesia—yet the underlying diagnosis is more difficult to identify.

Many children and adults wind up with a team of "-ists," having sought the advice and support of endocrinologists, cardiologists, neurologists, gastroenterologists, etc. Unfortunately, in many cases, the healthcare provider doesn't see the "big picture" for children and adults experiencing what appear to be a multitude of unrelated symptoms. So, while each symptom may be tested, described, and, to some extent, treated, the underlying genetic diagnosis of mitochondrial disease is often overlooked.

The History of Mitochondrial Disease

Many researchers and clinicians today would call Dr. Salvatore DiMauro of Columbia University one of the "fathers of mitochondrial medicine." In fact, Dr. DiMauro and his colleagues described and identified some of the first mitochondrial DNA mutations and diseases in the 1970s, approximately a decade after a Stockholm physician named Rolf Luft identified the first patient who had a syndrome that could be correlated to mitochondrial dysfunction in muscle cells.

Dr. DiMauro suggests that the history of mitochondrial diseases can be segmented into two periods: the pre-molecular era (1962-1988) and the molecular era, which continues to evolve today. During the early years of mitochondrial medicine, mitochondrial disease was considered very rare and very fatal. In that period, the diagnosis of mitochondrial disease was made by a handful of experienced physicians based on the person's symptoms, blood and urine biochemistry, and muscle biopsy. Today, many people still feel that mitochondrial disease is rare and difficult to diagnose; however, the landscape of mitochondrial medicine today is a vast improvement from that of yesteryear. Significant advances in molecular mitochondrial medicine now offer patients a much greater scope of genetic sequencing and more specific diagnoses. As improvements in diagnosis occur, the spectrum of mitochondrial disease also widens significantly. Children and adults who were previously not identified or were misdiagnosed are now increasingly stumbling into a mitochondrial disease diagnosis. Whereas Mito was thought to affect a very small percentage of patients fifty years ago, today mitochondrial disease is considered the most common of all metabolic disorders.

In the 1960s, '70s, and '80s, research was focused on identifying and describing mutations in the mitochondrial DNA (mtDNA), and many syndromes were named, such as MELAS, MERFF, Kearns-Sayre, and Leigh disease. Subsequently, the identification in the mid-1990s of defects caused by mutations in nuclear genes opened the door for exponential growth in depth and quantity of research and review articles in the field of mitochondrial medicine. As evidence of the relationship between mitochondrial function, aging, and "popular" diseases such as diabetes, autism, Parkinson's disease, Alzheimer's disease, and heart disease continues to mount, mitochondrial disorders are increasingly becoming a "hot topic." (For more in-depth information on current mitochondrial disorder research see the Mitochondrial Medicine Society's website: www.mitosoc.org.)

Adult patients and parents of children who were diagnosed with Mito in the "pre-molecular era" were often told by their physicians that they were the only case (or one out of a handful) in the world. Today, the umbrella has opened even wider and encompasses everything from very ill babies to mildly affected adults. In addition, efforts of advocacy groups and foundations are finally able to be globally successful as the Internet offers new opportunities to raise awareness about Mito and create patient and family networks. The struggle for appropriate patient care, diagnosis, awareness, and a cure still exists for adults and children facing a mitochondrial disease diagnosis today; however, children and adults with recognized mitochondrial disease are a growing population and, consequently, efforts to improve treatment and patient care are emerging!

Who Has Mitochondrial Disease?

Making mitochondrial disease even harder to diagnose is the fact that it doesn't just affect specific groups. Mitochondrial disease can affect babies, children and teens, as well as adults of all ages. Some people are born with Mito (and show symptoms at birth), while others do not show symptoms until later in childhood, as teenagers, or as adults. Some people have a family history of mitochondrial disease (or strokes, muscle disease, or multi-system disease), while others have no history at all. Mito can affect boys and girls, men and women, and does not seem to discriminate between race or socioeconomic status.

We don't really have a perfect idea of how many people have mitochondrial disease, in part because the diagnosis is relatively new, and because obtaining a diagnosis is difficult (invasive, expensive, and requires expertise). World leaders in mitochondrial medicine agree that the incidence of mitochondrial disease is *at least* 1 in 4,000 (as common as cystic fibrosis). They also agree that there are probably many more people affected than currently diagnosed, and some speculate that the incidence is actually closer to 1 in 1,000.

Mitochondrial disorders are the most common type of metabolic disorder. Additionally, now that research has demonstrated that mitochondrial function has a significant impact on many other diseases, including cardiovascular disease and neuromuscular diseases, new therapeutic approaches are emerging that investigate how mitochondrial function can be improved with hopes of improving health for the general population.

What Causes Mitochondrial Disease?

Most clinicians agree that the term mitochondrial disease refers to a group of disorders wherein a person (child or adult) has symptoms that stem from some impairment of mitochondrial function. That impairment may be caused by too many mitochondria, a defect in the energy production process within the mitochondria, too few mitochondria, or mitochondrial dysfunction of some other type (i.e., spontaneous mutation). Mitochondrial disease is classified by the inheritance type as well as by the symptoms. (More in-depth information on this will be provided in Chapter 2 on diagnosis and causes.)

What Are Mitochondria?

How can a disease affect so many body systems and such a diverse group of people? Fundamentally, it's because mitochondria are important to *all* of us and *each* of us. Let's begin by learning more about the mitochondria and why these tiny powerhouses are so important.

Often, the mitochondria (single = mitochondrion) are called the powerhouses of the cell because energy production (i.e., the manufacturing of the body's energy molecule, ATP) takes place within the mitochondria. Hundreds or thousands of mitochondria are found in all human cells (except red blood cells) and are extremely important. Without some mitochondrial function, a person could not live. When there is a flaw, or defect, in the process of producing energy within the mitochondria, the result is mitochondrial disease. Such defects may be minor or significant, which helps, in part, to explain why the symptoms vary in degree and are so diverse among those who have mitochondrial disease. Not only are the mitochondria important for producing essential energy for the body, but the specialized function of each cell in the body is also dependent on the mitochondria. In other words, these tiny organelles are biological superstars, creating the necessary energy for a living cell's survival and communicating with our body so that essential functions can occur.

Interestingly, mitochondria were once bacteria that, over the last billion years, have evolved to become the most efficient mechanism of producing energy that exists for living things. Remember, there are many (millions) of mitochondria in our cells. Furthermore, there are different types of cells in our bodies that require different degrees of mitochondrial energy. For example, skin cells have relatively few mitochondria and require very little energy for their defined function. On the other hand, muscle cells have thousands of mitochondria and are constantly harnessing the energy produced by and stored within the mitochondria in order to yield the needed mechanical energy to "move." Not only are mitochondria involved in energy production, but these tiny organelles are also involved in processing and converting the food we eat into usable energy.

When we eat, our cells break the food down into usable "energy building blocks" called molecules. Two such molecules are glucose and fatty acids (other important molecules are amino acids and proteins). These molecules must then be broken down into a usable energy source, or, for our purposes, an "energy molecule." In healthy mitochondria, over thirty "energy molecules" can be produced from just one molecule of glucose! In addition, much like a battery, the energy created from these molecules can be stored if not needed right away. This energy is the fuel for the automatic functions of the body, like digesting food, breathing, walking, talking, hearing, thinking, keeping warm, using oxygen from the air we breathe, and pumping blood to our organs. When we increase our activity level or energy demand through physical activities like exercise, or when we are stressed, scared, hot, cold, sick, etc., more energy is needed in order for the body to remain stable. Our bodies are equipped with an innate sensor that works to always keep our bodies in balance (called homeostasis). Without even knowing it, our bodies are constantly adjusting the amount of energy released dependent upon our bodies' needs in a given moment. This is significant for people with mitochondrial disorders because their energy levels, and subsequently the degree of their symptoms, can fluctuate from moment to moment and so they are especially vulnerable during periods of increased energy demand, such as when they have a cold, a fever, or go too long without enough food or drink to fuel their cells.

What Do Mitochondria Do?

The biochemistry related to mitochondrial function is complex, and is described in great detail in Chapter 10. This section provides an overview of what the mitochondria do, and what the most important components are in energy production.

The primary energy currency that is produced by the mitochondria is ATP. ATP stands for adenosine triphosphate and is the usable energy molecule required by the body's organs to function. The key word in understanding energy production (and why any mitochondrial defect has such a significant impact) is *usable*.

Think of food as foreign currency that must be converted in the mitochondria into a usable form. Further, imagine that the foreign currency comes in two forms: cash and coins. For our analogy, cash is the glucose—the first molecule that is broken down from food. Coins are the other molecule, called fatty acids. Now, when you are holding the foreign currency in your hand, you can't buy anything with it until you deposit your cash and coins into a bank that can convert the money into legal tender. Only then can you go shopping and spend the money!

In a similar way, food is broken down by the body into several smaller building blocks, including glucose, amino acids, and fatty acids, that can be used by our cells. However, the body doesn't use glucose and fatty acids as the primary source of energy. Instead, the glucose and fatty acids from food—just like the foreign coins and cash—need to be converted into something that can serve as a usable energy supply. Our body's organs and systems need a constant supply of usable energy to function properly. That usable energy is ATP. Without the proper conversion of the food we eat into ATP, an energy shortage will exist. Because of the ongoing demand for ATP by our organs, our body is equipped with millions of mitochondria to serve as powerplants to manufacture enough ATP. Every cell is full of mitochondria, which take those components derived from food and, through a process called oxidative phosphorylation (OX-PHOS), convert the food into fuel that can be used throughout the body.

Why Do I Need to Know This?

It is important that as patients, parents, and caregivers we try to understand the science of Mito. This introductory chapter will give you an understanding of the basics. Knowledge is empowering, and while the process of oxidative phosphorylation, for example, isn't part of the outward manifestation of the disease, understanding the terms and the "why" helps us to be better advocates for ourselves and our children. You'll find it useful to be able to explain mitochondrial disease to others, comprehend the reasons for use of the supplements in the "Mito Cocktail," and be able to make measured decisions about clinical trials and potential therapies in the future. Be patient as you are learning—this is a journey! When you're ready to digest it, the complicated biochemistry of mitochondrial function is described in depth in Chapter 10, along with visual aides.

Oxidative phosphorylation describes the incredibly efficient series of reactions that occur in living things to produce energy. In order for our bodies to function optimally, we rely on our mitochondria to do their job effectively and efficiently, producing a steady supply of usable energy currency in the form of ATP. There are many potential defects that can occur during this process, especially along the pathway where most of the OX-PHOS reactions take place (i.e., the electron transport chain, or ETC for short, where complexes I-V are found).

Oxidative phosphorylation (OX-PHOS) and the electron transport chain (ETC) refer to the process and the place where energy is made, respectively. OX-PHOS is the series of metabolic reactions that create energy and the ETC is the primary pathway in the mitochondria where energy (in the form of ATP) is generated. Complexes I-V are biochemical groups that are linked together to form the ETC. (Sometimes OX-PHOS is referred to as cellular respiration, and the electron transport chain is also known as the respiratory chain.)

What's In a Name?

The term "mitochondrial disorder" (or disease) conventionally refers to a defect somewhere along this energy-building pathway. Consequently, patients are sometimes given a name to their syndrome such as "complex I & III deficiency." Others, however, are diagnosed based on a clinical presentation and characteristic constellation of signs and symptoms, such as "MELAS" (Mitochondrial Encepholopathy, Lactic Acidosis, and Stroke). For many people, their mitochondrial disease still doesn't have a formal name or a gene that can be identified as the cause, although this is rapidly changing as the field of mitochondrial medicine advances. Likewise, although these names are helpful from a disease classification standpoint, they are also inadequate. These names are descriptive based on the syndromes and symptoms often associated with these subtypes of mitochondrial disease. It is important for patients and primary care clinicians to realize that the names are incomplete descriptions. Patients may "look" different and have different symptoms and outcomes, even when they have the same "diagnosis." For that reason, while it is helpful to classify mitochondrial disease diagnoses, it is also useful to approach Mito from an "energy metabolism defect" perspective, knowing that the fundamental issues for all people with Mito often cross the boundaries of classification that we know today.

Mitochondrial Function, Aging, and Disease

Mitochondrial diseases, as we know them today, are likely only the tip of the iceberg. In fact, experts such as Dr. Christoph Westphal, who study mitochondria's role in diseases of aging, suggest that many people in the general population suffer from

The terms used to describe mitochondrial disease and its biochemistry are confusing, and sometimes two terms are used interchangeably, such as these terms below:

Mitochondrial disease = Mitochondrial disorder = Mito = mt dz = mt disease = MD = "energy metabolism disorder"

Oxidative phosphorylation = OX-PHOS = Cellular Respiration

Electron Transport Chain = ETC = Respiratory Chain = Complexes I, II, III, IV, V

Citric Acid Cycle = Kreb's cycle

Have you visited the glossary in the back of this book yet? The glossary is an excellent resource, offering simple definitions for all of the medical and scientific words in this book. Check it out!

mitochondrial diseases that are either not yet diagnosed or not yet classified. As our understanding of mitochondrial function improves, we are beginning to see a connection between the health of a person's mitochondria and the health of his body. In particular, there is a great deal of evidence that demonstrates that neurodegenerative diseases, including Alzheimer's disease, Parkinson's disease, ALS, and Huntington's disease, are caused to some extent by a mitochondrial dysfunction. Also, oxidative stress caused by free radicals contributes to diseases of aging and the aging process. In addition, defective or dysfunctional mitochondria have higher rates of oxidative damage than healthy mitochondria.

So, aside from primary mitochondrial disease, what are some causes of defective or dysfunctional mitochondria? One cause is getting older! Indeed, studies that examine the mitochondria in the elderly as compared to younger people with known mitochondrial disease note many similarities between the two otherwise unrelated groups. Type 2 diabetes is also considered a mitochondrial disorder amongst academics, and the role of mitochondrial health in heart disease is gaining traction as well. For adults and children with mitochondrial disease, there is a message of hope within all the science. As what we know about the role that mitochondria play in common disease processes and aging becomes clearer, so will our understanding of mitochondrial diseases. The opportunity for treatment and therapeutic agents will evolve as improved mitochondrial function becomes the focus of researchers and pharmaceutical companies around the world. There is even some theory that exercise, a well-known "anti-aging activity," increases energy production by multiplying the number of mitochondria within a cell (even in people with mitochondrial disease). In the meantime, those who are living today with mitochondrial disease can know that they are part of a pioneering group of patients who are advocating for better health for everyone in the future.

Key Points from This Chapter

■ ATP is in demand throughout the body. The most energy-hungry organs/body systems are the muscles, gut, brain, eyes, and heart. Symptoms of mitochondrial disease tend to be more frequent or more problematic in these areas, and may manifest in subtle ways such as fatigue, muscle cramps, weakness or pain, slurred speech, shaky hands, erratic blood pressure, etc.

■ Oxidative Phosphorlyation (OX-PHOS) describes the series of metabolic reactions that take place in the cell's mitochondria to make energy. The electron transport chain (ETC) is a group of five protein complexes where most of that usable energy is actually created in the form of ATP.

■ Although people with mitochondrial disease have a known defect or dysfunction that ultimately generates less ATP, the mitochondria are still effective to a degree. In other words, a 100 percent defect in the mitochondria would be incompatible with life.

■ Mitochondrial function is vital to all human beings, regardless of age, race, class, gender, etc. The mitochondria are important to ALL people because they provide the essential energy that is necessary for health and survival. In this way, mitochondrial disorders, like aging, affect all of us!

SPECIAL INSERT

State of the Union on Mitochondrial Medicine

Mark Korson, MD

Tufts Floating Hospital for Children, Boston MA

When I am with a patient or family for whom mitochondrial disease is a new diagnosis or a new consideration in a diagnostic journey, I usually encounter a measure of confusion and a sense of being overwhelmed. And the more questions asked—there is frustration, as well. This is mitochondrial disease, a relatively new field of medicine; there is so much that is unknown. I generally sigh and sometimes I say something like, "Well, twenty years ago we wouldn't have had much to talk about, and I am hoping that ten years from now I'll be able to give you many more answers."

Patients and families, clinicians and providers face the same challenges that characterize mitochondrial medicine in 2011: the need to clearly delineate the many clinical presentations of mitochondrial disease; the lack of a suitable, clinically-relevant classification system; the absence of a diagnostic test that can reliably identify all cases; the lack of available, effective therapies. And the list goes on….

If we look at all we don't know and don't understand, the obstacles before us are incredibly daunting. However, many patients do show similar patterns of symptoms that allow us to be aware and anticipate their problems. Now evolving is DNA testing on which we are learning to rely to confirm a diagnosis rather than use less sensitive or specific testing methods. Even if we haven't specific therapies right now, understanding how the body's physiology appears to be misbehaving—not at the cell level but at the organ level—allows us to intervene in ways that can improve a patient's day to day life. And research in all areas of mitochondrial disease is moving the field forward—clinical recognition, pathophysiology, diagnostics, and treatment.

It is important to have faith that the process of medicine will bring enlightenment to this field like it has every other disease in history. Understandably, it is hard to be patient when it is your life that is affected or your child's future is at risk. I have no answer for this. It is too close and personal. As a physician, it is at this point in the conversation when I have to leave the realm of science and sit helpless—hearing your worries, listening to your anger and frustration, offering to support and advocate… and talking about 2021.

2

The Journey to Diagnosis and Understanding the Causes

Your doctor has told you that you, a family member, or your child *might* have a mitochondrial disease. Chances are, you have never heard of this condition before. You may have been a healthy and active person your entire life, only to be baffled by the onset of new symptoms in your teen or adult years. Your baby may be sick, not growing well, and missing important developmental milestones. Or, your child might be showing more and more concerning symptoms, some of which are getting worse, like difficulty walking, feeling tired all the time, and trouble with digestion.

Mitochondrial disease, or the specific type of mitochondrial disorder that you are dealing with, might be a new and shocking diagnosis. Or, this might be the end of a long line of misdiagnoses. This might finally be the answer after trying to interpret many puzzling symptoms for months or years. You might even still be seeking a diagnosis, wondering about the possibility of mitochondrial disease and trying to explain your symptoms and get your physician's support for further testing. Even if you have waited months or years to figure out what has been going on with your own health, your child's, or someone you care for, a mitochondrial disease diagnosis is always emotionally overwhelming and frightening. You may even be confronted by people who doubt you and your symptoms (or your child's symptoms). They may even question the diagnosis of mitochondrial disease, assuming that you are overreacting, a hypochondriac, or manipulating the system. When faced with so many questions and an uncertain future, it's only natural to wonder, "What happens now?"

Many of us go right to the Internet when we get new information like this. We want to understand: How is the diagnosis made? What does it mean? What was the cause? What's the cure? What does the future look like? While a wonderful resource for support and information, the Internet is liable to provide some misinformation and has no filters for those of you facing a new diagnosis! Mitochondrial disease is a "young" disease, only first described and published in the medical literature in the 1980s. The medical literature often describes and reports the most progressive cases, describing a litany of symptoms and effects on many organ systems as well as mortality rates. If you are a spouse, adult patient, or parent of a child facing a Mito diagnosis and you have read these articles, is it any wonder that you feel crushed and hopeless? Currently, there is no "cure" for Mito, but there are very good management options and therapeutic recommendations (see Chapters 4 and 5). Stop the information overload and take this process of obtaining and learning about a mitochondrial disease diagnosis one step at a time.

Testing for Mitochondrial Disease

Whether we recognize it or not, we are consumers, even when it comes to healthcare. We come to a hospital or clinic with a certain, unspoken expectation that we will be treated with respect, examined carefully, tested, and diagnosed. Our culture believes that some diagnosis is better than no diagnosis. A test is better than no test, some information is better than no information, etc. We also operate on the premise that, if a diagnosis can be found, then there is an opportunity for treatment. We unconsciously expect treatment options to be presented to us, and accept and recognize that they may not be easy, but we're willing to rally. We may be fully prepared to fight or suffer through the treatment because we are always hoping and striving for a cure. We immediately set a goal in our mind of *removing* the diagnosis just as soon as we have received it.

Do I really need to know? Some people need a diagnosis—for themselves or their family member. They need information, and want the truth even if it is difficult to bear. They feel that a diagnosis offers definition, closure, and options. On the other hand, some people don't want or need to know. They may not want to face a diagnosis if there isn't a cure. They may not be interested in tests and test results if the outcome and treatment strategy don't change. Often, these two different emotional responses to testing and diagnosis occur in the same family, and require patience and compromise as families and parents struggle to make decisions about testing. Equally frustrating is the situation that arises when a patient or family would like a diagnosis, but are unable to proceed due to financial limitations, travel requirements, restrictions related to their primary physician, hospital, or insurance, etc.

Most mitochondrial specialists now recommend that their patients undergo additional testing to determine a molecular diagnosis, which offers specific genetic information about the type of defect behind the mitochondrial disease in your family. However, while this may be optimal, this is still not always possible because not every gene mutation for mitochondrial disorders has been identified. There are <u>many</u> different syndromes and classifications that fall under the larger umbrella of mitochondrial disease—MELAS, MERFF, Kearn's Sayre, Complex II, etc.—and each occurs as a result of a specific gene mutation. Some have clearly defined corresponding symptoms (such as MELAS) and have been studied more thoroughly through research and clinical trials. Others are still not well understood. A decade ago, the majority of patients had a "suspected" or "clinical" diagnosis of mitochondrial disease because the tools for testing and conclusive diagnosis were both cost-prohibitive and limited in accuracy. Today, as diagnostic technology improves, more and more families are undergoing extensive testing in hopes of arriving at a specific diagnosis.

Detailed information about your mitochondrial disorder can help you and your family understand the genetic risk to other family members, may influence treatment approaches, can facilitate insurance coverage of treatment, and may allow you to participate in clinical trials targeting your specific diagnosis. On the other hand, the journey to a diagnosis remains difficult, cumbersome, and frustrating for most patients, parents, and families. There are very few centers in the world that provide "expert" diagnostic services for mitochondrial disease (see Appendix B for a list). Testing can be very expensive, time-consuming, and potentially invasive (i.e., muscle biopsy, spinal tap). Arriving at a diagnosis is stressful and can take months from start to finish. Despite these challenges, there is an increasing expectation amongst the medical community that a definitive diagnosis is strongly preferred; consequently, more people are receiving more testing and more detailed information as part of their diagnosis. However, how patients can and will use this information for their own benefit remains to be fully seen.

Metabolic and Genetic Testing

For many years, muscle biopsy was considered the gold standard when diagnosing mitochondrial disease and still provides an unparalleled level of detail in many cases. Unfortunately, muscle biopsy comes with many challenges. For children, a tissue sample is taken by a surgeon while your child is asleep under an anesthetic. Adults may be able to have the procedure done with a local numbing anesthetic in an outpatient environment. Both adults and children typically have the muscle biopsy taken from the upper thigh, and results can take weeks to months to complete. In addition, there are only a few centers and laboratories around the country that have appropriate expertise for mitochondrial diagnostic testing from muscle tissue. Further disadvantages of muscle biopsy include expense, pain, risk of infection, risk associated with anesthetic, and risk for potential inaccuracy of results if the biopsy is mishandled or interpreted incorrectly. On the other hand, muscle biopsy gives the most detailed information about potential defects, offering both insights into how the electron transport chain is operating as well as the genetic mutations that may be causing the disease.

As technology and research improve, new and improved testing options are emerging. Now mutations in both the mitochondrial DNA and nuclear DNA can be detected via molecular (genetic) testing (buccal swab, saliva, blood), offering a somewhat less expensive and definitely less invasive option for those with suspected mitochondrial disorders. Unfortunately, even these tests are not completely definitive in the majority of cases. To that end, muscle biopsy testing (or biopsy and testing of other tissues, such as liver or brain) still plays a very important role in delineating potential defects in the electron transport chain (Complex I-V defects). This is true even when molecular (genetic) testing is negative or inconclusive, because not all of the genes that cause mitochondrial disease have been identified yet. Further, sometimes the information about defects in the electron transport chain from tissue biopsy influences the specific molecular tests called for. Molecular testing is a vast field; finding a specific DNA defect can be like looking for a needle in a haystack. The information from a biopsy might provide clues that help focus the DNA sequencing. In other words, the information determined from both types of tests is important and influences full understanding of the diagnosis. However, because there is not a single standard approach to diagnosing mitochondrial disease, the entire process is confusing. Patients and parents can begin by really learning about and understanding each test, how they are used, and what the results may mean.

Mitochondrial disease is typically diagnosed from a three-pronged approach that includes a) symptoms and clinical presentation, b) biochemical, metabolic, and/or physiologic testing (such as blood tests for lactate, pyruvate, amino acids, organic acids, as well as MRI and MRS imaging), and c) molecular and histological testing (such as DNA sequencing from blood, skin, or tissue biopsy, along with studies that describe the microscopic appearance of the tissue).

Before tackling a description of each of the tests that can be used to help diagnose mitochondrial disease, it is important to understand that a mitochondrial disease diagnosis is not based on test results alone. Mitochondrial disease is typically diagnosed from a three-pronged approach that includes a) symptoms and clinical presentation, b) biochemical, metabolic, and/or physiologic testing (such as blood tests for lactate, pyruvate, amino acids, organic acids, as well as MRI and MRS imaging), and c) molecular and histological testing (such as DNA sequencing from blood, skin, or tissue biopsy, along with studies that describe the microscopic appearance of the tissue). Molecular and histological testing also can provide information about the number of mitochondrial DNA that are defective. For example, people may have mitochondrial disease that occurs from a defect or from having too many, too few, or malfunctioning mitochondria (associated with diagnoses of mtDNA depletion, deletion, and duplication). Any one of these abnormalities could be suggestive of mitochondrial disease, yet a diagnosis is most accurately determined when findings in each of these areas are consistent with the abnormalities characteristic of Mito.

In most practices today, patients with clinical symptoms suggestive of mitochondrial disease are tested for basic metabolic abnormalities indicated in the blood and urine. For example, many people with mitochondrial disease have abnormally high levels of lactic acid and other metabolic by-products in their blood and urine, all of which can be detected by fairly basic metabolic tests. When the patient's lab results are suggestive of mitochondrial disease, the diagnostic physician may order additional tests such as MRI, MRS, tissue biopsy, and DNA sequencing (see Table 2.1).

Is the Testing and Diagnostic Process the Same in Children and Adults?

While the results may ultimately be the same, the process of obtaining a diagnosis does differ between children and adults. A review of the medical literature suggests that children are more difficult to diagnose for the following reasons: a) "classic" symptoms may or may not be present, b) there is greater variability of symptoms in children, and symptoms may change rapidly, c) the majority of pediatric Mito diagnoses result from nuclear DNA mutations, which are more difficult to identify, d) accuracy of testing may be more questionable in children (i.e., child is struggling during a blood test, which can cause the results to be falsely elevated), and e) histology from muscle biopsy is more frequently found "normal" or "nonspecific" in children. In both adults and children, proper handling and processing of blood tests is important, which is discussed in Table 2.1.

Adult and teen patients more typically present with what can be called a "classic mtDNA syndrome" that, to a physician experienced with mitochondrial disease, is very recognizable. Muscle weakness in adults is more often able to be positively associated with ragged red fibers (RRF) (usually found in mtDNA syndromes) when the muscle is tested in a laboratory. In addition, adults with mitochondrial disease are more likely to have a specific genetic mutation that can be more easily identified on the mitochondrial DNA (mtDNA) through molecular blood testing. Since there are only thirteen mtDNA genes, compared to thousands of nuclear genes, testing is in some ways more straightforward for adults. On the other hand, some adult patients and their families would argue that an adult Mito diagnosis is *more* difficult to obtain. Adult patients are often not taken seriously when complaining of nonspecific symptoms such as muscle weakness, headache, upset stomach, etc. In addition, adult patients often face greater financial barriers and are self-advocates who don't have the caregiver support to help organize and travel to medical appointments, diagnostic centers, etc.

For adults and children, the greatest challenge to obtaining a diagnosis is that there is not a consistent "abnormal" finding that indicates mitochondrial disease. However, diagnostic criteria have been developed within the last decade that help clinicians better identify and diagnose suspected mitochondrial disease in adults and children by implementing a comprehensive scoring system. Although there is still a lack of standardized diagnostic criteria, these two published sets of criteria (see Table 2.2) have been widely adopted and can help distinguish between mitochondrial disease and other disorders with multi-organ involvement. It is difficult to rule out mitochondrial disease even with these criteria, because they are not very discriminating.

Table 2.1 Tools and Tests Used in Making a Diagnosis of Mitochondrial Disease

Diagnostic tool or test	Examples of findings associated with mitochondrial disease	Good to know...
MRI & MRS (Brain imaging)	■ Increased lactate (also called a "Lac peak") in brain tissue (MRS) ■ Bilateral or symmetric lesions on the brain (MRI) ■ Atrophy of the brain (MRI)	■ MRS and MRI should be used in tandem as part of a mitochondrial disease workup because metabolic information can be gathered. ■ Children are often sedated for an MRI or MRS, which can present risks.

Muscle biopsy	■ Can provide descriptive data about the histology (size, shape, number, or structure of the mitochondria), e.g.,
	  ● Ragged red fibers (RRF)
	  ● Mitochondrial proliferation or depletion.
	■ Can provide information about the efficiency of the energy production pathways, and identify defects in the pathways, e.g.,
	  ● Defect in the electron transport chain (ETC), listed as Complex I, II, III, IV, and V
	  ● Defective oxygen phosphorylation (OX-PHOS)
	  ● Specific enzyme defects, such as PDH (pyruvate dehydrogenase complex) or fatty acid oxidation dysfunction
	  ● COX deficiency (cytochrome c-oxidase)
		■ May be fresh or frozen, which refers to the way the tissue was handled after biopsy.
		■ Fresh muscle biopsies are able to provide a greater level of detail than frozen muscle biopsies; however, both are used for diagnosing mitochondrial defects.
		■ Patients have rights—take your time and ask for detailed discussion before committing to a muscle biopsy. It's a big decision, and one that you should feel confident about!
		■ There are several diagnostic centers in the United States that specialize in muscle biopsy testing. Patients are more likely to receive more accurate results by going to a specialized center for this test.

Skin biopsy (Fibroblasts)	■ Elevated lactate ■ Elevated pyruvate ■ Specific enzyme defects, such as PDH (pyruvate dehydrogenase complex) or fatty acid oxidation dysfunction	■ While a skin biopsy is less invasive than a muscle biopsy, it is not as informative and is often normal, even in patients with mitochondrial disease. Muscle is more energy dependent (more mitochondria per muscle cell) and more commonly affected.

Molecular blood tests	■ Can identify specific mutations in mtDNA genes, such as those associated with:
	  ● MERFF
	  ● LHON
	  ● MELAS
	  ● many others, found at www.NORD.org (The National Organization for Rare Diseases)
		■ There are thirteen genes that encode structural parts of the electron transport chain (ETC) that can show a mutation. These are called mtDNA mutations. Also can be called tRNA mutations.

| Molecular blood tests cont. | ■ New sequencing tests can detect heteroplasmy and identify mutations on many of the nuclear genes (nDNA), such as the POLG gene, which affects mtDNA transcription and therefore mtDNA quantity (i.e., depletion).

■ Some genes, which are associated with specific Complex I, II, III and IV defects, can also be identified now by molecular blood tests. | ■ It is estimated that there are more than 1,000 nuclear genes important to mitochondrial structure, function, replication, and other organelle biologic needs. Most mitochondrial disease is expressed through nuclear DNA mutations.

■ Heteroplasmy is important in determining how many mtDNA in the same cell have a normal or mutated sequence.

■ When a patient presents some specific symptoms associated with mtDNA syndromes (including muscle weakness, exercise intolerance, hearing loss, vision loss, stroke, and multiple organ involvement) or there is strong family history suggesting maternal (mtDNA) inheritance, molecular blood testing may used as part of the initial diagnostic testing, even before muscle biopsy. |
| **Bio-chemistry from blood and urine** | ■ Amino acid profile demonstrates elevated alanine or other suggestive abnormalities

■ Urine organic acid analysis abnormalities

■ Carnitine deficiency

■ Coenzyme Q10 deficiency

■ Elevated lactate

■ Elevated pyruvate

■ Elevated lactate to pyruvate ratio (may vary depending on exact type of diagnosis; electron transport chain defects are often correlated with elevated lactate to pyruvate ratio and elevated lactate)

■ Blood/urine acetylcarnitines | ■ These blood tests can be ordered and interpreted by a neurologist, geneticist, or metabolic specialist. In many cases, the physician sends the blood to a reference lab for testing.

■ Many, but not all, patients with mitochondrial disease have an elevated lactate level.

■ Lactate levels are more likely to be high when a Mito patient is sick or in a "metabolic crisis."

■ Readings of lactate and pyruvate levels are often inaccurate due to the specimen being taken incorrectly or mishandled. Blood for this test MUST be taken properly without a tourniquet and should be put on ice immediately. The assay should be run within 20 minutes for accurate results.

■ The most important element for accurate lactate/pyruvate testing is good blood flow. In other words, the blood should flow freely into the collection tube from the vein (usually in the forearm) without clotting or stopping and starting.

■ Pyruvate also requires deproteinization in a special tube, which should be noted and handled by the laboratory.

■ These tests are considered "screening" tests that would suggest additional testing if abnormal in the presence of other mitochondrial symptoms. |

Say What? Making Sense of the Different Terms Used in Testing for Mito

Molecular testing (DNA analysis): Examination of specific genes to detect abnormalities, from blood or tissue.

Biochemical testing: Measuring the amount or activity of a particular enzyme, metabolites (such as lactic acid), or protein in a sample of blood, urine, or other tissue from the body.

Muscle Biopsy (or biopsy of other organ tissue): Biopsy of a piece of muscle about the size of the tip of your pinky finger that is typically removed from the thigh while under anesthesia in a hospital. This small piece of muscle allows for the visual evaluation of the structure of the muscle fibers as well as molecular and enzymatic analysis of mitochondrial function.

Histological or histochemical study: A microscopic examination of tissues, such as muscle or skin. In this manner, a muscle biopsy is used, in part, to provide the opportunity for histological or histochemical (examining the biological products found in the muscle or skin) study. Tissue is most commonly obtained via a surgical procedure where a small biopsy sample is taken from the muscle or other organs.

Enzymology testing: Testing to understand the biological activity of enzymes, such as the study of the efficiency of enzymes that are important in energy production in the body. For example, these enzymes can be part of the electron transport chain, fatty acid oxidation, or carnitine transport. Enzymology testing can be done on blood, muscle (fresh or frozen), skin, and occasionally the liver, and can help determine how the mitochondria use oxygen as well as how much ATP is being produced.

While the number of centers for mitochondrial medicine and mitochondrial specialists are growing, there is still a gap between the number of patients seeking a diagnosis and the opportunity for them to be evaluated appropriately.

Where Did This Come From? Understanding the Genetics of Mitochondrial Disease

At some point during the process of testing, you have asked, "How did this happen?" What causes mitochondrial disease? If you are a parent of a child with the diagnosis, you may be fearful that you passed on the disorder to your child, and may be additionally frightened about the risk to your other children. Conversely, teens and adult patients are sometimes baffled by the sudden onset of symptoms and by the subsequent diagnosis, as well as the explanation of inherited mitochondrial DNA muta-

Buccal swab: A method of collecting cells for extraction and testing using a sample taken by swiping a cotton swab inside the mouth to collect cheek cells. Some nuclear and mitochondrial gene mutations associated with mitochondrial disorders can be identified this way.

Heteroplasmy: Medical term describing the presence of a combination of normal and mutated mitochondria in the same cell and in mosaic fashion in organs and the body. Heteroplasmy explains why a mother with few or no symptoms of Mito may have a child with significant clinical mitochondrial disease, or why siblings may have varying degrees and extent (by organ systems affected) of the disease. It also explains why some tissues in a mitochondrial patient may function normally while others are severely affected. Accordingly, the severity of disease presentation in this case depends on how many healthy and "unhealthy" mitochondria were randomly given to each egg in fertilization and to all daughter cells during fetal development. (Refer to Figure 2.4.)

Myopathy: Medical term describing muscle cell dysfunction as a result of disease that primarily affects the function of the muscle fibers. Mitochondrial myopathy may present as weakness, exercise intolerance, and fatigue.

Nuclear DNA (nDNA): More commonly called "chromosomal DNA," this is the DNA that makes up the twenty-three chromosomes inherited from each parent and is most typically associated with genetic diseases. The majority of mitochondrial diseases, especially in children, are in fact inherited from the nuclear DNA (making up twenty-three chromosome pairs) from both parents.

Mitochondrial DNA (mtDNA): A small piece of DNA, unique to the mitochondria, that makes (encodes) only thirteen structural proteins, which are part of the electron transport chain. These mtDNA mutations are maternally inherited and are more commonly associated with late childhood, teen, or adult onset mitochondrial disease, but can present in childhood.

tions after being relatively healthy for fifteen to fifty years! Mitochondrial disease may result from the genes that you or your child has inherited—from your mother, or in combination from your mother and father. In some cases, we can't identify the genetic defect; those patients are thought to have a spontaneous mitochondrial defect.

Your Secret Code—DNA, Genes, and Chromosomes

DNA stands for deoxyribonucleic acid and is a molecule made of two individual strands paired together. These strands contain a code composed of units called bases (nucleotides). The bases must match together between strands perfectly to form base pairs that are the same in every human being. The specific sequence of base pairs results in a specific genetic code that functions like the instruction manual (code) for our bodies. Even one alteration in this base code can interfere with the genetic code and cause a major dysfunction in the body's ability to work properly.

Table 2.2   Mitochondrial Disease Diagnostic Criteria

Criteria Set #1:
Points assigned for clinical signs and symptoms in three major areas:
    I. Clinical signs and symptoms (max. four points)
        A. Muscular Presentation
        B. CNS Presentation
        C. Multisystem Disease
    II. Metabolic/Imaging Studies (max. four points)
    III. Morphology (histology) (max. four points)

A score of eight to twelve is associated with "definite mitochondrial disease"; based on sixty-one children with multi-system disease and a suspected oxidative phosphorylation disorder who underwent muscle biopsy and genetic testing. While designed for children, the criteria can be applied to adults as well.

References (abstracts available on www.pubmed.gov):
- E. Morava, MD PhD et al; *Mitochondrial disease criteria: Diagnostic applications in children.* Neurology. 2006 Nov 28;67(10):1823-6.
- Wolf NI & Smeitink JA; *Mitochondrial disorders: A proposal for consensus diagnostic criteria in infants and children.* Neurology. 2002 Nov 12;59(9):1402-5.

Criteria Set #2:
Detailed major criteria and minor criteria are listed and scored from six sub-areas:
    1. Clinical
    2. Histology
    3. Enzymology
    4. Functional
    5. Molecular
    6. Metabolic

A definite diagnosis is determined from the identification of two major criteria or one major plus two minor criteria. This scale is useful for diagnosing adult patients because the sensitivity to respiratory chain defects is greater for enzyme and functional studies.

Reference (abstract available on www.pubmed.gov):
- FP Bernier et al; *Diagnostic criteria for respiratory chain disorders in adults and children.* Neurology. 2002 Nov 12;59(9):1406-11.

* Patient and family note: The diagnostic criteria for these two scoring systems are not listed in detail here because of length and complexity. Patients and families can self-advocate by sharing the references cited here with their primary care physicians who can request the full-text articles from their medical library.

When millions of base pairs combine together as a long piece of DNA with some proteins, a chromosome is formed. Every chromosome contains thousands of genes. Genes are arranged in a specific way that results in the instructions for how to make proteins (chains of amino acids). These proteins have very specific functions in the body and are important for cells to work properly. Proteins are made up of amino acids, and the order of the amino acids determines the form and function of that particular protein. For example, some proteins are called enzymes and are absolutely neces-sary for energy production and metabolism. Other proteins are hormones, antibodies, or signaling molecules that allow cells to communicate with each other so that basic body functions, like digesting food, can occur.

Why do we think of certain diseases as genetic, or caused by genes? Remember, sections of the DNA code are called genes. Many thousands of genes are contained on a chromosome. Normally, humans inherit forty-six chromosomes from their parents (twenty-three from each). All of these chromosomes contain the nuclear DNA (nDNA) that is found in the nucleus of the cell and contains inherited genes from our mother and our father. In every cell, there are a number of mitochondria which, as you know, make energy for the cell. Mitochondria have their own DNA, called the mtDNA. When there is an error in *any* of the DNA (genetic or in the mitochondria), this is called a mutation and is the cause of many diseases (in this case, your or your child's mitochondrial disease).

Mitochondrial DNA (mtDNA)—Inherited From Mom

For some families, a long family history of unexplained strokes, deafness, dia-betes, weakness, neurological issues, etc. in parents, siblings, aunts, and uncles, and so on suddenly "makes sense" when the broader umbrella of mitochondrial disease is suggested. In this case, it is possible that this diagnosis is a relief, as it gives a name and validity to the symptoms and struggles that you or your family members have faced for many years. As one adult patient, who was diagnosed only after her second child was diagnosed with Mito, shares, "All I can remember as a kid is my Mom napping on the couch, and that I was tired all the time too. My teachers thought I was lazy—I thought I just wasn't very athletic. I watched my mother struggle with depression, pain, and fatigue for all of my young adult life, and then when I had kids and I started to feel the same way, I thought I was crazy. I get it now—it's mitochondrial disease, and none of us ever knew." In these cases, mitochondrial disease in the family has been inherited from an mtDNA mutation that has been passed down through generations of women.

As we see in Figure 2.3 on the next page, we know now that each cell has many mitochondria, and those mitochondria have their own DNA (which is different than the rest of the cell's DNA). All of our mitochondria are inherited from our mother's egg; therefore, diseases carried on the mitochondrial DNA are only passed on from mother to child. If the mother is a carrier or affected by mitochondrial disease at the time of conception, each fertilized egg will contain both normal and mutated mitochondrial DNA (mtDNA), which are randomly passed to her children in such a way that any unborn child has the potential to acquire the mutation. As the embryo develops from successive steps of cell division and replication, cell lines may then have variable ex-pression of mutated and normal mitochondria. These cell lines subsequently make up the tissues in our bodies such as muscle, nervous, and gastrointestinal tissues, which define the organs commonly affected by mitochondrial disease. From here we can be-gin to understand the concept of heteroplasmy, defined as the presence of diseased and functional mitochondria in any given cell or tissue.

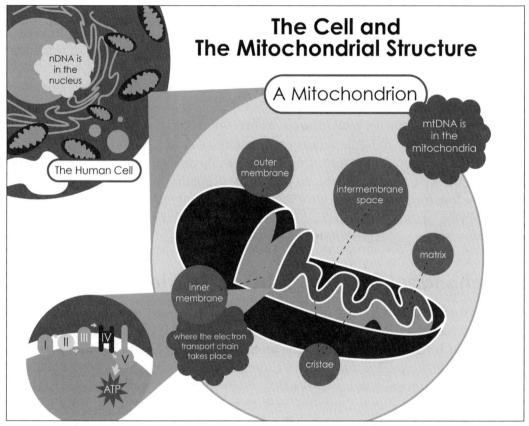

Figure 2.3: Cell containing a nucleus and many mitochondria.   *Image by Jane Adams*

Heteroplasmy implies that there are healthy and unhealthy mitochondria in the same cell (see Figure 2.4). The mitochondrial cells of every person with Mito contain a mosaic of normal and abnormal DNA. An mtDNA mutation may affect a large number of the mitochondria, making the chance of the mother passing the mutation on to her child during fertilization of the egg more likely. On the other hand, even if a woman has only a few unhealthy mitochondria and very mild or no symptoms of Mito, there is still a likelihood of passing on the mtDNA that carries the defect. Keep in mind that mtDNA defects can affect boys and girls, but are only passed down through the women in a family.

Let's imagine that you have twenty-four apples in a brown paper bag. Half of the apples are rotten and half are freshly picked. If you line up four bowls on a table and randomly reach into the bag and place six apples in each bowl, what is the likelihood that one bowl will be full of only fresh apples, while another bowl is full of only rotten apples? The likelihood cannot really be predicted because it is random and based on chance. Maybe one bowl has five fresh, or "healthy," apples and one rotten, or "mutated," apple. In that case, you still have five good apples to use to make a pie! On the other hand, another bowl may have randomly gotten five rotten apples and only one good apple. Now the likelihood of your pie being affected is very high. But it was based on chance.

Now imagine that your bag contains twenty rotten apples, and only four fresh apples. The likelihood of having a rotten apple in all four bowls is 100 percent because you

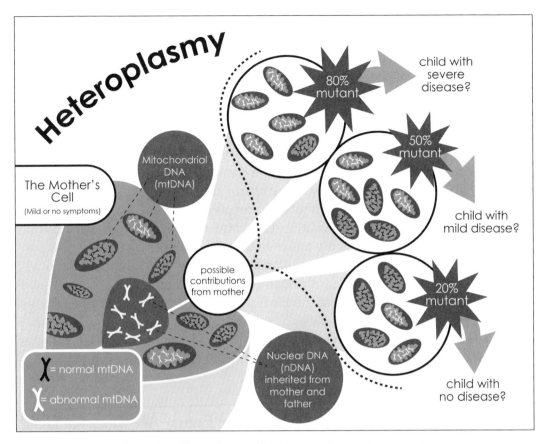

Figure 2.4: Heteroplasmy: healthy and unhealthy mitochondria in the same cell.

Image by Jane Adams

only have four fresh apples to pick from! Similarly, if a mother has a higher proportion of mutated mtDNA to healthy DNA, the likelihood of having a child with Mito disease (and potentially more severe disease) is higher. On the other hand, if your bag contains mostly fresh apples and only has a couple that are rotten, the likelihood that you will wind up with one bowl that contains *all* of the rotten apples is very low. In this case, a mother who only has a few mutated mtDNA may have no symptoms, and may have children with no disease, or multiple children who are healthy or have only moderate disease. It all depends on chance and the number of mitochondrial DNA that are altered.

An mtDNA disease may occur if there is a point mutation, deletion, or depletion of the mitochondrial DNA. While patients with mtDNA inherited diseases may be affected in a variety of ways, the clinical features tend to be characteristic of the classic mtDNA syndromes and can potentially be more easily recognized by clinicians than other types of mitochondrial disease. However, as mentioned previously, not all patients "fit the bill" of those characteristic syndromes, so diagnosis remains elusive. Nonetheless, features of classic mitochondrial inherited disease that are considered most common include stroke or stroke-like episodes, seizures, vision or hearing problems, ragged red fibers (RRF), muscle weakness, lactic acidosis, and heart problems. A list of some mitochondrial disorders is provided on page 29, although it is worth noting that the characteristic features and defining criteria (including known genetic defects) are very complex. The National Library of Medicine website offers the most comprehensive description and listing of each of the different mitochondrial disorders via the OMIM database (Online Mendelian Inheritance in Man, http://www.ncbi.nlm.nih.gov/omim).

Also of importance in this discussion is that many more people carry an mtDNA mutation than those who have actual "clinical disease." In fact, a study led by Patrick Chinnery and researchers in the United Kingdom suggests that one in two hundred people carry an mtDNA mutation, implying that a large percentage of the population has the potential to develop or pass on an inherited mitochondrial disease. What we don't know is at what rate disease develops and is passed on, since, like the apples in the bowls analogy, the potential to have an egg with more dysfunctional mtDNA than healthy mtDNA is based completely on chance. In addition, the symptoms of mitochondrial disease can vary or be quite mild, and Mito is often under-recognized or misdiagnosed.

In addition to inherited forms of mitochondrial disease, there can be sporadic DNA mutations that occur during a person's lifetime and may lead to spontaneous expression of mitochondrial disease. In this manner, a healthy person's mitochondrial DNA can become damaged due to toxicity from medications or the environment, trauma, or physiologic stress (such as a surgery or prolonged illness), which could then cause mitochondrial disease. In fact, this is presumed to be the cause of mitochondrial disease for many adult Mito patients.

Nuclear DNA (nDNA)—Inherited From Mom and Dad

What about the rest of your DNA? Your nuclear DNA (your chromosomal DNA) was acquired from your mother and father. Most childhood cases of Mito are caused by a defect in the nuclear DNA. There are many more proteins encoded in the nuclear DNA than the mtDNA which have important and complex functions that are essential to cellular energy production. In fact, we know that there are more than 1,000 genes in the nDNA that are directly important in mitochondrial function! Many of these are crucial for the electron transport chain (see Chapter 10) to work properly. So, even though the nDNA is outside of the mitochondria, it still plays a very important role in energy metabolism and mitochondrial function.

But how can two healthy parents have a child who is very sick from mitochondrial disease? To understand the risk of inheriting a mitochondrial disease, we have to understand a little about heredity. The way that nDNA is inherited is called "Mendelian inheritance," which means that a copy of each gene comes from each parent (refer to Figure 2.5). Diseases that are caused by a mutation in a person's genes (a.k.a, genetic diseases) can be inherited several different ways:

1. **Autosomal Recessive (also called "Recessive inheritance")**— Autosomal recessive inheritance means that BOTH parents must have passed on the specific genetic mutation in order to cause the disease. In this situation, both mother and father are "carriers" of the same defect on one of the hundreds of nuclear genes that are important for

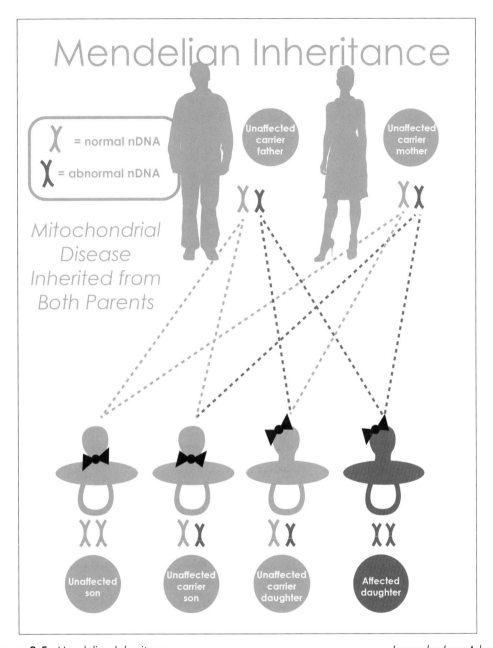

Figure 2.5: Mendelian Inheritance   *Image by Jane Adams*

mitochondrial function. Carriers do not usually have any symptoms of this autosomal recessive disease; however, when these two parents have a child, the child has a 25 percent chance of being born with the disease. In this case, there is also a 25 percent chance of having no disease, and a 50 percent chance of being a carrier (without symptoms) of the genetic mutation. This inheritance pattern accounts for the majority of mitochondrial diseases in children, especially those that are apparent since birth. Keep in mind, the chance of having Mito from this type of inheritance does not correlate with the severity of the disease. Severity and presentation of symptoms is related to the specific gene mutation. Many other genetic diseases in children are caused by recessive inheritance, such as cystic fibrosis and PKU.

2. **Autsomal Dominant (also called "Dominant Inheritance")**—In some circumstances, only one parent has to pass on the altered gene in order for the child to have mitochondrial disease. This is called autosomal dominant inheritance. Dominant genes are frequently associated with a family history of a disease. If one parent has a mutation on a gene that is responsible for a protein that is important for energy production in the mitochondria and passes on that mutated gene, the child will probably have mitochondrial disease. People who have a dominant gene mutation for a mitochondrial disorder usually will have some symptoms of the disease, even though they may be quite mild (and may have been unrecognized). In this case, mothers *or* fathers can unwittingly pass on the mutated nDNA responsible for the disease in their children. The risk of a child developing Mito in this scenario is 50 percent. However, for mitochondrial disease, this form of inheritance is much less common than recessive inheritance.

3. **X-Linked**—The final way that genetic diseases may be inherited is called X-linked. X-Linked diseases are far more common in men than in women because of the way that chromosomes are inherited. Women have two X chromosomes, while men have only one (their other sex chromosome is a Y). Mothers contribute the X chromosome and fathers contribute a Y chromosome to boys or an X chromosome to girls. In this case, X-linked diseases are passed on from mother to her son or daughter on the X chromosome—there is no transfer from father to son. Hemophilia and color blindness are examples of X-linked genetic disorders. X-linked mitochondrial disease is rare, with the exception of pyruvate dehydrogenase complex deficiency, which can be X-linked.

4. **Mitochondrial inheritance**—This is a mutation in the mtDNA (maternally inherited DNA), which is believed to account for about one-fourth of all mitochondrial disease cases in the population. We talked about this in detail above. Remember, until larger population-based studies are employed, many of these statistics about incidence remain as estimates.

M itochondrial disease can be inherited from a person's mother (mtDNA), from both parents (nDNA), can occur spontaneously, or may be acquired as a result of exposure to toxins, medications, or other environmental triggers.

There are some known mitochondrial diseases, clinically referred to as syndromes, caused by mtDNA and nDNA mutations. However, not all patients fit the descriptions exactly, making definitive diagnostic criteria for these syndromes a challenge. In addition, while some syndromes are known to be associated with mtDNA mutations, others may be caused by either mtDNA or nuclear DNA mutations, may be sporadic, or may be unknown. A partial list is offered below of the most commonly identified syndromes; however, many patients have mitochondrial diseases or subtypes that are not listed below! In addition, some of the names can be deceptive as there may be greater or fewer features than those included in the syndrome's name. Finally, it is important to recognize that only a fraction of all of the nuclear genes that may cause mitochondrial disease have been identified.

Most Common Known Mitochondrial Diseases Caused by mtDNA Mutations:

LHON (Leber's hereditary optic neuropathy)
MELAS (Mitochondrial Encephalomyopathy, Lactic Acidosis, and Strokelike Episodes)
MERRF (Myoclonic Epilepsy and Ragged-Red Fiber Disease)
NARP (Neuropathy, Ataxia, and Retinitis Pigmentosa)
POLG Mutation (mtDNA mutation, but without characteristic clinical features)
DAD (Diabetes and deafness)
KSS (Kearns-Sayre Syndrome)
CPEO* (Chronic Progressive External Ophthalmoplegia Syndrome)
Leigh Disease* or Syndrome (also called MILS: Maternally Inherited Leigh Syndrome)
Alpers Disease* (Progressive Infantile Poliodystrophy)
Pearson Syndrome* (Sideroblastic anemia, bone marrow and pancreatic dysfunction)

Most Common Known Mitochondrial Diseases Caused by nDNA Mutations or Sporadic Mutation:

MEMSA (Myoclonic Epilepsy Myopathy Sensory Ataxia) (also referred to as MIRAS: Mitochondrial Recessive Ataxia Syndrome)
Alpers Disease (Progressive Infantile Poliodystrophy)
Pearson Syndrome* (Sideroblastic anemia, bone marrow and pancreatic dysfunction)
Leigh Disease* or Syndrome (also called MILS: Maternally Inherited Leigh Syndrome)
CPEO (Chronic Progressive External Opthalmoplegia Syndrome)
MNGIE (Myoneurogastointestinal Disorder and Encephalopathy)
FAOD (Fatty Acid Oxidation Disorders)
MIRAS (Mitochondrial Recessive Ataxia Syndrome)

* may also be X-linked, autosomal recessive, or spontaneous

Other Mitochondrial Disorders, With Both mtDNA and nDNA or Unknown Genetic Causes:

Carnitine deficiency
Co-enzyme Q10 deficiency
Mitochondrial Cytopathy
Mitochondrial DNA Depletion
Pyruvate Carboxylase Deficiency
Pyruvate Dehydrogenase Deficiency
SCAD (Short Acyl-CoA Dehydrogenase Deficiency)
VLCAD (Very Long Chain Aycl-CoA Dehydrogenase Deficiency)
Complex I, II, III, IV (COX) and/or V Deficiency (usually Mendelian, although may also be maternally inherited)(Patients may have one or more defects in the five ETC complexes)

Source: Patrick Chinnery, Mitochondrial disorders overview. US National Institutes of Health Bookshelf http://www.ncbi.nlm.nih.gov/books/NBK1224/ and OMIM® Online Mendelian Inheritance in Man http://omim.org/

Diagnostic Trends in the Field of Mitochondrial Disease

A molecular diagnosis gives insight into the inheritance type that has caused mitochondrial disease in you, your child, or your family. As outlined in the chart of "Tools and Tests" (Table 2.1), molecular diagnosis can be completed via muscle biopsy, skin fibroblast testing, or gene sequencing of the blood, but the type of testing as well as the results (including the need for further testing) depends on several factors. Diagnosing physicians may suspect a specific genetic defect based on your clinical picture. In addition, mitochondrial defects may not be present in all tissue types, even in a person with known mitochondrial disease. For example, blood or skin may not have the same degree of abnormality as more energy-dependent tissue like muscle, brain, or heart, but will be tested first because skin and blood are easier samples to obtain and would be the first step in testing to begin to identify the mitochondrial defect.

Again, understanding the three-pronged approach to mitochondrial disease diagnosis is important: a) symptoms and clinical presentation, b) biochemical and metabolic testing, and c) molecular and histological testing. Family history and clinical symptoms are just as important as diagnostic tests! The challenge today is for patients and families to be able to obtain a diagnosis within the confines of a general lack of awareness and knowledge about mitochondrial disease. In addition, because molecular testing is a newer technique and is very expensive, it is frequently denied by many health insurance companies on the first request. You should and can expect to appeal this decision by submitting physician letters of necessity that document the importance of a detailed diagnosis in order to assess family risk and to begin appropriate treatment/supplementation. Complex Child e-magazine (www.complexchild.com) offers a comprehensive resource section on insurance appeals, including sample letters, state assistance programs, and suggestions for obtaining coverage for everything from tests to hospital beds.

Nonblood requiring tests such as buccal swab (cheek cell swab) and saliva testing are new options for DNA genome sequencing that are less expensive and less invasive for patients than traditional muscle biopsy. From a simple cheek swab sample (a cotton swab is rubbed inside the cheek to collect buccal cells), buccal swab testing can actually identify mtDNA mutations, complex I and IV defects, and nuclear DNA point mutations can be identified. Buccal swab testing is especially useful in families where there is positive family history and clear clinical symptoms that allow a physician to confirm a diagnosis through the test.

Genomic sequencing can be performed using a buccal swab, or saliva or blood sample to identify changes in many mtDNA and nDNA genes that have been identified by researchers as linked to mitochondrial disease. Sometimes more detailed molecular testing from a blood sample can be used in order to determine the likelihood of a mitochondrial disorder when there are multiple unrelated symptoms (such as headache, vomiting, and poor growth) and abnormal screening tests such as blood lactate and alanine levels. In other cases, molecular testing may be used to confirm that which your family history and symptoms suggest.

Common Misdiagnoses in Children Who Have Mitochondrial Disease

Children with mitochondrial disease are often a puzzle, even to specialists in well-known hospitals. As awareness of and understanding about mitochondrial disease improves, so do diagnosis rates and diagnostic methods. However, there are other diseases that can masquerade as Mito, and many children still are misdiagnosed, or are first diagnosed with one of the following conditions:

- autism spectrum disorder (ASD)
- pervasive developmental disorder (PDD)
- seizure disorder
- cerebral palsy
- intellectual disability (formerly mental retardation)
- kidney disease (renal tubular acidosis)
- poisoning or toxin exposure
- meningitis, encephalopathy
- metabolic or genetic disease of unknown origin
- fatty acid oxidation defect
- short bowel syndrome
- immunodeficiency
- leukodystrophy

The following is a list of "red flags" that would indicate a need for additional testing for a potential mitochondrial disease. These are signs and symptoms that would NOT typically be present in the other conditions listed above. Keep in mind, this is not a complete list of possible symptoms associated with childhood Mito, but is a list of "cues" that may indicate further testing is needed.

- Elevated blood lactate or elevated lactic acid
- Seizures, especially with abrupt onset and in the presence of an infection or fever
- Symptoms that are worse when your child has an illness
- Difficulty recovering from an infection, especially one with a fever
- Growth problems, failure-to-thrive
- Unexplained or sudden hearing loss
- Strokes or stroke-like episodes
- Shaky or jerking muscles (myoclonus)
- Lack of coordination (ataxia)
- Severe constipation or dysmotility
- Exhaustion with exercise or exertion
- Difficulty waking up from anesthesia
- Low muscle tone or weakness with no explanation or obvious cause
- Acute or unexplained muscle pain

Other Causes of Mitochondrial Disease

Some cases of mitochondrial disease may be secondary. That is, there is an abnormality that is caused by some other disease that affects the body's energy production capacity. Depending on the primary disease and its inheritance patterns, other family members may or may not be at genetic risk. Examples of primary diagnoses that have secondary mitochondrial dysfunction include Prader-Willi syndrome, Rett's syndrome, and organic acidemias. In other cases, mitochondrial disease occurs as a result of a condition that depletes the mitochondria, such as malnutrition, ischemia (not enough blood getting to an organ, such as the heart, brain, or muscles), and long-term use of some medications. Furthermore, some children and adults may develop mitochondrial disease as a result of exposure to a toxin, such as a medication that has a damaging effect on the mitochondria. For example, a number of adults develop mitochondrial myopathy due to long-term use of a medication class called "statins," which are commonly used to control cholesterol (hyperlipidemia/hypercholesterolemia). Similar toxicities can occur as a result of drugs used to treat AIDS or, more rarely, diabetes, or depression.

There can also be an environmental event that causes a person to become physiologically overwhelmed and exhausted. For example, severe viral or bacterial infection or illnesses, severe gastrointestinal illnesses, and surgery requiring a period of pre-op fasting and recovery have been known to "trigger" the onset of symptoms in a person who already had an underlying (but asymptomatic) genetic mitochondrial disorder. In this case, perhaps the patient had a predisposition to develop an acquired form of mitochondrial disease because there were a number of defective mitochondria that already existed in that person's cells (heteroplasmy).

The threshold then for developing Mito disease or symptoms is much lower if there are already a large number of dysfunctional mitochondria in the cells. In addition, it makes sense that the organs and tissues that need a lot of energy to work properly, such as the brain, heart, and muscles, are more affected by stressors such as illness, surgery, or drug toxicity. This premise helps also explain, in part, variant age of onset and the apparent sudden appearance of clinical problems.

Despite all of these potential ways that mitochondrial defects can be inherited, a child or adult can still have Mito even when a genetic defect on the nDNA or the mtDNA cannot be identified. In those cases, Mito disease may have been acquired (i.e., secondary to damage caused by medications or toxins) or perhaps developed spontaneously.

Help! What Does All of This Mean for My Family?

If your child has just gotten a diagnosis of mitochondrial disease or you suspect she might get one, you may be feeling a whole slew of emotions and are likely grieving the loss of your dreams for your child's future. If you are an adult patient, or your spouse is going through this diagnosis, you also may be grieving the loss of your previous reality. Everything that you knew and thought to be true feels uncertain now. Anxiety, sadness, depression, anger—and every emotion in between—are normal responses to the stress associated with "the diagnosis." The words "a disease without a cure" penetrate the very existence of many parents and patients so that the prognosis seems hopeless. Often, after the shock of receiving a mitochondrial disease diagnosis comes the insult of being expected to interpret it, advocate for ourselves and our loved ones, and survive the disease.

Giving in to the rollercoaster of emotions can blind you from focusing on being a good advocate and a good listener. It is very important to begin now by being in tune with your body, or your spouse's or child's needs. The journey to a diagnosis is typically long and fraught with stress. This process requires endurance and patience.

REBECCA, MOM TO LEAH
(TEN YEARS OLD LIVING WITH MITO)

When Leah was diagnosed, she was just a baby. The doctors told me she wouldn't live to be three years old. She was so sick, and I was so heartbroken. All I could think of was how I imagined her future—she would never get married, she would never have babies, she would never drive a car, or have a sweet sixteen birthday party...the 'she'll never' was all I could see. It actually took me about a year before I recognized how much I was missing right now by always thinking about and grieving her future. I couldn't appreciate anything sweet and special that she WAS doing because I was so focused on what she couldn't do. I suppose I was grieving, and that's normal when you face a diagnosis that is so uncertain like this. But now that she is ten years old, and has outlived her prognosis, I have learned to appreciate every day, and every moment. I love her and live for her right now, because who knows what the future brings? Maybe she will do those things, or maybe she will do something totally different that I can't expect or imagine.

The first step in understanding a diagnosis of mitochondrial disease is acceptance. Acceptance is not the same as defeat! Acceptance is acknowledgment of this new challenge, and acknowledgement that you and your family may face a new reality now than what you had before or had expected for the future. Do not give up hope, and never let anyone—physician or otherwise—predict the future for you, your child, or your family.

Genetic counselors are an enormously helpful part of your healthcare team. They are trained to support you and your family and explain the potential risks of passing on mitochondrial disease to future children, and what risks those children and other family members should be aware of. They can answer your questions as well as connect you to clinical diagnostic or confirmatory testing, clinical care professionals, support groups, and clinical trials that are excellent resources for you and your family. The National Society of Genetic Counselors has a comprehensive listing of genetic counselors online, http://www.nsgc.org/.

Despite the devastating cases that have been described in the medical literature, there is a new and growing population of patients with mitochondrial disease that are outliving their prognoses and are finding a great quality of life in new and meaningful ways. The spectrum of people living with mitochondrial disease is quite broad and changing rapidly, especially as the connections between mitochondrial function and other diseases are made.

Remember, although difficult, learning the diagnosis is only one part of your journey. Start now, as much as you can, to focus on that which is possible and practical. More about coping and learning to live fully with Mito is covered in Chapter 3.

Key Points from This Chapter

- The journey to a diagnosis of mitochondrial disease can take months or even years for some people, and is potentially expensive, invasive, and exhausting. Despite this, more physicians are referring patients for full diagnostic workups when mitochondrial disease is suspected, as a specific genetic diagnosis is now strongly preferred over a "suspected" or "clinical" diagnosis only.

- Improvements in diagnostic testing now offer diagnosticians the technology to sequence DNA from blood, cheek (buccal) cells, and saliva, as well as other tissues such as skin, liver, and muscle. This allows mutations related to mitochondrial disease to be identified in more (but not all) people.

- There are about forty mutations in the mtDNA and three hundred mutations in the nDNA that have been identified and linked to mitochondrial disease; however, it is likely that there are many more that have yet to be discovered.

- No one test can offer a definitive diagnosis of mitochondrial disease; rather, diagnosis is made from a three-pronged approach that includes a) symptoms and clinical presentation, b) biochemical, metabolic, and physiologic testing, and c) molecular and histological testing.

- Patients often undergo several studies as part of their diagnosis, including blood tests, DNA sequencing studies, MRI and/or MRS, muscle or tissue biopsy, and urine biochemistry.

- Mitochondrial disease can be inherited from a person's mother (mtDNA), from both parents (nDNA), can occur spontaneously, or may be acquired as a result of exposure to toxins, medications, or other environmental triggers.

SPECIAL INSERT

Mitochondrial Disease–Past, Present, and Future

Katherine B. Sims M.D.
Nancy Slate, research coordinator
Mitochondrial Disorders Clinic, Massachusetts General Hospital

The term mitochondrial disease was coined in the 1980s and followed the long recognition of the mitochondria as organelle and the growing biochemical understanding of the role this organelle played in cellular energy metabolism. Initial human disorders identified were those with clinical syndromes [MELAS, MERRF, LHON] that were later shown secondary to mitochondrial DNA (mtDNA) mutations. Over the last decade, additional mtDNA mutations, as well nuclear DNA (nDNA) mutations, have been identified in those with multi-system clinical features of cellular energy failure. Although much progress has been made in identifying and cataloging the molecular mutations, both mtDNA and nDNA, the biochemical understanding of the cellular consequences of defects in oxidative-phosphorylation or the other cellular processes potentially disrupted in mitochondrial dysfunction, and the consequences to the whole person, remains poorly understood.

A mitochondrial diagnosis is usually suggested by clinical symptoms but requires additional testing to identify other biochemical, physiologic, or molecular abnormalities which allow for more definitive diagnosis. Tissue biopsy remains a mainstay of diagnostic evaluation as direct analysis by light microscopy, electron microscopy, electron-transport chain (ETC), carnitine biochemical, and coenzyme Q10 analysis may yield positive results. This can be helpful even if molecular testing is unremarkable. A number of diagnostic clinical criteria have been published (UA Walker et al 1996; FP Bernier et al 2002; NI Wolf and JAM Smeitink 2002; F Morava et al 2006) and allow semi-quantitative assessment of a person with signs and/or symptoms suggesting a mitochondrial energy metabolism disorder. Each of these criteria has their strengths and weaknesses but do assist in diagnostic clarification. It remains, however, for future research to delineate better criteria which can make diagnosis easier and more certain.

Following the diagnosis of a possible or definitive mitochondrial disorder, the mainstay of treatment is symptomatic management. Depending on the extent and details of the clinical problem (e.g., presentations with gastrointestinal, cardiac, neurologic, ophthalmologic, audiologic, endocrine, renal or hepatic, amongst many) a patient's management can vary widely. A general mainstay of treatment, however, is to develop strategies to decrease metabolic stress. These include avoidance of illness or early treatment, avoidance of extended fasting, dehydration and/or metabolic acidosis, adjustment to physiologic limits (e.g., exercise intolerance), rest, good nutrition, and treatment of organ-specific dysfunction. The empiric use of vitamins ("mitochondrial cocktail") is also commonly prescribed. This is a mixture of vitamins, often formulated, which are biochemical co-factors that operate in the mitochondrial pathways, as well as a variety of antioxidants, which presumably help protect the mitochondria from stress and damage.

Amongst one of the greatest challenges, for patients and families, is a daily one—how to maintain optimum health and to avoid illness. Because of the lack of a standard treatment of care, many patients may feel adrift and care may vary from provider to provider. The diagnostic evaluation of mitochondrial disease presents a number of options and constraints. There is the decision about whether or not to undergo a muscle biopsy and if one elects to do so, should it be a frozen biopsy done near home or a fresh biopsy, that usually involves travel. Should the physician, patient and/or family consider a molecular test in hopes of avoiding the more invasive muscle biopsy? If so, which of the myriad of molecular testing options to order and will insurance coverage be obtained? Should testing be deferred and a less "perfect" diagnosis accepted (but similar management options put in place) until newer diagnostic techniques are developed? There are also the hurdles with insurance which arise, for coverage of the mitochondrial cocktail and monitoring labs in addition to diagnostic testing. Even after all of the testing or labs, the currently available treatment or management options will still be essentially the same.

Research is ongoing in the field of mitochondrial disorders and it offers the best hope for future treatments and diagnosis. Researchers are developing better sequencing tools to uncover more causal genes and are also analyzing metabolites in the hope of finding more diagnostic markers. Cell studies are evaluating channel signals and protein interactions. All of these research projects may potentially help with development of future disease treatments and management guidelines. Genetic counseling and family planning depend on molecular diagnosis and currently this is available only for the minority with mitochondrial disorders.

The future holds promise. New technologies and more global research partnerships allow for more scientific collaboration. Scientists are using many different and sophisticated scientific approaches to learn more about the mitochondria and mitochondrial function. The research communities are very willing to share this knowledge with clinicians to help improve patient care and patient/family support groups are encouraging care providers to work to establish a standard of care. The multi-level involvement of clinicians, researchers, patients, and patient families' has enabled mitochondrial disease to become more widely recognized. It is our hope that this awareness will stimulate more funding and research efforts to help elucidate, treat, and manage mitochondrial disease.

3

Accepting the Diagnosis and Learning to Live WELL with Mito

"Be who you are and say what you feel, because those who mind don't matter, and those who matter don't mind."
—Dr. Seuss

Mito is, in some ways, like other chronic conditions; it is a lifelong diagnosis that will have a ripple effect on you, your family, your job, your finances, your education, your relationships, and your everyday activities. Learning to live a "normal life" again after getting a diagnosis of mitochondrial disease, for your loved one or yourself, can be a little bit like learning to live on a different planet. While you occasionally venture out into the new world, you are more timid and feel disoriented. You feel confined because you don't understand the roadmaps, the people, and the language. Things that were easy to do before are now challenging, and you are constantly required to adjust your expectations. Other people don't understand what it's like to live as you do, yet you don't have the energy to try to explain. Some days are really emotionally and physically hard.

Then, one day you meet someone else like you and you are so grateful. You begin to learn the language and eventually begin to speak for yourself again. You learn to adjust your expectations and to change your routine so that you can find your way on your own. One day, you realize that you actually feel thankful, and that even though your life is quite different than it was before (and quite different than the life you had imagined), you are happy. You realize that there are things that you have learned and that you have overcome that you would have never expected of yourself, and you are surprised to find that you can laugh and feel happy in this new place that was so frightening before.

Initially, it might feel like your life is over when you, your child, or your loved one gets a diagnosis of mitochondrial disease. We begin to live again when we can recognize and accept that this diagnosis is not about predicting the future or fighting a battle, it is about dealing with major change *right now*. The journey that you take to arrive at a diagnosis of mitochondrial disease marks a pivotal beginning of a new chapter in you and your family's life. It may not be what you expected, but it can be rich nonetheless.

Reacting to the Diagnosis

There are many people in our world today who live with chronic illnesses, which can be catastrophic, require lifestyle adjustments, or are life-threatening. Children, parents, spouses, and adult patients each face their own unique challenges and reactions to unexpected diagnosis; however, research actually suggests that, at least at the time of diagnosis, people have some similarities in their initial reactions:

1. Shock, i.e., "This can't be happening to me."
2. Disbelief, i.e., "The doctors/tests must be wrong. This isn't for real."
3. Grief about the future, i.e., "Now I (or my child) won't ever be able to…."
4. Sorrow, i.e., "I'm too sad to do anything."
5. Anger, i.e., "My child doesn't deserve this. This isn't fair and I will fight this even to the end."
6. Isolation, i.e., "No one understands how I feel and what we are going through."
7. Denial, i.e., "If I don't do anything, maybe he'll be ok. Maybe he'll just get better on his own."

Take note of how *emotional* the reactions are above. Learning to live with Mito is easier if you can learn to recognize and forgive yourself and others for the normal emotional responses that occur as part of coming to terms with a new diagnosis. Sorting through your feelings and giving yourself (or your spouse or family) a break helps you move closer to the stage that will enable you to begin *living* again: acceptance.

Now What? Steps to Accepting the Diagnosis

When our daughter was first diagnosed, we experienced all of the emotions (at different times) that are listed above. We also devoured information about Mito like we were starving. We read everything we could get our hands on, and, honestly, understood and absorbed very little of it. Our daughter's condition was really not any different now that we had a name for her particular set of symptoms and setbacks, but the name, "mitochondrial disease," was just so powerful. It consumed our thoughts and controlled our reactions to *everything*. For a long time, I couldn't look at my daughter without hearing the doctor's words in my head. One day, it just hit me when I looked at her. She was the same precious little girl that she was before this diagnosis, the same little girl who loves strawberries and stuffed bears and for me to blow kisses on her bare belly. Acceptance began for us only when we stepped back and realized that we had to learn to see that this new diagnosis was going to be a *piece* of our life, not the whole.

Learning to *live* with the diagnosis of mitochondrial disease is our ambition. When you look back, over the months or years that Mito affected you or your child's life, will you be resentful? Could you be grateful instead? We can look to others who are parents, family members, and adults who live graciously with mitochondrial disease as our teachers. Our purpose is to redefine what we want, what brings us *real* happiness, and how we can live again in spite of the Mito diagnosis.

How you hopefully arrive at a state of peace and acceptance about this disease is so individual. However, there are many parents, adult patients, teens, kids, and spouses who have walked this road before us who can offer their insight and advice. The following "steps" are lessons learned from our Mito community.

1. Take the Time You Need

Even if this was a diagnosis that you were expecting or had been pursuing for a long time, you still probably felt shocked when the diagnosis was confirmed. In addition, most people have difficulty processing information and remembering any details when they receive such overwhelming news. Don't be afraid to take the time to process this new information and ask more than once for help or for information to be repeated (or better yet, written down for you to reference later). Follow-up appointments should be frequent right after the diagnosis so that you and your family have time to absorb the details and formulate new questions to ask. Typical clinics won't prompt you to do this, but are usually responsive if you ask for a quicker follow-up.

I found that I always needed to take a small pocket recorder to my daughter's appointments, and with the physician's permission, would record the "plan" portion of our appointment so my husband and I could remember the details later and talk about our decisions. We also learned never to make decisions on the spot during an appointment unless there was an urgent need, because we simply couldn't process the details as well when we were feeling frightened or emotionally overwhelmed. Keep in mind, I am a nurse and my husband is a physician and even with our medical backgrounds, we still found that we needed that extra time to absorb new information about our daughter's diagnosis. Hence, you have permission to take the time that you need! Better to take pause and feel good about your decisions than to wrestle with unnecessary confusion and emotional stress later.

2. Allow Yourself to Be Overwhelmed

It is normal to be overwhelmed. It is understandable when successful people who are accustomed to being able to make good decisions and control the consequences feel as if they have been punched in the stomach by surprise with the Mito diagnosis. As mentioned in the list of typical reactions above, it is "only human" to feel angry, sad, detached, depressed, afraid, or any combination of these! Even the most successful and resourceful patients, parents, and families who learn to find joy, hope, and quality of life despite the diagnosis of mitochondrial disease still find themselves at rock bottom once in a while. I say all of this not to create further despair about your life now that there is a Mito diagnosis on the table. In fact, no physician, family member, or expert can predict the future for you, your child, or your family. But to pretend that by just knowing the diagnosis we can all feel better and get back to life the way it used to be would be dishonest, so I feel obliged to unpretentiously and humbly admit that yes, this new life will be hard. I have yet to meet a family or patient with mitochondrial disease who is not exhausted and humbled by the effort of living with the daily challenges inherent to the diagnosis. On the other hand, I have encountered numerous parents, adult patients, and families who really do live each day to the fullest. They are compassionate and hopeful, and they are joyful and inspire others. They work hard and make tough decisions. Many of these patients and families were told at the point of their diagnosis that there was little hope for their future. Some of them are profoundly physically affected by the disease and others have symptoms that are invisible to the outside world. Yet ALL of them have felt truly lost at one point or another during this crusade, as if they had been dropped into an alien country without knowing the language or the landmarks. Allow yourself to be overwhelmed, and give yourself the space to see beyond those feelings.

3. Find Support in Others Who Understand

When asked what helps them cope, almost all of the patients and parents in our Mito community respond with two things: information and support. (How to access more information on mitochondrial disease is detailed in Step #10.) Finding support from others who have Mito (or more broadly, special needs or chronic illness) can be the lifeline that you need when you are at the end of your rope. Use the resources around you and be persistent in trying to forge worthwhile connections. Many parents report that they felt uncomfortable or sad when they first attended a support group, but that they are very glad that they didn't give up, as those groups helped them to develop long-lasting friendships. Social media sites like Facebook, telephone or web-based seminars, and support groups offered by nonprofit organizations, online bulletin boards, Yahoo! Groups, and specialized email listservs are great (free and easy) places to start. (See Appendix C for a list of informative websites and support networks.)

4. Recognize When You Are Overstressed

For many, when we receive a devastating and emotional diagnosis like mitochondrial disease, we instinctively feel right away that we should be "ready to fight." This is a normal reaction! Think about it. As a culture, we believe and put great faith in the battle to "beat cancer," "defeat autism," "battle MS," etc. In addition, as human beings it is actually our innate instinct to want to fight anything which threatens us. Our bodies are "prewired" with an inborn response to anything that we perceive as a threat. This inborn reaction is called "fight or flight" and is an instinct that we carry today and that has helped the human race survive! When any human or animal is faced with perceived danger (note the word perceived—not necessarily real danger, but that which they *feel* is a threat), the body's sympathetic nervous system activates, preparing them to respond either by fighting or escaping. When a lion is chasing a deer in the African tundra, the deer, who was happily grazing before being pursued by the predator, is able to mobilize his muscles quickly and run very fast to escape. Similarly, humans undergo a reaction causing us to become aroused and alert during a fight or flight response. Historically, this was useful so that we wouldn't be eaten alive by saber tooth tigers and could be ready to fight a predator or take flight (escape quickly) from dangerous situations. Today, there is a great deal of psychological theory that asserts that our society lives in a chronic state of fight or flight. We are all stressed all (or most) of the time, and this chronic state of heightened adrenalin and arousal can actually wear us down, aging us prematurely. The instinct is obviously very useful, but is also obviously supposed to take place just once in a while. Imagine though, if the average person today is overcompensating for the stimulus around him with a stress response, what does that mean for those of us who are living with or caring for someone who suffers from a chronic disease like Mito?

So how about you…are you ready to fight, flight, or freak out? Both children and adults with mitochondrial disease have a tendency to become trapped in a chronic state of "fight or flight." Just because you feel tired and don't have the energy to run like a gazelle does not mean that your body is not revved up and stressed! Let's take a closer look at the inventory of reactions that occur in the body during a heightened stress, or fight or flight, state:

- Pupils dilate. We freeze, so we can acutely hear and see better. Our breathing gets more rapid.
- Our mind feels overwhelmed and we have a very strong urge to run away from our problems or the clinic, school, etc. where the stressors lie (this is the "flight" part of fight or flight).
- "Unnecessary" body processes slow down or stop completely, such as digestion, growth, tissue repair, or reproduction.
- Blood pressure and heart rate increases. Oxygen demand increases. Blood vessels to other organs, such as the kidneys, constrict, shutting down "nonessential" systems.
- Glucose and fats are mobilized in order to fuel the muscles. A massive amount of energy is redirected from storage to be used immediately, if necessary.
- Bowels and bladder loosen (might have an accident), and sweat glands are activated. Blood vessels to the skin constrict to conserve blood flow (so the skin becomes pale and clammy).
- The adrenal glands release hormones called catecholamines (like adrenalin), which contribute to the biochemical reaction in the brain and body causing the stress response.

You may feel that you, as a parent, patient, or caregiver, should be fighting the disease at all times. You might feel this so instinctively that it influences your decisions without your recognition. Others might make you feel this way also. For example, even if family and friends are trying to be supportive, wishes such as "You can beat this" add to our already overwhelming feelings of stress and contribute to our perception that we are preparing for battle.

When you are overstressed, you may be instinctively reacting to this urge to "fight or flight" without conscious recognition. This is especially true in stressful circumstances (such as a hospitalization or procedure), or when given new information about your or your child's condition. The mother of a school-aged child with Mito, Sharon, shares this example:

> The morning is going ok. My daughter's tube feeding is complete and I'm getting her ready for school. Then the phone rings. I get a little anxious just hearing the ring, and then I panic inside when I see on the caller ID that the hospital is calling. It's the cardiologist. The results from my daughter's recent tests on her heart are in and they are abnormal. Not life-threatening (in fact, probably not a new condition but just newly identified for her). I can't help it—I freak out when I get off the phone! My coffee and breakfast are left untouched. I frantically get my daughter off to school and am on the Internet seconds after. Next thing I know I have forty pages of material printed out and I've sent emails to all of her doctors. It's noon—I didn't eat any breakfast, missed my morning exercise class, the kitchen is a wreck, and I missed the opportunity to do everything I had scheduled that day. I feel nauseous and exhausted. Looking back, this has happened to me so many times that I wonder when I will figure out how to pace myself and not get so excited with every new piece of bad news!

Theresa points out that although her daughter's tests were abnormal, they were NOT life-threatening, and were probably confirmation of symptoms that had been present for awhile. If Theresa can learn to recognize the distress and symptoms in herself of the "fight or flight" reaction to this type of news, she can not only make better, more rational decisions, but she will also protect herself from the effects of this type of chronic stress.

Psychologists agree that people with over-reactive stress responses are much more likely to suffer from anxiety, depression, and anger. You can imagine how our instinct to survive can work against us when we are trying to just live as an adult patient or care for a child with mitochondrial disease. The exaggerated physical response to constant stress actually creates a vicious cycle that makes us physically and emotionally sicker. You feel stressed, you aren't able to make good decisions, and your body shuts down nonessential systems in order to be prepared to fight. You then feel poorly later, worse than you would have otherwise, due to the consequences of the increased energy demand and redirection of energy from digestion and tissue repair. You are then slightly compromised when the next threat occurs—it could be a confrontation with a nurse, doctor, or teacher, a letter of denial from the insurance company, or even the sound of sirens while on the highway. Your body overreacts again because you are already in a heightened state of stress, and you feel frazzled. You may be tearful or angry and agitated. For adults with mitochondrial disease, this cascade of responses contributes significantly to daily symptoms, including nausea, fatigue, headaches, and muscle pain. For caregivers, you may find yourself wearing out, so that everything seems to be more than you can handle (also called "caregiver burnout").

Children, both children with Mito and their healthy siblings, are not immune to stress either. Kids with Mito may have symptom flare-ups or more erratic presentation of symptoms during periods of chronic stress (chronic can mean months or years). Siblings and healthy kids suffer too. Realistically, we can only minimize the stress of our lives and our diagnoses to a degree. However, we **can** recognize when we are over-stressed and try to slow down our body's instinctive fight or flight response by learning to take note of our body's stress signals.

I'm a Wreck!

Stress Signal Alert! Are you...

- Irritable, with a tendency to snap or say things that are out of proportion to the situation?
- Tired? You sleep a lot but the sleep is not regenerating. (Even for people with Mito, sleep should be regenerating for at least a short period of time.)
- Avoidant? You don't want to talk to people, go to meetings, or be in places where you have to interact with people.
- Constipated, nauseous, gassy, or have diarrhea? The result of your body shutting down blood flow to digestive organs and slowing peristalsis.
- Procrastinating? Junk piles up, bills are overdue, nothing gets done, and the demands that people make of you (even friends or family) seem overwhelming.
- Depressed? You feel unmotivated to do the things that you used to enjoy.
- Emotional? You are tearful even in inappropriate places (like the post office or the reception desk at the clinic).
- Or you are angry and yell or overreact even in situations that aren't stressful? Or both?
- In pain? Symptoms (for kids and adults with Mito) are worse. For caregivers, headache, backache, stomachache, muscle ache. Muscles may be shaky.

And a few other signs just for kids...

- Acting out? Tantrums, pushing, shoving, biting, yelling.
- Sleepy in inappropriate places or despite the opportunity for rest periods?
- Avoidant? Avoids eye contact, avoids talking.
- Withdrawn? Doesn't want to participate in activities—even those that he enjoys.
- Crying, tearful, anxious, begging, whining, fussing?

5. Give Yourself Permission to Grieve

Grieving is fundamental to acceptance of the diagnosis. Learning to live with mitochondrial disease is a process. Grief is part of that process, whether you are a parent, a family member, a caregiver, a teen, or an adult patient. Often we don't allow grief to be part of the process of learning to positively cope with the diagnosis of Mito. In part, this is a consequence of being hyper-focused on the difficulty of obtaining the diagnosis and the medical complexity that is inherent to mitochondrial disease. It may have taken months or years of effort, multiple doctor visits and travels to out-of-state medical specialists, hundreds or thousands of dollars, and a crash medical education before finally receiving the diagnosis. For many, the next logical step after the diagnosis is to get more information, to try to see more doctors, and to throw the family into the process of responding to the medical needs of the person who is affected. In truth, these steps are critically important, but too often are at the expense of working through the fundamental grief that you are *allowed* to feel as you uncover the impact that this diagnosis will have on your life, your self-esteem, and your dreams (for you or for your child).

Grieving can allow us to let go of and accept some of those fears. Grieving gives you the freedom to be sad for the loss of some of our dreams for the future. Let me be clear, grief and acceptance are not about passively lying down and letting Mito take over your life. It is NOT giving up! Acceptance, of grief and of the diagnosis, is about dreaming *new* dreams, looking around for *new* opportunities, and seeking different perspectives from a new point of view. Your vantage point has changed, so we must begin taking control of the little things that make you or your child and family feel better *now* so that you begin to be able to consciously direct your energy in ways that make you feel well, both physically and spiritually. However, when we don't stop and allow ourselves to recognize these feelings of grief and to give ourselves (and our other family members) the time to feel sad, to be in denial, to be angry, etc. we can get stuck on an endless loop of frenetic searching.

My dear friend Tom lost his wife to MELAS a few years ago. He is a successful businessman and his wife, Sally, was always "the life of the party" —social, energetic, and extremely involved and supportive of him and their children. He shares with us this story:

> When Sally first became sick, I knew what it was before the doctors did. I spent hours upon hours reading on the Internet, looking up scores of information related to her every symptom. When I read about MELAS and mitochondrial disease, I said, "This is it! This is what she has." I knew I was right. When she was diagnosed shortly thereafter, I continued my crazed search for answers. I didn't sleep. I worked all day, took her to multiple specialists around the country, and spent nights reading everything I could find online. I have no medical degree, but I threw myself into understanding how to fix her disease with a vengeance. I stumbled

upon a trial in mice in the Netherlands where they were manipulating the mitochondria. I was so excited—this would cure my wife! I recall bringing the articles to her physicians—finally, one of them looked at me and said, "Where is Sally now?" I was flustered by the physician's lack of interest in the mouse study. "She's at home," I said. Sally's doctor said, "Go be with her. That's what you should be focused on." It was like I was hit over the head with a ton of bricks. Sally was at home alone and I had been so focused on the idea that I could fix her disease that I hadn't even really been there for her in a true emotional and caring way.

6. Prioritize & Organize

When you, your child, or your family member has mitochondrial disease, one of the best skills that you can learn is to prioritize and organize. Prioritization and organization applies to both physical spaces as well as our mental clutter. There are many books, websites, and tips on tackling clutter and getting organized. Take advantage of these resources! When your physical space is clean and uncluttered, you will be able to think more clearly. Further, learning to prioritize is critically important for anyone who has multiple specialists and reams of medical records as part of their medical care and history. One of the worst things that a patient or parent can do is to arrive at a semiannual clinic visit with the mitochondrial specialist and, due to lack of prioritization before the appointment, "dump" everything into the nurse or physician's lap! Often, patients or parents want to save everything for that all-important appointment and immediately launch into a description of the details of various symptoms, several concerning episodes, questions about labs and test results and follow-up appointments, and concerns about new issues. The physician or nurse in the clinic is overwhelmed with the amount of information and spends more time trying to sort through which of the symptoms and questions is the most treatable or threatening, while being unable to really appropriately respond to most of the family's concerns or questions.

The solution to this frustrating scenario is to prioritize. Literally, keep track of symptoms, episodes, questions about medications, etc., in a designated notebook and jot down details along with questions and the date. Likewise, if you are concerned about symptoms, track them. For example, how often do you or your child get headaches? What time do they begin? Are they related to food, medicine, light, sleep, temperature, etc.? Now, armed with this information, take the time BEFORE the appointment to organize the information. What questions are most pressing? What medicines need to be refilled? Which labs are outstanding? Preparing for the appointment this way allows you to have a much more productive visit, and empowers you to feel calm and in control in order to get the most out of your visit. Learning to be organized and to prioritize is a skill and a discipline that takes persistence and practice! However, honing these abilities can be an extremely effective method to manage the multiple challenges that are "normal" for anyone living with Mito.

DAD & HUSBAND'S PERSPECTIVE

My name is Dave, and I am the dad of a daughter with mitochondrial disease, and the husband of a lovely woman who also suffers from Mito. When our daughter Haley was diagnosed, I was a senior VP at a major financial investment firm in a major city. Like everyone else there, I worked long hours. I was on track to become a partner in the firm in the next five years. I had a stellar education and a MBA from a well-known and well-respected (and very expensive) university, and I was known for my ability to coordinate multiple projects and lead several different groups of people. Relationships and commitments to clients are important. There was no question that I was a future partner in the firm. I would easily be making six figures and have a solid portfolio in a year or two.

I want people to understand how a diagnosis of mitochondrial disease takes away more from a family than perfect health. When my wife was pregnant with Haley, she became very sick. She didn't get an actual Mito diagnosis until our daughter Haley was born and was struggling even in her first few months of life. Obviously, during those months I couldn't be at client dinners. I gave up opportunities to lecture and to attend networking lunches. I only went to the appointments that were crucial for me to keep my job afloat and I did 80 percent of my work from my phone or laptop between doctor's appointments and home. After Haley's initial diagnosis, there was an expectation in my firm that I would be "back to myself." But I wasn't the one who was sick! Instead, I was now the sole provider and caregiver for my family, and their needs were greater than I could ever meet. Months went by where I stayed up all hours of the night trying to catch up and keep a pace somewhat equivalent to the firm's expectations. I was absolutely exhausted. My wife was exhausted. My daughter was sick, and not getting better but not getting worse either. I couldn't be thankful because I was so overwhelmed. A year later I got a 20 percent pay cut—the financial impact on our family was huge. We were already strapped from the medical expenses and out-of-pocket costs for adaptive equipment for both my wife and daughter.

Over the following year, there was less and less talk amongst partners in the firm about my success. They didn't give me big clients and I didn't ask for them. My ability, as an individual, was so different than what I was realistically able to do. It's tough to sacrifice your success and financial career potential for a disease that we didn't ask for and didn't see coming. I will not be a partner in the firm. Realistically, I won't be there much longer and we'll have to move somewhere else in the country with a less competitive job market and lower cost of living. I struggle with the fact that I wish my co-workers recognized that this isn't a choice; it's just a side effect of the disease on our whole family.

7. Remember to Remember

One of the best tips I learned from an adult Mito patient is to "remember to re-member" by taking advantage of the technology offered by today's computers and cell phones. Smartphones are especially great tools for managing hectic schedules by of-fering calendar functions with alarms and alerts that you can customize. Set the timer or calendar reminder features so that you can be automatically reminded to take or refill medicines, call for appointments, submit insurance appeals, etc. In addition, you can use the "notes" feature on smartphones to keep track of important information, such as medical record numbers, names of your medications, test results, etc. The way that my friend Wendy—an adult with Mito—described it to me is this:

> I was sitting there in the hospital, and because I have such bad short-term memory now I couldn't remember anything that I had done prior to ending up in the ER. And I really couldn't comprehend what the doctors were asking me to remember to do when I got home. My husband said to me (because I had asked him to remind me of this when I got confused), "Remember to remember." That triggered my memory that I had everything in my iPhone, so all I had to do was look at my notes and my calendar to know what I had been doing, what meds I took, etc. And I could just ask the doctor to help me type in his instructions, so that when I got home I could remind myself!

I find that one of the best ways to find peace with an overwhelming diagnosis is to use tools that help me stay organized, and online calendars (free Google calendar is especially good), notes, lists, reminders, alarms, etc. can help take away some of the pressure we feel when we get overwhelmed!

8. Establish Routines and Simple Rituals

What can you realistically do every day that you enjoy? Can you have a special cup of coffee or hot tea every morning in a favorite mug? Can you sit down for a moment in the afternoon or evening while you look out the window at a garden or birdfeeder? Do you enjoy reading the newspaper or a book, listening to a book on tape, or exercis-ing? Can you cuddle with a pet, read books to your kids, or rub peppermint lotion on your feet? Can you try yoga, meditation, or journaling? Begin to establish routines and simple rituals by first identifying simple things that you enjoy. Make a list—does your family look forward to fresh bread or bagels from the bakery on Sunday morn-ings? Often, we already have little routines that we take for granted; however, if we enjoy them, we can allow those existing routines to become sources of happiness for us. Instead of mindlessly having your coffee or going to the library, become cognizant of this activity and be very aware of the details. How do you like your coffee? Use your favorite mug, buy your favorite beans, sit down for the first sip. Peppering an otherwise stressful day with little routines and simple rituals such as a cup of tea or reading the paper can help us to feel grounded, and gives us something to look forward to even when we are feeling very sad or overwhelmed.

Routines and simple rituals are very important for children as well, including healthy siblings and kids of adults with mitochondrial disease. Can Sunday night be a night for movies and ice cream? Can you establish a special bedtime or morning routine that can be repeated, even when away from home? Can you leave notes on the mirror or in a lunchbox every day? When we are overwhelmed with big problems, little things are easier to control and can help us learn to find joy in the simplest of pleasures.

9. Keep a Journal

If you are resistant to the idea of keeping a journal, you are not alone! Many people resist the idea, complaining that they just don't have the time or energy to keep a journal, especially because they are dealing with mitochondrial disease and all of its challenges. However, it is especially important for parents, teens, and adult patients who live with mitochondrial disease to keep a journal, and to enjoy the benefits of this simple tool! It is worth it to yourself to give it a try for a month—you might find that journaling is not only satisfying and rewarding but also gives you the peace and perspective that you need. There are many reasons to keep a journal, and here are just a few:

- You can be free and open about your feelings, sharing things in a journal that you might not be ready to share aloud.
- You can track your life, literally, which is really important for any child or adult living with mitochondrial disease. Are certain times or seasons better for you? When did that symptom really begin, and when did it get better or worse? How do I feel during holidays or when I'm stressed?
- Journaling allows you to "try on" decisions before making them by writing about them and considering the pros and cons.
- Journals are a great place to write down questions as you think of them, which can be referenced for future clinic/doctor visits.
- Journals do not judge; journaling gives you personal freedom to express yourself fully. It is documented that journaling relieves stress in children and adults.
- Journaling is a ritual that can be completed anywhere in just ten minutes a day.
- Journaling helps you feel that you have completed something. When you finish journaling, you feel that you have done something good for your mind and your soul.
- Journaling helps you set and adjust your goals, and gives you space to air your anger or frustrations without damaging relationships.
- Journaling is compared to meditation because of the tendency for one to relax when writing freely.

10. Become Empowered by Knowledge

You cannot feel in control when you don't understand what's happening. Parents, you may be watching your child suffer, fail to gain weight, have confusing or erratic symptoms, and be exhausted, and no matter what you do, sometimes you cannot make it better. Patients, you may be struggling to keep up with the demands of your own daily care and feel that you are climbing an impossibly tall mountain where the top is always out of reach. You will be able to put yourself in the driver's seat more often, and you will be more confident in yourself as an advocate (for yourself or for your child) when you are armed with knowledge. Knowledge is empowering. Understanding the nuances of your diagnosis and your symptoms allows you to plan better and prioritize your medical needs. You can tease out what's most threatening in your own set of symptoms when you understand what's happening in your body where an energy metabolism defect is present. Patients, families, and parents all agree that, especially during the initial year of receiving a diagnosis, information is vitally important.

Unfortunately, describing and understanding mitochondrial disease is difficult! Most of us don't have a degree in biochemistry and might only vaguely remember something about the mitochondria from high school. Think about learning about mitochondrial disease and your specific diagnosis in the same way that you would approach training for a new job. Would you be emotional and react to information at a job train-

Here's a scenario that most of us who are mothers can relate to. This is an example of how controlling our response to information is difficult to do, but obviously important.

Erin is three years old and she has just gotten a diagnosis of Complex I & IV mitochondrial disease. Erin's mitochondrial doctors are located in a different state so her parents are really trying to advocate for her locally with their pediatricians and other specialists. Erin's mom has been reading about mitochondrial disease. She reads that children with mitochondrial disease can get hypoglycemic (low blood sugar) more easily, and that they should never go a long period of time without food or drink (fasting). Fasting can cause increased lactic acid levels and in some children can contribute to seizures. Erin's mom remembers the time that Erin underwent a procedure at the hospital when she was a baby and they had her fast for eight hours (NPO the night before). Erin's mom starts to breathe fast and her heart rate quickens. She feels panicky. What if that period of fasting caused her daughter's current condition? What if they had recommended she not fast— would she still be suffering from chronic seizures and developmental delays right now? Then Erin's mom remembers the time last week when Erin's preschool teacher allowed Erin to go without snack all morning. Erin's mom is now in a fury. How could everyone fail to acknowledge how serious this is? What should she do?

ing with fear, anger, or sadness? (Hopefully not.) The point is to try to separate yourself emotionally from the opportunity to learn objectively about mitochondrial disease and about the symptoms or secondary issues that affect you or your child or spouse.

Revisit the chapters on diagnosis (Chapter 2) and biochemistry (Chapter 10) in this book again and again, allowing the information to sink in and make sense slowly over time. In addition, the list of useful websites in Appendix C offers a comprehensive list of patient-friendly websites and support networks. Many now have videos that tell the story for you!

Seek information *on purpose.* A thoughtful, controlled approach to learning about mitochondrial disease can help you to feel empowered by knowledge and prevent you from becoming more stressed by what you learn! In general, there are some dos and don'ts to being a good information seeker:

- **DO** use the Internet—it's free and it's fast.
- **DON'T** believe everything you read on the Internet. Go to trusted sources first and most frequently (such as support groups, organizations, and non-profits dedicated to supporting people with mitochondrial disease).
- **DO** learn to use www.PubMed.gov, the free medical online database. Look for articles that are "review" articles, as those will usually summarize the most recent and relevant research. Ask your local hospital to help you obtain full-text articles through their medical library.
- **DON'T** begin reading thirty-seven research articles on your first search. Find articles that are written by well-known physicians who are clinical leaders in the field. If in doubt, ask for help from friends or trusted organizations.
- **DO** use a little time each week to read and learn more.
- **DON'T** get in the habit of spending hours at a time on the computer.
- **DO** take advantage of groups where you can learn more and ask questions.
- **DON'T** believe that everything you hear is going to happen to you.
- **DO** keep yourself reasonably up-to-date about clinical trials and new research that might impact you or your child. For example, you can subscribe to email alerts from www.clinicaltrials.gov.
- **DON'T** spend hours a week looking for such trials. Rely on the organizations you trust to pass on this type of important information.
- **DO** recognize that there is a cost-benefit to educating yourself. Read and educate yourself so that you can be empowered, more confident to make decisions, and better equipped to ask questions of your medical team.
- **DON'T** attempt to become an expert at everything. Your job is not to become a medical or research authority. Practice moderation.
- **DO** give yourself a pat on the back for trying to be a great advocate!
- **DON'T** beat yourself up if you don't know everything. Remember, this is a process and on this journey you will always be learning.
- **DO** ask for help!

11. Learn to See Yourself or Your Child Beyond the Diagnosis

"This is what I have, but it is not who I am."
—Teen Mito "survivor"

Our next step in learning to *live* with Mito is to make a conscious choice: "I am willing to accept the challenges and the pain that I might face because of my/my child's Mito diagnosis, but we will live and be happy anyway."

Here's the important distinction. *Mitochondrial disease is something that you have, it's not who you are.* Let me say it again for parents: *Your child has mitochondrial disease, but the diagnosis does not define who he or she is or what he or she will become.* Had you imagined that your son would be an all-star athlete? Maybe he will. Maybe he'll do something else amazing that you can't even imagine. Had you and your spouse planned to retire on a houseboat on the coast? Maybe you'll find a way to take a cruise together now and have invaluable memories without waiting until your retirement. Did you imagine that your family would be together for Christmas last year, only to find that the holiday was spent in the hospital? While so devastating, you also found a family of support in the friends and nurses who connected with you during that hospital stay. Letting go of our preconceived ideas of happiness is, for most people, extraordinarily difficult. However, it is one sure-fire way that you can begin to positively adjust to this new (and wonderful) life ahead of you despite the challenges that you will face from this illness.

It is easy to get caught in despair and to feel defeated when that which we expected doesn't happen. Margaret is a nurse practitioner who helps many patients with mitochondrial disease and she notes that there are many reasons why families who deal with Mito may feel stressed or unhappy. "There is so much potential for disappointment, not to mention stress from the ambiguity of the disease. But the patients and families who seem to cope with this the best are those that have a very conscious calmness about them. They are determined but flexible, and they always seem to be able to step back and take a look at the big picture before reacting. They really know how to count their blessings. On the other hand, they hope for the best but are prepared for the worst, so that they are always fairly prepared and in control."

The challenges that will be placed before you as a result of your illness or that of your child are, for the most part, out of your control. However, your reaction and your response to those challenges are completely within your control. In addition, you should recognize that it takes practice to improve your reaction and your response, and that with every challenge you have the opportunity to become even better at staying calm and feeling empowered. Redefining what brings us happiness, our quality of life, what we *really want* for ourselves, our children, and our family—these steps can help bring us back to solid ground when we are floundering and feel lost.

LINDA

My husband and I came to terms with Robby's diagnosis and disabilities quite differently, as is common in couples. My husband was quiet and immediately accepting, with no need to research, learn, or grieve. I, on the other hand, struggled with depression for the first several years of Robby's life. I grieved a very long time for the child I thought I would have—one who would walk, talk, go to a regular school, graduate college, and get married.

I dealt with my emotions by learning as much as I could. I spent a tremendous amount of time researching mitochondrial disease on the Internet, seeking assistance from others on Internet support groups, as well as hitting the stacks in the medical school libraries. When Robby was two, I went back to school and obtained a masters degree in educational psychology—a degree that focuses on identifying and helping those with special needs. I will concede that our different approaches to dealing with Robby's disease and disabilities caused friction within our marriage. But we survived, and today are united in our steadfast devotion to and love for Robby. We both marvel at the amount of joy he brings to us and those around him. No longer do I struggle with the issue of "why us?" We just try to support each other on the continued journey of loving Robby.

I try very hard to stay in the moment with Robby, but find myself fearing the future. Doctors have never been able to give us a prognosis for him. It is possible that his disease will take a more degenerative course and that he will pass away before reaching adulthood. It is also possible that he will live well into adulthood with very extensive caretaking needs. Both scenarios frighten me. I am in no way ready to lose Robby—his smile, his gorgeous laugh, his hugs and kisses. But I am also not logistically or mentally prepared to take care of a grown man who is dependent on me for diapering, bathing, dressing, lifting, and transferring. We have never qualified for any kind of nursing or PCA help, and in the absence of outside help, I feel unsure about our ability to continue to do everything ourselves. Since Robby is now entering puberty, we will be spending the coming months making our home more handicap accessible, and seeking information about ways we can continue to take care of him at home as long as possible.

I derive a lot of solace from the relationships I have formed through Internet support groups. Some are specifically geared to parents of children with mitochondrial disease. Others are for parents of children with multiple disabilities caused by other syndromes or diseases. In the early days, when I was coming to grips with Robby's condition, I derived great benefit from weekly psychotherapy as well as antidepressant medication. I'm sure I would not have survived that difficult first year without intense professional support. There are still times I find myself brooding and wishing our lives were different. When this occurs, I find that spending quality time with my son will bring me out of it in short order. I think it is important to try as much as possible to let go of the disease, the diagnosis, the prognosis, the treatment, the therapy, the medication, and the rest of it—and just be with your child in the moment. When I do this, I experience joy that allows me to transcend the negatives.

12. *Choose your Friends Wisely*

Have you heard of a circle of trust? There is a circle of trust, described by experts, that we unconsciously project onto the people around us. In addition, psychologists propose that there are three fundamental criteria that must exist for someone to be "allowed" in the circle of trust: expertise, authority, and experience. In other words, we feel that people who are experts or who have similar experiences speak the truth. Note that "family member" is not listed in the circle of trust criteria. Neither is "friend" or "neighbor." Many parents of affected children and affected adults bitterly complain that family or friends are the least supportive and are even frequently hurtful with their comments or actions. Define your own circle of support very carefully.

Sometimes family members are not the best support group or resource! Kathy is an adult patient and mom who found that her spouse would become defensive and angry anytime she tried to discuss new symptoms with him, so she learned to talk it over with her friends who also have Mito and to lean on her spouse for other things that he was more comfortable with. In the same manner that we are learning to dream new dreams and redefine our view of success and happiness, we are also going to benefit from being consciously choosy about the people who we turn to in need and those whom we let in to our "circle of trust." The joy of this is that you can choose who you allow in! Again, these choices put us back in the driver's seat and give us much needed feelings of control. Perhaps there were friends who let you down but others who stepped up when you didn't expect it. Take note of this and be willing to share your anxiety, fears, or anger with the people who you can trust. On the other hand, for others, don't give them the opportunity to let you down! Choose how you relay information to them so that you are ultimately protecting yourself and your own attitude.

When I was a corporate trainer for Dale Carnegie many years ago, we used to talk about attitude and how we must invest a great deal of energy each and every day into our attitude. Our attitude needs attention and exercise just like our muscles! I believe this is especially true for any parent, caregiver, or affected teen or adult who lives with mitochondrial disease. I used to share an example in my classes that if you put a cut onion in a drawer full of apples, in a few days all of the apples smell bad and spoil. So... keep the onions out of your circle of trust!

Perhaps what offers us the most hope while living with mitochondrial disease is knowing that other people are living full and happy lives despite the disease's challenges. One mother of an affected teen shares, "Mito, for our family, is like the pink elephant in the room. Everyone is always wondering about it but afraid to ask. Sam's diagnosis changed our lives completely—but we don't know how to talk about it, so we just pretend it isn't there a lot of the time...even though we are always thinking about it! When I'm online chatting with other moms who have kids with Mito, it's like we don't *have* to talk about it because we all know what it's like!"

13. Choose the Right Care Manager

Every organ in the body is dependent on energy to function properly, and each organ must function well in order for the body to be healthy. For the person with an energy metabolism disorder, i.e., mitochondrial disease, every affected organ system may require a different sub-specialist. You could easily become lost in the system, bouncing from cardiologist to endocrinologist to neurologist to the ER while navigating tests and follow-ups and further tests before starting the cycle over once more. At some point, it helps to identify one healthcare provider that takes on the role of "manager." But who might that person be?

It's tempting to seek out a mitochondrial disease specialist as the cornerstone of your care, but there are real disadvantages to that approach. First, doctors, particularly specialists, are often busy and don't talk to each other. Clinic notes often lag behind what is happening in real time with the patient. Finally, as a result, the patient often becomes the primary provider of information, adding to the existing burden of actually living with the disease and the symptoms! Dr. Mark Korson from Tufts Floating Hospital for Children in Boston has over twenty years of experience caring for people with mitochondrial disease. He recommends that patients work hard at establishing an active partnership with their primary care provider (PCP) from the initial diagnosis, even if the PCP has no previous experience with mitochondrial disease. Table 3.1, based on Dr. Korson's ideas, shows the advantages and disadvantages of using each provider as your "manager."

As evidenced by Table 3.1, the challenge lies in the fact that while the mitochondrial disease specialist is more knowledgeable, he is less available. The best scenario is one in which a patient has regular visits (one to three times a year) with his mitochondrial disease specialist, and also has an involved primary care physician "at home" that is available to manage everyday challenges. For example, patients may adjust their "Mito cocktail" supplements once or twice a year with the Mito specialist, keeping their primary care physician up-to-date about the changes. However, if the patient has a virus or an infection and needs medical care, antibiotics, fluids, or follow-up, the primary care physician is the most appropriate resource. The PCP can see the patient more frequently, and as his experience with Mito grows, so will his ability to make recommendations for minor issues. In sum, one doctor cannot replace the other. Mito patients need a specialist experienced in mitochondrial disease as a guidepost; however, relying on that specialist to handle weekly or monthly issues is unrealistic and can be frustrating for both doctor and patient.

To be the best advocate for yourself, your child, or your loved one, it is important that you act as the "broker" between specialist and PCP. Navigating the medical system is challenging. You can follow these suggestions to improve coordinated care between multiple doctors:

1. Assess your PCP. Note that being knowledgeable (i.e., having prior experience with mitochondrial disorders) is less important than being conscientious and open to communicate. Some PCP's admittedly have very busy practices and simply don't have the time to engage in the detailed history of a Mito patient. To that end, sometimes the "best" doc-

Table 3.1 PCP or Specialist: Which is Better for Mito Patients?

PRIMARY CARE PROVIDERS	MITO SPECIALISTS (GENETICS, NEUROLOGY, METABOLICS)
Advantages: ■ Local ■ More available than specialty clinics ■ Number of PCPs is growing ■ Some are willing to be more involved in coordinated care ■ Competence increases over time ■ Can form a solid, long-lasting relationship with patient and patient's support network ■ Can help be an advocate for the patient at the local level ■ Can learn from Mito specialist by consulting when appropriate ■ Can better manage patient care during an acute event, such as a hospitalization or surgery because he has local hospital privileges	**Advantages:** ■ Excellent understanding of mitochondrial disease ■ Get the big picture and can help prioritize care options ■ Familiar and experienced with chronic disease ■ Have useful and practical experience ■ Are the most experienced with this population and can manage symptoms based on experience, even in circumstances in which there are few evidence-based treatment options ■ Are likely to have protocols
Disadvantages: ■ Lack of understanding of mitochondrial disease ■ May not grasp the big picture ■ Have busy practices and are unaccustomed to or unwilling to take on a complex patient ■ Not usually good at managing chronic disease ■ Don't have experience managing Mito symptoms in the office (reflex reaction to send patient to the hospital or specialist for everything)	**Disadvantages:** ■ Usually not local (often requires overnight travel) and not readily available to answer questions ■ Practice may be overwhelmed by complex patients ■ Number of practices is few, so choices are limited ■ May be less accustomed to helping patients navigate daily challenges involving school, work, disability, etc. ■ Unfamiliar with the patient services available in the place where you live ■ Visits are less frequent, i.e., quarterly, biannually, or annually and may involve expensive travel costs. ■ Visit may be out of network and not covered by insurance

tor or most popular physician in a community may not be the "best" for the person with mitochondrial disease, because he is too busy!

2. Propose that the PCP and Mito specialist/clinic share the title of "medical home." They need to be able (and willing) to communicate. Specialists are almost always willing to spend a few minutes on the phone or via email with a patient's primary care physician, especially if it saves

the patient a special visit to the specialist. Ensure from the beginning that your PCP feels comfortable reaching out to the specialist for advice. Ask permission to "introduce" them to one another via email or by sharing a card. Physicians are often more comfortable communicating with each other as they deem necessary rather than through you, the patient. For example, if a patient has a confirmed case of flu, the PCP may call the Mito specialist to let them know and get their recommendations. Ideally, the specialist would work with the PCP to briefly outline a plan, so that if the patient's needs became more acute, the PCP is prepared and the specialist is aware of the situation.

3. To help ensure that these professionals successfully communicate, seek out a cooperative (and organized!) contact person in each clinic setting, and shower that person with praise. Always go out of your way to show your appreciation when he keeps the line of communication flowing! The nurses, nurse practitioners, and office administrators are often more available to answer minor questions (or seek out the answers) than the physician, and they can help make your clinic visits much more successful and pleasant!

4. Parents and patients need to be good advocates. Be assertive, but always respectful, otherwise you may actually be obstructive to optimal communication.

5. Keep a medical record of notes, according to doctor. Consider bringing a handheld recorder to the appointment and with your doctor's permission, record the visit conversation so that you can make accurate notes later.

6. Carry with you important and recent documents, or carry a clinic visit book with summary impressions.

7. Keep a brief letter summarizing the medical problems, the diagnosis, and how it was made (check out www.ihealthrecord.org).

8. Ask the PCP or specialist to call the Mito specialist while you are in the office for important plan changes or when troubling new symptoms arise.

9. PRIORITIZE! Identify the most important needs and give those priority, otherwise understanding the "big picture" becomes even more overwhelming. Lack of organization and prioritization is probably the most frequent mistake that patients and families make. Go the appointment prepared and focused on what you hope to resolve immediately.

Coordinated care feels especially impossible to many adult patients whom I have known. The needs and numbers of the mitochondrial disease patient population are quickly outgrowing the existing medical networks that patients rely on in order to navigate their complex health needs. In addition, adult patients are often dealing with symptoms (nausea, pain, weakness, fatigue) while struggling to keep track of medical appointments and a lot of information. However, communication, planning, advocacy, and awareness are at the root of the solution, and we, the patients, parents, and care-givers, can begin to improve those areas today.

14. Keep Your Perspective

Those who don't live with a chronic illness may not understand why living with mitochondrial disease is stressful. It may appear to others that you (or your child) get a lot of support, have fewer demands (like a job, or expectations in school), and get to "lay around" a lot. In reality, the stress of living with Mito is both physical and emotional. Physically, it is frightening and tiring to endure even the most typical and nonthreatening Mito symptoms, such as fatigue, muscle pain, and nausea. Emotion-ally, for adult patients, living with Mito means learning to define oneself in a new way. Letting go of the things that before may have given you feelings of worth, like your athletic ability or ability to earn money and achieve career success, can be very stressful. For everyone who is involved with the care of someone with mitochondrial disease, the ongoing quest for information, support, and for interpretation of medi-cal tests and symptoms is stressful. Many parents feel that they are forced advocates, fighting for their child's rights in school, for medical care, for appropriate home sup-port. Many caregivers feel that no one but they are able to adequately care for their child, husband, or wife.

There is also legitimate fear that your or your child's condition will progress. This brings about fear and subsequently more stress that is a result of not being able to plan ahead and control the future (even the very near future, in many cases.) For parents and spouses, there is caregiver stress and caregiver fatigue that results from the "must-dos" of daily life—supporting the family, preparing meals, cleaning the house, and in many cases, being the twenty-four-hour nurse while tending to other family members' needs as well. For kids, there is stress from the unknown. Kids are understandably fearful of "what might happen," not limited to hospitalizations, invasive tests or proce-dures, disrupted routines, missed special events, and the memory or unpredictability of sickness. Older kids and teens can also suffer from stress related to hormones, pu-berty, and peer pressure. Kids and adult patients both can exist in a chronic state of stress because their bodies are out of their control. Changes in appearance, mobility, and independence can be traumatic, regardless of your age.

Perspective is our saving grace here. It is easy to get completely overwhelmed when you take on everything all at once. Tube feedings, doctor appointments, bills, insurance denials, school issues, work issues, financial constraints—there is more to be worried about than we can say in one breath! Keep your perspective and force yourself if necessary to compartmentalize the issues so you can tackle them one at a time. Going back to the idea of prioritizing is important. Facing ten challenges simultaneously feels much worse than tackling one. When you are overwhelmed, force yourself to stop and get perspective. Ask yourself, "Is this life or death right now? Do I have to make a decision about this right now? Will harm come to me or my child if I pause and clear my thoughts about this?" It can feel like the sky is falling, especially when we face so many significantly difficult and important decisions and challenges on our own. However, as adults and as advocates, we have to teach ourselves, our children, and those around us how to find and keep perspective. Here are some suggestions:

- Try to step out of yourself and look at the big picture. In the grand scheme of things, how truly significant is this?
- Make a list. What are you worried about? What can you do about it? What is beyond your control? What small steps could you take right now to improve this situation?
- Write this question down as well as the answer: "What is the worst thing that will happen if...?"
- Do something else—whether you enjoy baseball or bargain shopping, get out and do it if you can. It doesn't have to be the major leagues or an all-day affair, sometimes grocery shopping, a leisurely drive, or an extra long shower gives us a much-needed opportunity to regroup.
- Call someone who is good at listening, not judging.
- Know that you are not alone. Remind yourself that others are facing similar or greater challenges, just like you.
- Think about something else that gives you peace. What are you good at? What do you do well? What do you adore about your child? What do you treasure? What do you really want?
- Believe in yourself. You are amazing person who can do amazing things. Tomorrow will be different than today.

The other side of keeping perspective is learning to find humor and hope even in desperate situations. I know a dedicated mom whose daughter with Mito was in the hospital for three hundred days of the last year. Obviously, their family faced incredible demands and stress every day. However, this mom is amazing, and her ability to find humor and hope even when her daughter is sick for weeks at a time helps her daughter and her family tremendously. She always has perspective, and she is very, very honest. "At least Kimmie had the chance to see her friends when they visited this weekend," she'll say, even though they are disappointed to learn that Kimmie wouldn't be going home as soon as they had hoped. During a time when Kimmie was unable to eat any solid food, her mom froze water into fun shapes for her to enjoy as her "meal" with her sisters. They actually celebrated the different shapes of ice cubes and let Kimmie pick her favorite. Rather than being bitter and angry because she was unable to eat solid food, Kimmie was enthusiastic about licking an ice cube in the shape of a triangle. This family's perspective and ability to find a blessing in just about anything—

no matter how very small—amidst difficult situations has undoubtedly helped them cope over the last year of turbulent hospitalizations. One day, I asked Kimmie's mom how she found the personal strength to keep such a wonderful perspective. She said, "I choose to live with no regrets."

Some Unexpected Energy Drains

- Sitting up in a chair for long periods of time (the term "long" is relative to each child or adult)
- Recovering from any illness, even just a common cold and especially an illness with a fever or vomiting
- Recovering from a day with a lot of walking or activity
- Being in a noisy place or a place with a lot of people or other stimuli in the environment
- Walking from the parking lot or through a store
- Skipping a snack; not eating enough protein and complex carbohydrates at a meal
- Not drinking enough water or low-sugar fluids throughout the day
- Heat and humidity, even indoors
- Poor posture, which contributes to poor oxygen consumption (slumped in a chair or bed or too fatigued to sit up straight)
- Stress/anxiety (emotional)
- Cold temperatures (your mitochondria have to turn on to generate heat to keep your body temperature normal)
- Fever, even low-grade
- Reading, both books and on the computer (your eyes use a lot of energy!)
- Puberty, menopause, menstrual cycle, hormone fluctuations

15. Learn to Balance the Energy Budget

One of the most important lessons that any caregiver or patient with mitochondrial disease can learn is energy budgeting. Did you know that Earth has an energy budget? In order to stay in a constant state of balance, or equilibrium, the physical energy expenditures must be equal to or less than incoming energy transfers. In other words, the sum of the losses should be the same as the sum of the gains. Without disruption, this equilibrium happens naturally. However, emissions, greenhouse gases, and changes made by man to the earth's surface can significantly alter the energy budget of the world!

Similarly, a person with mitochondrial disease, regardless of age, has an energy budget that ideally should stay near equilibrium. On any given day, the energy demands (outgoing) should be less than or equal to energy stores. If demand exceeds available energy, a budget deficit is going to occur. Depending on your specific diagnosis and overall health, your energy account may be very rich or very poor. However, environmental factors, such as heat, illness, dehydration, stress, or poor sleep can burn through even the most solid energy reserves, again resulting in an overall deficit.

If we know that there is a finite energy supply to be used each day, can we decide how we are going to use it? Let me ask you this: If you won two million dollars in the lottery, would you just start spending it and giving it away randomly, or would you decide what you really wanted to buy with your winnings? In the same way, we have to accept that for a child or adult with mitochondrial disease, a limited energy supply is inherent to the diagnosis. If a child begins his day with ten units of energy, but it takes four units to ride on the hot bus to school, two units to carry his backpack and walk to his classroom, and one unit to wait the extra hour until snack, he is starting his day with only three units of energy left to learn, socialize, and grow! No wonder he is exhausted, his speech is slurring, he cannot focus, and he is inattentive, acting out, or sleepy by lunch. Using this example of energy currency can help teachers and employers understand that you as a parent or affected adult are trying to make wise use of a limited energy supply, and just like a budget, you have a finite amount of currency to work with. Use it wisely!

Learning to live with mitochondrial disease, as a person who is affected or who is caring for someone else, is a process. It is a journey that will challenge you and require more of you emotionally, physically, and spiritually than you may imagine is possible. After having worked with hundreds of families and patients, as well as cared for my own daughter with this disease, I want to impress upon you that there are bountiful blessings peppered in amongst the hardships on this journey. My hope is that we can learn our way by following advice from those inspiring parents and adult patients who show us every day, despite the challenges, how to live with Mito. As Rebecca, an adult patient and mom of two Mito-affected teens, has taped on her refrigerator, "Today, we are going to *live anyway*!"

Key Points from This Chapter

■ Recognize that information can be overwhelming, and give yourself time to absorb and process it. Take a friend, a family member, or a pocket recorder to your appointments.

■ Information is definitely empowering but can be equally overwhelming. Don't go overboard with online searches; do take advantage of support groups and disease foundations that help organize the information for you.

■ Take advantage of the technology that smartphones and online calendars can offer in order to help you get organized and to remember important information—from appointments to medication reminders.

■ Find joy in simple rituals that you can manage and control, like enjoying a cup of tea in a favorite mug or writing in a journal.

■ Recognize hidden energy drains and take steps to manage them. Even sitting in a chair reading a book takes a significant amount of energy!

■ Learning to live with mitochondrial disease is a process and everyone experiences different emotional responses to the diagnosis. Coping with the symptoms and with the disease is very individual, but is important as part of the road to accepting the diagnosis in a way that helps you find and focus on the positive.

4

Approaches to Treatment, Including Vitamins, Supplements, and Therapies

So you have a diagnosis. Now what? As patients in a consumer-driven health-care system, we expect the next step after a diagnosis to be a solution. Many families and adult patients share that they expected that they would be prescribed treatment, or that they or their children would endure more testing or intense therapy, but that they had hope, during this initial stage, that these treatments would offer them a chance to reverse the disease. They expected to be given a prescription, or at the very least—a plan.

Depending on where you received your diagnosis, the approach to therapy and treatment may vary, which is frustrating for many patients. There is not a standard of care (yet) for managing mitochondrial disease, so we see a wide variation of disease and symptom management approaches throughout the US, Canada, Europe, and Australia. Further, the process of diagnosis and treatment can be dramatically influenced by the referring doctor's knowledge of the latest clinical recommendations. The diagnosis phase is consequently the most confusing for patients and families, as they find themselves facing many questions: Should we seek a second opinion? When do we begin trying supplements? How much testing is necessary? How can I advocate for insurance coverage and school therapies without a diagnosis?

In reality, the best treatment approach to mitochondrial disease is focused on maintenance and emergency management. Maintenance means that there are things you can do to avoid a health crisis, and emergency management means that when a crisis does occur, there are ways to mitigate its effects. Think about your car. Do you wait until the engine blows up before you decide to fix it, even though you learned from the mechanic months earlier that there was an issue that could cause overheating? Managing the daily challenges of mitochondrial disease is much like routine maintenance of an automobile. It is our job as patients and parents to help ourselves and our children be as healthy and robust as possible so that, when an illness or an emergency presents itself, we have given our bodies as much reserve energy and support as possible.

Who Treats Mito?

One of the most common questions I hear from new patients, parents, and family members is "What doctor should I see?" Unfortunately, as you learned in Chapter 2 (The Journey to Diagnosis and Understanding the Causes), diagnosis of mitochondrial disease is complex! In addition, many patients find that the clinician or medical center where they received a diagnosis is not able to act as a long-term care provider or care manager. Consequently, many patients and parents are self-advocates, juggling multiple specialists and multiple medical centers while trying to be the gatekeeper of all of the information.

Treatment of mitochondrial disease is very important. While a cure for Mito is not available, management of the disease and the related symptoms is not only possible but necessary. If you are unsure of where to begin to find a physician who can help manage your mitochondrial disease, prescribe the Mito cocktail, and be available to help you in the event of an emergency, you can start at your closest University hospital. Most University hospitals will have a doctor who specializes in genetics (most frequently a pediatric specialist), several neurologists with various subspecialties, and perhaps a metabolic physician. Inquiries to those doctors about their experience with (and willingness to learn about) mitochondrial disease is a good starting point.

One could argue that the type of physician is actually less important than their clinical experience with mitochondrial disease patients. Some mitochondrial medicine specialists are doctors who were trained as metabolic doctors, and also follow patients with other metabolic disorders, such as PKU (phenylketonuria) or FOD (fatty acid oxidation defects). Likewise, some mitochondrial specialists are geneticists (due to the inherited nature of the disease, as explained in Chapter 2), and many are neurologists because of the wide array of symptoms that impact the brain and central nervous system. Any and all of these can be excellent care providers for you or your child. However, choosing the right team of physicians is important. Refer to the section entitled "Choosing the Right Care Manager" in Chapter 3, which offers tips about how to find a physician who can be your advocate and manage your treatment.

What is Used to Treat Mito?

Even though routine maintenance doesn't result in absolute remission of the disease, vitamin and supplement therapy does help many children and adults feel better and do more every day! The strides that have been made in understanding mitochondrial disorders in recent years instill confidence that someday there WILL be a solid and curative treatment option for children and adults. Today, however, therapy is focused on boosting the function of the mitochondria in the cell while supporting the body metabolically as much as possible.

Patient's responses to and use of treatments for Mito, including vitamins, supplements, and various therapies, are mixed. Sometimes parents may feel that there is no hope for their child once diagnosed with mitochondrial disease, and as a result, do not pursue much in the way of supplements or vitamins. Some physicians are strongly supportive of vitamins and supplements, while others may be indifferent or feel that there isn't enough evidence or research to support their use. Adult patients are typically the most eager to try various treatment options, but at the same time most often lack a consistent and organized plan or approach.

The "Mito Cocktail"

It's funny that the phrase that refers to the daily treatment regimen for kids and adults with Mito conjures up an image of a fancy drink in a chilled glass garnished with a cherry and an umbrella (Figure 4.1)! In reality, the "Mito cocktail" is the name given to the slurry of vitamins, antioxidants, supplements, and co-factors that are frequently recommended by physicians to increase mitochondrial efficiency and cellular energy production. Children and adults who have mitochondrial disease have an energy metabolism defect that takes place at the cellular level.

Although most of the ingredients in the Mito cocktail can be found in the vitamin section at the drugstore or health food store, it is important to understand WHY these ingredients can be helpful, and it is also important to be clear about dosage, side effects, and use (see Table 4.3). In addition, each patient will have a relatively unique supplement combination since the prescription is based, to a de-

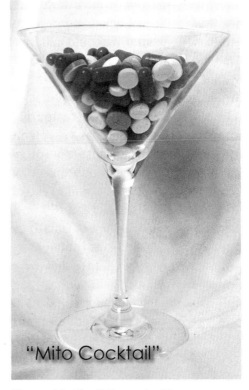

"Mito Cocktail"

Figure 4.1: The "Mito cocktail."
Image by Jane Adams

gree, on a person's mitochondrial disease diagnosis (for example, Complexes I and II are more responsive to riboflavin) and the presence of certain symptoms. Finally, since the dosing of these vitamins and supplements is much higher than the recommended daily allowance for healthy people (usually five to twenty times higher), buying bulk bottles of these vitamins and supplements over-the-counter isn't very practical or recommended.

The following is a description of the vitamins and supplements that typically appear in Mito cocktails. Always consult with your doctor before taking any medication, including vitamins and supplements, especially if you have mitochondrial disease. It's just not smart for anyone to self-prescribe their Mito cocktail!

Coenzyme Q10: The Energy Taxi

During energy production (ATP synthesis) in the mitochondria, electrons are moved from one station to the next along complexes that are part of the electron transport chain. Coenzyme Q10 (CoQ10) exists naturally in our cells and supports mitochondrial energy production in the electron transport chain by carrying electrons from cytochrome to cytochrome in order for ATP to be produced in the mitochondria. Without CoQ10, there is no electron transfer. In other words, CoQ10 is a carrier (or an electron taxi), and is necessary for electron transport. The biochemistry is obviously much more complex than described here (see Chapter 10 for more on biochemistry), but for simplicity's sake let's use the analogy of New York City on a busy rainy morning. Imagine if there were only twenty taxis available to do the job of shuttling all the people (i.e., electrons) who need to get to work in order to produce their daily quota (i.e., ATP). Now, what if we could call in a back-up fleet of fifty more taxis (i.e., coenzyme Q10 molecules) to come in and help? Theoretically, all of the people (i.e., electrons) would get to work, right? And if they got to work, then you could expect that everyone would be able to make their quotas (i.e., more energy).

Coenzyme Q10 is a co-factor that occurs naturally in the cell, but can also be purchased over-the-counter as a supplement. However, typical drugstore products contain 100 mg of CoQ10 per capsule or softgel, and are not considered pharmaceutical-grade, so their purity is not standardized. Evidence and research suggests that patients with mitochondrial disease should take a standard dose of 5-30 mg of CoQ10 per kg of weight per day. Therefore, a 100-pound person with a mitochondrial disorder would take about 250-1500 mg of CoQ10 every day. Hold on, that's as many as fifteen pills per day if purchased over the counter! Fortunately, there are some options for patients with mitochondrial disease that are much more effective, covered by insurance, and "easier to swallow."

Ubiquinone is the form of CoQ10 that is found in most over-the-counter capsules and softgels and is also sold in a pharmaceutical-grade powdered form that is used by compounding pharmacists. This premium grade sold by pharmacies specializing in mitochondrial supplements is thought to be the most effective, although it is perhaps not as effective as ubiquinol (which is described below). Pharmacists dispense the ubiquinone powder in a liquid-oil suspension or in capsules according to individual patient needs and the doctor's prescription.

Ubiquinone is the oxidized form of the enzyme, is insoluble in water (conversely called "lipid-soluble"), and is the most common ingredient in the Mito cocktail. There is very solid evidence in the medical literature from the last five years that supports the use of ubiquinone in treating mitochondrial disease. There does not appear to be an improvement in absorption or therapeutic benefit in very high doses (above 2400 mg/day in adults), suggesting that most patients will find the greatest benefit at a dose between 5-15 mg/kg/day. Ubiquinone is commonly known as "CoQ10," is the least expensive, is the easiest to obtain (especially via a compounding pharmacy), and is effective for many patients. (See Table 4.2 for a comparison of ubiquinone and ubiquinol.)

During energy production in the cell, the body converts ubiquinone into a reduced form, called ubiquinol, which is then used to assist cellular energy production. In order to actually increase blood levels of coenzyme Q10, the body must convert ubiquinone into ubiquinol. If someone is not able to do so adequately, she can take supplemental ubiquinol, which is now commercially available. Age also plays a role, as aging bodies may not as effectively convert the ubiquinone to its redox form, ubiquinol. Ubiquinol is also thought to be helpful for children; parents report that their children have more energy and are better able to recover from illness when taking ubiquinol. Ubiquinol is more expensive than ubiquinone and cannot usually be formulated as part of the cocktail by a compounding pharmacy. Most patients purchase ubiquinol from specialized vendors who produce the product (see list in Appendix E). Since ubiquinol is three to five times more easily absorbed, a lower dose is necessary for the same effect (2-8 mg/kg/day) as high-dose ubiquinone. Ubiquinol is generally agreed to be more bioavailable (better absorbed by the tissues) and is preferred by many clinicians who treat patients with mitochondrial disease. However, since it is more expensive and is not always able to be compounded with other medications, ubiquinol is not always the best option. In addition, the patient consensus isn't definitively in favor of one or the other, as the response to both ubiquinone and ubiquinol seems to be pretty individualized.

CoQ10 is best absorbed when taken with a meal or snack that is high in fat (like peanut butter or cheese). Many people are unaware that it takes weeks (to months) before energy and stamina may improve from taking CoQ10; unfortunately, many patients give up on it after a week because they don't notice a difference. Some patients also say that although they don't think they felt a noticeable difference while taking daily CoQ10, they felt much worse several days later if they stopped taking it. The most recent recommendation from the Mitochondrial Medicine Society is that daily ubiquinol or ubiquinone doses should be divided and taken twice a day; however, the second dose should always be taken at least six hours before bedtime in order to avoid possible insomnia or inability to sleep.

It is useful to note that both forms of CoQ10 (ubiquinol and ubiquinone) play an important role in health for everyone, not just people with mitochondrial disease. CoQ10 has been studied in relationship to improved heart, immune system, and brain function. In addition, since co-enzyme Q10 levels naturally decline with age, there is great interest in the general community about the potential anti-aging benefits of taking supplemental CoQ10. When you put these pieces together you can connect the dots to see the big picture! Perhaps one day we'll be able to get our boost of energy from supplemental CoQ10 in our orange juice and Cheerios, but in the meantime, it has been approved by the FDA for treatment of mitochondrial disease, is readily available online or through a compounding pharmacist, and is often covered by insurance as well.

So, in a nutshell, we have learned several things about coenzyme Q10. Firstly, that our bodies require it for energy production. It decreases naturally with age resulting in older people having less energy and more disease processes. Individuals with mitochondrial dysfunction suffer from symptoms similar to the natural consequences of aging, including lack of energy and susceptibility to organ dysfunction. And finally, that supplemental CoQ10 can help improve energy and overall well-being in everyone. (See Appendix E in the back of this book for recommended suppliers of CoQ10.)

L-Carnitine

Like CoQ10, levocarnitine is important for energy production. It helps to break down fat from the food that we eat by transporting fatty acids across the mitochondrial membrane before the Krebs cycle begins. Most of a person's carnitine comes from diet (the highest concentration is found in beef), though supplementation of L-Carnitine (levocarnitine, Carnitor®) for patients with mitochondrial disease is common. L-Carnitine has been FDA approved for use in metabolic diseases. However, primary carnitine deficiency is not characteristic of most mitochondrial disorders. Physicians recommend L-Carnitine as a supplement in the Mito cocktail in order to boost "free" carnitine in the cells, with the goal of improving energy production, and increasing muscle tone and strength.

Some patients cannot tolerate L-Carnitine due to stomach upset and/or diarrhea, and most patients complain of a fishy odor (especially consistent with higher doses) excreted through the sweat glands. The odor is caused by the natural breakdown of the carnitine in the digestive system and can be improved with a short course of antibiotics.

L-Carnitine should be used with caution in patients who have a long-chain fatty acid oxidation defect. Blood levels should also be monitored carefully in all Mito patients who take L-Carnitine. Although L-Carnitine is a common amino acid supplement, there are no studies that demonstrate evidence of the benefit of carnitine for patients with mitochondrial disease. Despite this, levocarnitine has been one of the mainstays of therapy for patients with mitochondrial disease for many years, and is often prescribed as an IV solution during hospitalizations. Similarly, some patients find that doubling their L-Carnitine intake during an illness helps them feel stronger and recover more quickly.

B vitamins

Some B vitamins are co-factors that facilitate important mitochondrial reactions. B vitamins are water soluble and can be found in many foods including turkey, tuna, whole grains, potatoes, and bananas. Because B vitamins are water soluble, the excess is flushed out of the system daily, and an effect from this supplement should

The 2009 publication by physicians from the Mitochondrial Medicine Society, "A Modern Approach to the Treatment of Mitochondrial Disease" in *Current Treatment Options in Neurology,* names CoQ10 as the "frontline" approach to treating mitochondrial disease. Since it is the most commonly used, most researched, and most often recommended supplement, it is the first building block for the Mito cocktail.

Table 4.2 Ubiquinone vs. Ubiquinol

Ubiquinone	Ubiquinol
Patients report increased energy and less muscle weakness and fatigue with long-term use	Is better absorbed than ubiquinone by measurable blood levels, but higher dosing doesn't necessarily translate into clinical improvements
Form found in most over-the-counter coenzyme Q10 products	Commercially available, but not found in most drugstores; typically ordered online
The oxidized form	The reduced or "redox" form
Insoluble in water, should be administered in an oil suspension (compounding pharmacists often use olive oil)	Can be made soluble in water; still recommended that it be taken with a meal with some fat content
Poorly absorbed in the GI tract	Best absorption of the two forms
Typical dose: ■ *Child*—10-30 mg/kg/day (by mouth), divided into two doses ■ *Adult*—300-2400 mg daily (by mouth), divided into two doses	Lower dose used because better absorbed; Typical dose: ■ *Child*—2-8 mg/kg/day (by mouth), divided into two doses ■ *Adult*—50-600 mg/day (by mouth), divided into two doses
Least expensive form ($50-100/month for 1200 mg/kg/day)	More expensive overall, even though a lower dose is required
Take with meals to avoid stomach upset and to potentially improve absorption. (Many patients take their CoQ10 with a breakfast that includes a little peanut butter because the fat in the peanut butter helps absorption)	Take with meals to avoid stomach upset and potentially improve absorption
Over-the-counter form not recommended; premium grade powdered form from a knowledgeable compounding pharmacist or company specializing in mitochondrial supplements is preferred	Not available over the counter and rarely offered by compounding pharmacies
Side effects: Wakefulness, sleep disturbance (insomnia—take in the morning to avoid this), possible stomach upset	Side effects: Same as ubiquinone, some parents report increased agitation or aggressiveness in children (especially children with ASD)
Safety concerns: more (extremely high doses) is not necessarily better and may contribute to muscle breakdown. Talk with your doctor if you take blood thinners such as Coumadin (Warfarin) as CoQ10 can lower their effectiveness.	Same safety concerns as ubiquinone
Symptom improvement may take four to six weeks or longer	Symptoms may improve more quickly than with ubiquinone but can still take several weeks

be felt right away. B vitamins are very bitter and can be difficult to take in liquid form unless specially formulated or flavored by an experienced compounding pharmacist. Some patients with mitochondrial myopathy benefit from taking a B50 or B100 supplement, which is a complex vitamin that includes all of the B vitamins. Very large doses are not recommended.

B1 Thiamine.

Thiamine assists in the metabolism of carbohydrates to create energy and, more importantly, is a cofactor for the pyruvate dehydrogenase complex. In patients with PDCD (pyruvate dehydrogenase complex deficiency) thiamine can improve lactate and pyruvate levels as well as provide increased energy and alleviation of some symptoms. Recommended dose is between 50-800 mg daily, by mouth.

B2 Riboflavin.

Riboflavin plays a key role in energy metabolism. It has been studied in greater depth than other B vitamins and is thought to be especially effective at mitigating fatigue in patients who have Complex I or Complex II deficiencies. Riboflavin is naturally a bright orange color and can cause a change in the color of the user's urine, and may trigger nausea and anorexia in high doses. It is very inexpensive, and the recommended dose for Mito patients is 50-400 mg daily.

Creatine

Creatine helps maintain muscle mass and increases energy for cells. The highest levels of creatine are found in the muscles and brain, which are tissues that have the greatest energy demand. Creatine phosphate has been used by body builders to improve high intensity exercise capacity because it helps create energy storage during muscle use. A few studies in adult and child mitochondrial disease patients reported similar benefits, and creatine supplementation is becoming increasingly more common. However, there are some remaining concerns about the use of creatine. Over-the-counter (powdered form) creatine phosphate is immediately changed to creatinine as soon as it is added to liquid (in water, juice, or in the stomach). Creatinine is a toxic by-product naturally produced in the muscles from exercise and filtered through the kidneys. Increased creatinine levels can cause headaches, decreased energy, and worse, kidney failure. As a result, many physicians are concerned about supplemental creatine, especially high dose usage without vigilant monitoring of kidney function. Some research suggests that creatine monohydrate does not have the same negative side effects as creatine phosphate (more common powdered creatine described above).

In any case, use of creatine monohydrate is recommended primarily for patients with mitochondrial myopathy and muscle weakness and should always be used in conjunction with careful monitoring of kidney function from an experienced physician. In addition to possible kidney dysfunction, side effects commonly include diarrhea, dehydration (water intake should be increased because creatine is a salt), and weight gain. A typical dose is 1-10 mg/day. Creatine is also used as an IV medication during periods of crisis in the hospital for mitochondrial disease patients who can benefit from the additional metabolic support.

L-arginine

L-arginine is an amino acid that is not usually taken as a supplement by healthy people. Most L-arginine can be obtained through the diet; great sources are dairy products, nuts, and seeds. However, because L-arginine is involved in the production of creatine and produces a natural compound that causes enlarging of the blood vessels (vasodilation), supplemental L-arginine has been found to be very useful during acute periods of stroke, especially in patients who suffer from MELAS (one form of Mito, characterized by mitochondrial encephalopathy, lactic acidosis, and stroke). Maintenance doses are most frequently prescribed for children or adults with MELAS; the typical daily dose is 150-300 mg/kg (divided into two to three doses/day).

EXAMPLES OF TWO "MITO COCKTAIL" PRESCRIPTIONS

Bob, fifty-four-year-old adult with mitochondrial myopathy
- Folic Acid - 320 mg
- Carnitine (as L-Carnitine Fumerate) - 1200 mg
- Creatine Ethyl Ester - 2 g
- CoQ10 (ubiquinone) - 1200 mg
- Alpha lipoic Acid - 600 mg

Jennie, nine-year-old girl with Complex I and II
- CoQ10 (ubiquinol) - 120 mg (divided: 60 mg at 7:00 am, 60 mg at 1:00 pm)
- Riboflavin (B2) - 200 mg
- Vitamin C - 125 mg
- L-Carnitine (Carnitor®) - 600 mg, divided 3 x day
- L-Creatine (Solace brand Cytotine) 3 g

Antioxidants

Antioxidants are known as "free radical scavengers" and are thought to prevent and repair cell damage incurred by free radicals. Free radicals are the naturally occurring by-products of the oxidation process that occurs in the cell. Free radicals are thought to be produced in greater amounts as we age, causing "oxidative stress" to the body. Antioxidants help "clean up" those free radicals by neutralizing them, thereby stopping cell and tissue damage, which can contribute to disease.

For people who have mitochondrial disease, there is the potential for an increased amount of free radical damage due to an increase in the by-product free radicals coming from an ineffective energy metabolism process. Antioxidants are thought to be beneficial to the body in many ways including slowing the aging process and boosting the body's immunity system. Fruits and vegetables are great sources of antioxidants; in fact, nurses advise that patients "eat a rainbow" (i.e., fruits and veggies of varying colors) whenever possible to get extra antioxidant benefit through diet. Antioxidants such as vitamin C, vitamin E, selenium, and alpha lipoic acid are frequently prescribed by mitochondrial disease specialists in hopes of helping protect the body from free radical damage. Antioxidants also play a role during periods of acute illness and are often recommended during the winter months to help boost your or your child's immunity. In addition, a diet that includes foods that are high in antioxidants, such as blueberries, spinach, salmon, nuts, beans, cranberries, and pomegranates, is helpful.

Kellie has pyruvate dehydrogenase complex deficiency (PDCD) and began showing symptoms when she was a baby. Her parents waited two years after her diagnosis before trying CoQ10 or any other ingredients of the Mito cocktail.

KELLIE

When Kellie was little, it took so much effort just to get her to eat that I couldn't imagine giving her all of these awful supplements on top of everything else. Plus, I didn't know where to go to get this stuff, and my doctor wasn't very knowledgeable. A few years ago when we began to see a neurologist who is a specialist in mitochondrial disease, my husband and I decided that we would give thiamine a try for Kellie. Honestly, I had my doubts. I am a scientist and there is very little evidence to support the claims that these supplements change the course of the disease. Despite our lack of enthusiasm and at our doctor's urging, we went ahead and began with a moderate dose of thiamine prescribed by Kellie's neurologist. We found a compounding pharmacy who was experienced about mitochondrial disease and who offered free shipping. After a few months, we realized that Kellie was making significant improvements, both in her energy level and in her overall cognitive and physical abilities. Shortly thereafter, we added coenzyme Q10 to Kellie's daily thiamine dose. For a while, I struggled with it because it was so thick and oily and just pained me to give it to her, and I couldn't tell a difference. It was about six months later, when we were at Disney World on Kellie's Make-a-Wish trip, that we realized, "Wow!" We felt like there was suddenly a HUGE difference in her overall stamina and energy level. Even her teachers and therapists at school commented about it. I guess you could say now I'm a believer!

Compounding Pharmacists: Great Partners for Mito Patients and Families

Compounding pharmacists are great advocates for people with mitochondrial disease. A compounding pharmacist assists patients by creating a customized, "compounded" medication that combines the exact ingredients and dosages for them into one or two products. There are many benefits to working with a compounding pharmacist! For example, a compounding pharmacist can reduce the required volume of liquid medications or the number of pills to be taken each day by combining the vitamins and supplements prescribed into one formula. Compounding pharmacists also help ensure that the compounded medication is offered in the most palatable and easily administered formula for each patient. For example, some children have allergies to artificial colorings, sweeteners, or additives, or are unable to swallow capsules, so the pharmacist can offer liquids without additional additives. Compounding pharmacists also typically flavor liquid medications, making them tastier and easier for children to take. They work closely with the patient's physician and take into consideration the patient's dietary restrictions as well as the overall treatment plan.

Each compounded medication is unique and specific to each patient, and requires a prescription from a physician. The formula is based on multiple variables, including the prescription, the patient's symptoms, the patient's diagnosis, weight, allergies, physician recommendations, etc. The goal is for the physician, pharmacy, and the patient to work as a team in order to develop an ideal mix (or "compound") of these vitamins and supplements that offers the patient the most ease of use and the fewest side effects.

Since the monthly cost of coenzyme Q10 and additional supplements can be hundreds of dollars per month for someone with mitochondrial disease, cost is often a primary concern for patients and families. Compounding pharmacies are becoming increasingly savvy and knowledgeable about insurance reimbursement and are rather committed to helping their patients obtain coverage for the compounded vitamins and co-factors.

Exercise as Therapy

As discussed in Chapter 5, many people with mitochondrial disease believe that they cannot exercise. In fact, exercise intolerance is a hallmark characteristic of mitochondrial disease. As a result, many people shy away from exercise because they "feel worse" and ultimately have a very low activity level. Hopelessness associated with feeling fatigued and "just not able to do anything" seems to be more of a problem for teens, young adults, and adults, although kids can suffer similarly as well.

Interestingly, and of great importance, is that even though exercise leaves someone with Mito feeling tired, research has demonstrated that exercise actually improves

Table 4.3 Mito Cocktail: Ingredients, Dosages, and Side Effects

Note: Dosages of the following vitamins and supplements are individual based on age, weight, symptoms, and other factors. Please, never begin taking any of these compounds without the advice and involvement of a physician. In addition, keep careful records of your prescription and update it frequently.

Ingredient	Dosage (Typically Recommended Range)	Possible Side Effects
Thiamine (B1)	50-800 mg daily, by mouth	Allergic reactions (rash, hives), stomach upset
Riboflavin (B2)	100-400 mg daily, by mouth	Bright orange urine
Niacin (B3) (nicotinic acid)	50-100 mg daily, by mouth	Stomach upset, flushing in the face and neck, headache, and liver problems
Pyroxidine (B6)	10-250 mg daily, by mouth	Increased sensitivity to light, rash, stomach upset, allergic reactions, and tingling or numbness in the hands or feet
Cobalmin (B12) (cyanco-balamin)	100-1000 mcg daily, may be taken as an injection	Itching, diarrhea, headache, anxiety
Vitamin C (abscorbic acid)	100-500 mg up to three times daily	Nausea, stomach upset, diarrhea, kidney problems
Vitamin E (tocopherol)	200-400 IU (international units) daily	Nausea, diarrhea, bleeding, bruising easily, headache, fatigue; high doses not advised for people with diabetes or heart disease
L-Carnitine (levocarnitine, Carnitor®, carnitine)	30-100 mg/kg/day by mouth	Stomach upset, diarrhea, body odor, rash, increased risk of seizures in people with a history

mitochondrial function. The benefit of exercise as a treatment approach to mitochondrial disease is two-fold.

1. Exercise improves overall endurance and strength and can keep the mitochondria functioning more effectively.
2. Exercise helps the spirit. Not only are endorphins (happy hormones) released during exercise, but a consistent exercise routine really does help children and adults with mitochondrial disease overcome feelings of anxiety, depression, and helplessness.

It seems that even for people with mitochondrial disease, the fatigue from exercise is short-term but the benefits are long-term. Consistent, low intensity exercise can actually improve a person with Mito's overall baseline. Normal muscle fatigue is to be expected—you will feel tired after exercise. It is an important distinction that, for the child or adult person with Mito, fatigue of the muscles is different than exercise

Alpha lipoic acid (thioctic acid)	60-200 mg up to three times daily by mouth	Nausea, vomiting, rash, headache
Selenium	25-50 mcg daily	Risk of selenium toxicity in higher doses
Biotin (vitamin H)	2.5-10 mg daily	Stomach upset
Sodium succinate (Na succinate)	6 g daily	None reported
Vitamin K1 (phytonadione or phylloquinone)	1-25 mg daily by mouth	Jaundice, allergic reactions (rash, hives, swelling of the airway); contraindicated for use with blood thinners (Warfarin)
Coenzyme Q10 (ubiquinone)	5-15 mg/kg/day by mouth	Nausea, stomach upset, headache, loss of appetite, dizziness; benefits may take months to appear
Coenzyme Q10 (idebenone) (a synthetic product similar to CoQ10)	90-300 mg daily by mouth	Stomach upset, nausea, vomiting, diarrhea, headache, dizziness, confusion
Creatine	Up to 5 g, divided, twice daily	Stomach upset, nausea, muscle cramping
Ribose	15 g up to four times daily by mouth; may also be used with exercise to prevent muscle cramping	Stomach discomfort, nausea, diarrhea, headache, hypoglycemia (low blood sugar)
Uridine	150 mg	Stomach discomfort, diarrhea
Folic acid	1-10 mg by mouth daily	Stomach discomfort, diarrhea
Folinic acid (leucovorin)	400-800 mcg	Stomach upset

Adapted with permission from "Mitochondrial Cocktail Information Sheet," provided by America's Compounding Center (www.accrx.com). Patients and families should note that this is not a complete list, but a sample of the most commonly prescribed compounds.

fatigue felt by a healthy person. People with Mito describe heaviness in their muscles, and may say things like "I can't lift my legs to get up." Often these symptoms improve after a period of rest, although a sure sign of overexertion is prolonged weakness, muscle cramping, muscle spasm, and feelings of confusion or "brain fog" that generalize beyond the muscle groups that were exercised.

Because research studies have specifically examined the benefit of exercise to mitochondrial function in people with documented mitochondrial disorders, clinicians are increasingly in favor of exercise as a treatment approach for children and adults with almost all presentations of the disease. In fact, exercise is one of the few proven methods to actually improve mitochondrial function, even in people who have some unhealthy, or dysfunctional, mitochondria. However, moderation is absolutely crucial; a person with mitochondrial disease will never benefit from being pushed to the point of exhaustion.

Suggestions for Including Exercise as a Treatment Approach

- Plan rest periods before and after exercise.
- Eat and drink before and after increased activity. Many people benefit from a "fuel the fire with kindling" approach. Eat a snack and drink plenty of a low-sugar beverage about a half hour before and after exercise. Drink during the activity as well—don't wait to be thirsty, if possible.
- Keep it short. A little bit every day or even twice a day is always better than over-doing it (even if you feel ok!)
- Start slow and build up g...r...a...d...u...a...l...l...y. (Two minutes is better than one minute, and eight minutes is better than five minutes. Twenty minutes is average, and it may take a year of consistent effort to get there.)
- Don't be discouraged! The key is to know when you're tired and don't overdo it. Kids will benefit from long-term relationships with their physical therapists who can read subtle fatigue cues that the child may not recognize or be able to communicate.
- Adults: Know your body. Parents: Help your child learn how to express and recognize the need to rest.
- Partner with a physiotherapist if possible.

The key to exercise as an effective therapy is to think of it as therapy. In other words, a little bit every day is ideal; "take" your exercise just as you would take your Mito cocktail! Children with mitochondrial disease always benefit from physical and occupational therapy, which is frequently offered by the child's school. Even very high functioning children should have a physical therapy session at least once a week so that ongoing physical exercise, strength training, and conditioning are part of their individualized health plan. Adult patients often don't realize that they may qualify for and benefit from physical therapy as well; in fact, many adults (and kids) really enjoy warm water swimming offered in rehabilitation or hospital settings. Not only is pool therapy an excellent form of exercise for anyone with Mito, it also is frequently covered by insurance when prescribed by one's primary care physician for low muscle tone (hypotonia).

Muscle pain can be worse when lactic acid is elevated in the blood, and for many kids and adults with Mito, elevated lactic acid (or lactic acidosis) is an ongoing problem. In the case of a person with a mitochondrial disorder, lactic acidosis is not caused by exercise but is rather a result of inefficient energy production resulting in too much lactate as a by-product of the energy metabolism process. Exercise can actually reduce lactate production, improve mobility and endurance, and is a very simple and straightforward opportunity to improve your or your child's baseline. The Adult Metabolic Disease Clinic at Vancouver Coastal Health in British Columbia has created an excellent, illustrated step-by-step guide to stretching and strengthening exercises, which can be found at www.MitoAction.org/exercise.

Eat, Drink, Sleep...Repeat.

The real cornerstones to treatment of mitochondrial disease are nutrition, fluids, supplements, and rest along with daily energy conservation and management. As mentioned at the beginning of this chapter, maintenance is as critical as proper care in an emergency. Chapter 3, "Accepting the Diagnosis and Learning to Live WELL with Mito" and Chapter 5, "Managing and Preventing Symptoms" offer detailed explanations and examples of how to incorporate these fundamentals into everyday life for kids and adults with mitochondrial disease.

Key Points from This Chapter

■ The combination of supplements, antioxidants, vitamins, and co-factors that improve mitochondrial function are called the "Mito cocktail."

■ Several studies have been published that examine the effectiveness of the different components of the Mito cocktail. CoQ10 is used most frequently for adults and children with mitochondrial disease.

■ A compounding pharmacist is a wonderful resource and is able to combine pharmaceutical-grade formulas of prescribed ingredients into capsules or liquid.

■ Every person's Mito cocktail prescription and formulation is unique, and is based on her specific diagnosis, weight, age, allergies, tolerance to certain additives, ability to swallow capsules, and so on. The articles noted in the bibliography in Appendix F are helpful for patients who would like to discuss the Mito cocktail with their doctor.

■ Exercise is considered a treatment approach for mitochondrial disease, although exercise intolerance is a hallmark characteristic of Mito! Start very slowly and focus on small amounts of consistent exercise, such as warm water swimming, walking, or using a recumbent bike.

■ Nutrition, hydration, and energy conservation are as important as the Mito cocktail when we think about overall management of mitochondrial disease.

SPECIAL INSERT

Therapeutics for Mitochondrial Disease
Guy Miller, MD Ph.D.

Edison Pharma

The genomics revolution in medicine has brought our understanding of disease to a new level. Children once categorized by virtue of physical or development impairments are now being defined on the basis of single genetic defects. Nowhere is this more illustrated than in the newly emerging area of "mitochondrial medicine." In the last decade, we have defined names for many genetic diseases of childhood that hereto lacked both a diagnosis and cause. That many neuromuscular diseases have their origins in how cells make and regulate energy is not a surprise, but now armed with this data a new frontier is upon us.

Basic scientists can avail themselves of this information to reverse-engineer the criticality of such genes and proteins in the synthesis and regulation of energy metabolism. Clinicians now possess a diagnostic tool with which to classify these diseases, define their true natural history, and devise metrics to evaluate promising therapeutics. And lastly, drug developers can gain insights from our basic science and clinical colleagues to devise new therapeutic approaches leveraging an understanding of disease mechanism and novel translation approaches to therapeutic design and evaluation.

There is great promise, but what cannot be understated is the arduous road ahead. Today, some estimates place drug development from diseases of the brain at nearly a twenty-year venture, with an abysmal success rate of approximately 6 percent of those drugs that enter clinical development. Our challenge is to shorten this timeline, and to do so we need new diagnostic technologies and a clearer understanding of clinical metrics to de-risk early clinical trials where valuable therapeutic and disease information is gained.

The era of a first mitochondrial-targeted drug is upon us. Advances made by the R&D community will be critical: first and foremost to the children and adults who so desperately need treatment; to the scientists and clinicians who will use a first drug as a tool to understand energy metabolism; and to extend our basis of understanding of the role of energy metabolism, its regulation, and the mitochondria and disease. While the vision of mitochondrial medicine is lofty—understanding biology in terms of energy metabolism and regulation—its immediate rewards are proximate: treatment of those in need.

5

Managing and Preventing Symptoms

What Does Mitochondrial Disease "Look Like?"

One of the most difficult things for people to understand about mitochondrial disease is that no two patients "look alike." In fact, two people with the exact same genetic mutation might manifest different symptoms. Some symptoms are considered "classic," because they are symptoms that have been identified in a majority of patients since mitochondrial disease was first described in the medical literature. Classic Mito signs and symptoms include fatigue, muscle weakness, seizures, stroke, and other neurological involvement. However, even amongst "classic" features, there is great variability. In addition, as the spectrum of understanding about mitochondrial disorders widens, so too will the umbrella of signs and symptoms that we can consider classic.

It is important to pause here and note that every Mito patient will not currently have or develop all of the symptoms described in this chapter. Each patient has a unique presentation, and furthermore, many of a person's symptoms are also dependent on environmental factors, such as age, climate, history of illness, emotional/social supports, use of supplements, etc. You could even say that children and adults who have mitochondrial disease have more similarities on the inside (i.e., underlying cause of metabolic disorder) than they do on the outside (i.e., symptoms manifested)! Regardless, let's try to approach the symptoms of mitochondrial disease from the per-

The Most Common Signs and Symptoms of Mitochondrial Disease:

- Fatigue
- Seizures
- Developmental delay
- Muscular symptoms, including muscle pain, weakness, spasms, cramping, and low muscle tone (hypotonia)
- Gastrointestinal disorders, including dysmotility, gastroparesis, malabsorption, chronic constipation
- Dysautonomia (disorder of the autonomic nervous system), including digestive issues, erratic blood pressure, dizziness, and heat intolerance
- Immunodeficiency, including difficulty recovering from illness
- Persistent nausea, cyclic vomiting syndrome
- Autism spectrum disorders, including PDD-NOS
- Sensory processing disorder (SPD)
- Pain, including muscle pain and nerve pain
- Cognitive delay and neuropsychological issues, including memory loss, difficulty thinking, and problem solving
- Vision/hearing loss, optic nerve atrophy, sensorineural deafness
- Migraines/headaches
- Low stamina
- Sleep issues, sleep disorders
- Ataxia (tremor) and motor/movement disorders
- Pancreatic insufficiency
- Kidney dysfunction, urinary retention

spective of the adult patient, parent, or caregiver. Rather than provide detailed medical explanations, we'll focus on understanding each potential symptom, learn about some of the most common causes of the symptom, and tackle the practical advice and approaches that can help you manage these symptoms day to day.

It should be noted that the explanations in this chapter DO NOT replace the advice of an experienced physician involved in your or your child's care. Instead, as many patients, parents, and families seek information to interpret numerous symptoms that can manifest in people with mitochondrial disease, this chapter provides practical explanations and suggestions to improve overall management and understanding. Finally, I suggest that patients and parents refer to the additional resources offered in the Appendices, as well as the "Clinician's Guide to the Management of Mitochondrial Disease" and sample emergency protocols available at www.MitoAction.org/guide.

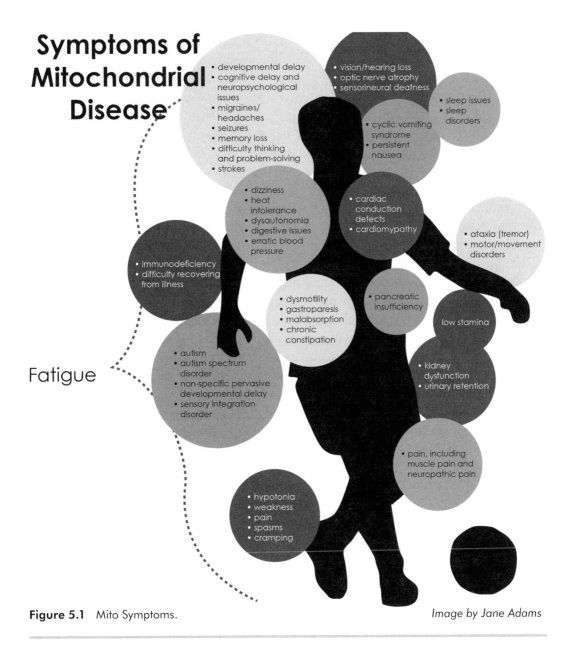

Symptoms of Mitochondrial Disease

- developmental delay
- cognitive delay and neuropsychological issues
- migraines/headaches
- seizures
- memory loss
- difficulty thinking and problem-solving
- strokes

- vision/hearing loss
- optic nerve atrophy
- sensorineural deafness

- sleep issues
- sleep disorders

- cyclic vomiting syndrome
- persistent nausea

- dizziness
- heat intolerance
- dysautonomia
- digestive issues
- erratic blood pressure

- cardiac conduction defects
- cardiomypathy

- ataxia (tremor)
- motor/movement disorders

- immunodeficiency
- difficulty recovering from illness

- dysmotility
- gastroparesis
- malabsorption
- chronic constipation

- pancreatic insufficiency

low stamina

- autism
- autism spectrum disorder
- non-specific pervasive developmental delay
- sensory integration disorder

- kidney dysfunction
- urinary retention

Fatigue

- pain, including muscle pain and neuropathic pain

- hypotonia
- weakness
- pain
- spasms
- cramping

Figure 5.1 Mito Symptoms.

Image by Jane Adams

Part 1: General Suggestions for Managing and Preventing Symptoms

Tracking Your Baseline

What does it mean to be above or below "baseline?" Baseline is not some magic number or formula for people with mitochondrial disease, but rather is a clinical term that helps to describe a person's unique level of "normal." In other words, it might be considered "normal" for a typical, healthy adult to be able to run on a treadmill for ten minutes. However, for an adult with Mito, that's not likely to be "normal!" Instead, an adult with Mito might have a "normal" baseline of being able to walk up and down the stairs in his home with little difficulty. This would be considered his "baseline," or a point of reference against which his energy level may be compared day to day. On a bad day, walking up the stairs might be more difficult. This would indicate that on that day, the adult person with Mito is feeling "below baseline." Similarly, it is important to recognize periods of time when we feel "above baseline." Why? Is it the weather? Better hydration? More rest? Less stress? New medicines or supplements? Without charting (literally, writing it down regularly) one's baseline, it becomes almost impossible to pinpoint when changes occur in the way we feel. "When did my child start having to nap every afternoon after school? It wasn't always that way...." It becomes hard to remember what happened and when it started (because it likely happened very gradually). When did you realize you just couldn't manage grocery shopping trips like you used to? Again, when changes are subtle and happen gradually over time, it becomes difficult to pinpoint exactly what happened, when. However, from a symptom management perspective, and from the point of view of the most valuable person on your healthcare team (you!), the ability to objectively report and track changes to your baseline or that of your child is tremendously helpful and important. Often, because Mito brings with it a mess of confusing symptoms and challenges, we can become very focused on the little details and kind of lose sight of the big picture of how we are really doing. Taking that step back and charting the baseline is a helpful way to gauge changes and can serve as a key player in your or your child's symptom management strategy.

Hydration

One of the most overlooked areas of symptom management and support for mitochondrial disease is hydration. Hydration is the clinical word to describe the amount of fluids that you drink or otherwise consume per day. Your hydration status is an assessment of how positively or negatively balanced your body fluids are at any given time. Most people (who are not using IV fluids or following an oral fluid intake regimen) tend to be a little bit on the "dry side" as compared to what is recommended. For people with Mito, good hydration is especially critical. Your body needs adequate fluids to function properly; in fact, water is essential to proper metabolism in the cells. Approximately 60-70 percent of our body weight is water, and for children and adults with mitochondrial disease, hydration is not only critically important but should also be considered a baseline supportive treatment strategy.

It is often surprising to parents and patients when they find that a simple hydration protocol can dramatically improve symptoms, and can offer metabolic support during times of stress (as in during a period of illness). Many people have heard of the USDA's recommendation that an adult consume eight glasses of water per day (sixty-four ounces, about 1.8 liters). For most adults with mitochondrial disease, this would be considered a great starting point, although some patients require even more hydration to really feel their best.

What Are I's and O's?

In medicine, a patient's fluid balance is assessed by his fluid intake and fluid output, also called "I's and O's." When we assess I's and O's, the numbers should be pretty close to one another. In other words, what a patient is consuming (input) (by mouth, by IV, by g-tube) should approximately equal the patient's output (by urinating or vomiting) in a twenty-four-hour period. In the hospital, nurses measure a person's I's and O's as a method of assessing hydration status. When measuring and tracking intake and output at home, it is helpful to know the following fluid measurements and conversions.

Abbreviations
- oz—ounce
- fl oz—fluid ounce. *Note: Fluid ounces are different than ounces by weight, so it's important to use a syringe, dropper, measuring cup, baby bottle, graduated cylinder, etc. when measuring fluid ounces.*
- ml—milliliter (this is the measurement noted on dosing syringes and droppers); the same amount as a cubic centimeter
- cc—cubic centimeter, the same amount as a milliliter (ml)
- L—liter
- tsp or t—teaspoon
- Tbsp or T—tablespoon
- Kg—kilogram; equivalent to 2.2 pounds (lbs)
- lbs—pounds

Conversions
- 1 fl oz = 30 ml (30 cc's)
- 1 fl oz = 2 Tbsp or 6 tsp
- 500 ml = .5 liter = about 17 fl oz (the size of an IV bag in the hospital)
- 1000 ml = 1 liter (1 L) = about 33 fl oz
- 1 cup = 8 fl oz = 240 ml (240 cc's)
- 1 tsp = 5 ml (5 cc's)
- 1 Tbsp = 15 ml (15 cc's) or 3 tsp
- 1 kg = 2.2 lbs

How Much Hydration Do You or Your Child Need?

When thinking about daily fluid management for kids and adults who live with Mito, how much hydration is needed? We first need to know how much is currently consumed as a baseline. Begin by taking a snapshot over a period of a few days of your or your child's fluid intake to determine the average amount of fluids that is consumed. (Note: for children and adults who use specially formulated formulas or fluids by mouth, IV, or g-tube, you likely are already on a hydration protocol; please stick with your doctor's recommendations. However, you can always follow and chart the amount consumed per day for good measure.) To get an accurate idea of your or your child's actual baseline fluid intake, you'll need to pay close attention to and record everything that is consumed by mouth, IV, or g-tube for about seventy-two hours. Doing this is really important, because without a starting point, you really cannot accurately begin to adjust hydration in order to improve symptoms. Use a simple chart like the one in Figure 5.2.

Figure 5.2: Example of a Daily Food and Fluid Log

DATE: Jan 27	FOOD EATEN	DRINKS CONSUMED	TOTAL OUNCES
6 am – 8 am	Cheerios with 4 oz milk; peanut butter toast	3 oz Gatorade; ½ cup (4 oz) chocolate milk	11 oz
8 am – 10 am	Popsicle (3 oz); crackers	1 cup (8 oz) milk; 4 oz water	15 oz
10 am – 12 pm	egg salad sandwich	1 cup (8 oz) green tea	8 oz
12 pm – 2 pm	cheese stick; strawberries	6 oz water; 1 cup (8 oz) sugar-free lemonade	14 oz
2 pm – 4 pm	cottage cheese; ½ granola bar	8 oz apple juice	8 oz
4 pm – 6 pm	chicken soup (6 oz); grilled cheese sandwich; carrots with dip	10 oz water; 8 oz milk	24 oz
6 pm – 8 pm	½ cup (4 oz) vanilla ice cream; banana	6 oz water	10 oz
8 pm – 10 pm	rice pudding	1 cup (8 oz) tea	8 oz
10 pm – 12 am		2 oz water	2 oz
12 am – 2 am		4 oz water	4 oz
2 am – 4 am			0 oz
4 am – 6 am		4 oz water	4 oz
TOTAL OUNCES			108 oz total (108 oz divided by 8 oz/cup = 13½ cups)

Note that some foods in Figure 5.2 that are primarily liquid-based, like Jello, broth-based soups, ice cream, Popsicles, and watermelon count as fluid intake in terms of hydration measurement. For adults and children who have a hard time reaching recommended fluid requirements, including these types of foods in your snacks and meals can add an additional ten to twenty ounces per day of good hydration!

"Maintenance fluid requirements" describe the amount of fluids that an individual needs each day to maintain his hydration baseline, and are slightly different for children based on the fact that they typically weigh less than adults. Physicians and nurses use the Holliday-Segar formula to calculate maintenance fluid requirements in children (see Table 5.3). Parents, you can use this formula, too, to estimate the goal amount of fluids that your child should take in during a twenty-four-hour period.

Table 5.3 Holliday-Segar Formula for Maintenance Fluid Requirements by Weight in Children

Weight (in kg)	ml of liquid per day
0-10 kg	100 ml of liquid per kg of body weight
11-20 kg	1000 ml + 50 ml per kg of body weight for each kg >10 (greater than 10 kg)
>20 (greater than 20)	1500 ml + 20 ml per kg of body weight for each kg >20 (greater than 20 kg)

To illustrate how to use the chart in Table 5.3, consider the example of Mateo. Mateo is a child who weighs forty pounds. What are his maintenance fluid needs? Forty pounds divided by 2.2 gives us his weight in kilograms = 18 kg, which falls within the 11-20 kg category of the Holliday-Segar chart. Therefore, Mateo needs 1000 ml per day for his first 10 kg of weight. He *also* needs an additional 50 ml for each kilogram of weight above 10 kg. Since Mateo weighs 18 kg, we need to calculate additional fluids for 8 kg (18 -10 = 8). Using the formula, 8 kg x 50 ml/kg = 400 ml/day. So, Mateo needs 1000 ml + 400 ml/day = 1400 ml/day of fluids (water, juice, Gatorade, Jello, milk, etc.)

How many cups is that? Remember, 1 cup is 240 ml. So, 1400 ml divided by 240 = about 6 cups. There are eight ounces in a cup, so yet another way to say this is that he needs 48 ounces per day. Therefore, for Mateo, a child who weighs forty pounds, he needs to be drinking at least 6 cups (or 48 oz) of low-sugar fluids every twenty-four-hour period to stay appropriately hydrated. That's a total volume equivalent to about three large water bottles per day.

However, **if** Mateo were sick, with a fever, an illness, was going to be in a warm/hot/humid environment (above 78 degrees), or was going to be active (playing outside, going to physical therapy, swimming, taking a field trip, etc.), his maintenance fluid requirements would need to *increase* to compensate. In addition, it's important to also think about the concept of "insensible fluid losses." This is a clinical term that describes the water that leaves our body without our knowledge each day through breathing and through the skin. An average healthy adult "loses" about 800 ml (100 oz) of water per day through "insensible fluid losses." Children and adults with mitochondrial disease have a tendency to breathe faster, shallower breaths when they are sick, active, in pain, or stressed. As a result, their insensible water losses may also be higher. Higher body temperatures (fever) also increase fluid requirements considerably. Obviously, illnesses that include vomiting or diarrhea would dramatically increase a person's fluid needs, and for an adult or child with Mito, would also require immediate medical attention. Finally, understand that infants and young children have a very low threshold to become dehydrated (i.e., they can become dehydrated more easily) since their overall body mass is lower, their metabolic rate is higher, and a greater percentage of their body mass is water. Consequently, if your child goes for more than six hours refusing all fluids, you should be concerned and seek the advice of your pediatrician immediately. Table 5.4 shows the range of recommended fluids for children based on weight.

Adults can follow a more general rule when calculating maintenance fluid requirements since there isn't the degree of variation in weight and size in adults as

Table 5.4 Holliday-Segar Method for Calculating Fluid Requirements

Holliday-Segar Method for Calculating Fluid Requirements	
Body Weight of Child	**Water/Free Liquids Required**
5 kg (11 lbs)	500 mL (16.67 oz)
6 kg (13.2 lbs)	600 mL (20 oz)
7 kg (15.4 lbs)	700 mL (23.33 oz)
8 kg (17.6 lbs)	800 mL (26.67 oz)
9 kg (19.8 lbs)	900 mL (30 oz)
10 kg (22 lbs)	1000 mL (33.33 oz)
11 kg (24.2 lbs)	1050 mL (35 oz)
12 kg (26.4 lbs)	1100 mL (36.67 oz)
13 kg (28.6 lbs)	1150 mL (38.33 oz)
14 kg (30.8 lbs)	1200 mL (40 oz)
15 kg (33 lbs)	1250 mL (41.67 oz)
16 kg (35.2 lbs)	1300 mL (43.33 oz)
17 kg (37.4 lbs)	1350 mL (45 oz)
18 kg (39.6 lbs)	1400 mL (46.67 oz)
19 kg (41.8 lbs)	1450 mL (48.33 oz)
20 kg (44 lbs)	1500 mL (50 oz)
More than 20 kg (>44 lbs)	**1500 mL + 20 mL per kg over 20 kg**
25 kg (55 lbs)	1600 mL (53.33 oz)
30 kg (66 lbs)	1700 mL (56.67 oz)
35 kg (77 lbs)	1800 mL (60 oz)
40 kg (88 lbs)	1900 mL (63.33 oz)

Conversion Chart
1 kg = 2.2 lbs
30 mL = 1 oz

Source: Holliday & Segar, 1957

there is in children. *Generally, adults should calculate 35-50 ml of liquid per kg of body weight per day to estimate their base fluid requirements.* For example, a 125-pound person weighs about 57 kilograms (125 lbs divided by 2.2 = 56.8 kg). Therefore, his maintenance fluid requirement, or the minimum amount of liquids that he should try to consume each day, is between 1995-2850 ml per day (57 kg x 35 ml = 1995; 57 kg x 50 ml = 2850). Divide this by 30 to estimate ounces, so about 67-95 oz, or 8-12 cups. If making exact calculations is confusing for you, consider instead trying to drink one to two cups of water or other beverage every hour while awake (excluding nighttime, although some patients find that a few ounces during the night can make a big difference in their morning energy level).

When discussing hydration with parents and patients, many people have reservations about *how* to increase their daily fluid intake. Some children and adult patients feel nauseous, especially when they have a full belly, so they don't feel like drinking (and can even be resistant). Children may be picky about what and when to drink, and parents tire of trying to force their children to drink more than they want. However, since we know that hydration is critically important for metabolic functions to take place, and we know that hydration can help improve energy and even manage symptoms, we need to be creative about finding ways to improve our hydration status. First, spreading the intake of fluids out over the day is much more beneficial than trying to "catch up" by chugging twelve or twenty-four ounces in a few minutes. It is also easier on the belly to take in an ounce or two at a time, as opposed to a large volume. Use your food and fluid log (Figure 5.2) to meet small fluid intake targets every couple of hours so that, at the end of a twenty-four-hour period, you have reached your overall daily fluid goal. Electrolytes are also an essential part of hydration management. Electrolytes refer to naturally occurring salts in the body, such as potassium and sodium. Generally, children and adults get enough electrolytes through the minerals in the foods that they eat. However, during periods of illness, or when increasing water intake, it is possible for electrolytes to become imbalanced or diminished. A simple strategy to help balance electrolytes is to incorporate a few cups of readily-available beverages that are electrolyte-balanced. Look for low-sugar varieties of vitamin-electrolyte enhanced water and avoid any that have sugar content greater than ten to fifteen grams per cup. High sugar drinks provide less hydration than water or low-sugar beverages because the carbohydrates slow the absorption of water into the cells. Also be wary of "energy drinks," which don't provide energy from water and electrolytes but contain undesirable caffeine and stimulants.

Finally, it is worth mentioning in this discussion about hydration that physicians recommend that most people with mitochondrial disease avoid use of lactated ringer's ("LR") solution. LR is an IV solution often used in emergency rooms or after surgery. The lactate in LR can worsen or elevate lactic acid levels in Mito patients and can be detrimental. Many metabolic and mitochondrial disease specialists recommend use of a "D5 ½ NS" dextrose-based saline solution during emergency/maintenance IV hydration instead (essentially, a balance of salt and sugar in sterile water).

Tips for Staying Hydrated:

- At the beginning of the day, fill the number of water bottles (some even have measurements marked right on the bottle) with your low-sugar beverage of choice and keep one with you all the time to sip. You can keep track of your progress, knowing that by bedtime, you should be working on your last bottle.

- Keep a clean cup next to the kitchen sink and next to the bathroom sink (for children, you can do this at school or in the classroom). *Every time* you or your child goes to the bathroom, insist on drinking an ounce or two of water right after washing your hands. (This works, because, the more you drink the more often you are in the bathroom!) Likewise, whenever you are preparing for a meal or an activity and are at the kitchen sink, stop and drink an ounce or two, depending on your needs.

- Enjoy a variety of drinks and liquid-based snacks, such as Italian ice, frozen yogurt, Popsicles, Jello, melon, sorbet, low-sodium broth, hot decaffeinated tea, iced herbal or flavored decaf tea, lemonade, juice (diluted with water to reduce the sugar content), Gatorade (especially G2, which offers the benefit of electrolytes with lower sugar), vitamin water, flavored water, seltzer, milkshakes, blended icees, smoothies, etc. Chocolate milk is a great pick-me-up and offers hydration as well as nutrition (fats, proteins, carbohydrates)—great for kids and for adults! Incorporate your favorite beverages into your routine in addition to water.

- For children, avoid the use of "sippy cups," or modify them by taking out the valve. Sippy cups use a one-way valve to prevent spilling; for children with Mito, the energy required to suck the liquid out through the valve prevents them from really getting the volume that they need. Try cups with better flow, try a straw, or try having your child drink a couple of ounces at a time out of plastic medicine cups.

Common Mito Symptoms that Are Helped by Hydration

Heat intolerance, exercise intolerance, low stamina, headache, constipation, gastroparesis (slow digestive motility), dysautonomia (dysregulation of the autonomic nervous system), dizziness, pain, low blood pressure, dry skin, fatigue, dry mouth, and muscle weakness are just a few of the more common Mito symptoms that may be improved by increasing fluid intake. Children and adults with mitochondrial disease have a very low threshold to become dehydrated. In fact, some metabolic physicians feel that clinical signs of dehydration (dry mouth, fewer wet diapers/fewer uses of the bathroom, darker urine, increased heart rate, skin that "stays" when pinched together) are "too late" to indicate dehydration in Mito patients. Instead, rely on subtle cues to let you know that it's time to increase fluids, such as weakness, difficulty focusing, headache, fatigue, thirst, and mild nausea. Often, you can literally see a person with Mito "droop" like a wilting flower when they begin to get out of fluid balance. Likewise, you can see him perk up after getting hydrated. Adult patients describe a "fog" that comes over them when they begin to need food, fluids, and rest. It is so important to learn to not only recognize theses subtle cues in yourself, your spouse, or your child, but also to stay on top of hydration status every single day. This is an area that is worth extra teaching effort and advocacy for kids and teens at school, and should be a priority for adults managing their own symptoms. If symptoms can be improved by something as simple as a smart hydration approach, then your efforts will be well worth it!

Rest

Even if you are not new to this diagnosis, you might still be figuring out how to balance the energy in = energy out equation. Rest is another important factor that, like hydration, is often overlooked and taken for granted when, instead, it should be considered a cornerstone of mitochondrial disease management. How much rest you or your child needs is very individual and is also dependent upon environmental factors (illness, weather, medications, stress, symptom flare-ups, activity level, etc.). A huge crux of this patient and family handbook is to help us, as parents, patients, and advocates, understand how to incorporate energy conservation into our daily lives so that we can really have the energy to do the things that we want the most. Nonetheless, accomplishing this gracefully is challenging, especially when symptoms and energy levels fluctuate from day to day (even moment to moment). Begin by incorporating these basic suggestions from patients, parents, and clinicians:

1. **Define rest for you or your child.** What type of rest is really *restorative* for you or your child? For example, you might think that sitting on the sofa watching TV is restful, yet it is not restorative. Why not? Think about the energy required to do that "resting" activity—your muscles are working to help you sit upright, your eyes are working to focus and watch the television, your ears and nerves are working to hear the sound, your brain is working to process the concepts….Is this really recharging your body's battery or just using a little less energy? It's important to specifically identify the types of rest that are most helpful for you or your child. Consider lying down whenever possible, as a half hour reclined may be more restorative than an hour sitting up. Many children and adults with Mito enjoy audiobooks, as listening to a book can be relaxing and allow you to lie down with your eyes closed. For kids who are in school, rest periods should not only be incorporated into their school day (and noted in their IEP), but also made available to them as needed. Taking the time to recharge before our batteries drain completely can help us or our children with Mito stay closer to our optimal baseline.

2. **Slow down during periods of illness, fever, or stress.** We simply cannot have the same expectations of our bodies (and our minds!) during periods of fever, illness, or stress, as the mitochondria are work-

ing at an even greater disadvantage during these times. Our reserves are literally wiped out and our body is trying to compensate and keep up when we are sick, dehydrated, overheated, or overwhelmed. One of the best ways to conserve energy during these difficult periods is to simply stop moving or at least slow everything that you do significantly, and allow for the opportunity to recharge. Keep in mind that it is not uncommon for kids and adults with Mito to need weeks or even months to recover from illnesses, especially those involving a fever.

3. **Be prepared to make adjustments to schedules** (work, school, activity level) **and to your own and others' expectations** during and after an illness, especially an illness with a fever. Likewise, a child or adult with Mito may not be able to do as well as he would "normally" do when fatigued, and the fatigue can have a snowball effect if appropriate rest isn't allowed. In addition, incorporate rest periods based on levels of activity. For example, after exercise or physical therapy, kids and adults need to build in extra time for a period of rest (ten minutes to an hour). And don't forget to hydrate as well!

4. **Plan for recharge periods.** Too often, adult patients in particular share the same story. "I was busy with my family, busy during the holidays, skipped the rest time and the snack that I usually have, and then crashed the next day and couldn't get out of bed." Prevent the dreaded next-day crash! Anticipate that your body needs a rest and rest before you are so tired that you can't get back up to your normal baseline.

5. **Pace yourself (or your child).** Pacing in everyday life requires that we constantly adjust to the moment as well as think ahead. This is actually a tall order for parents of children with Mito and for adults who are managing their symptoms. A hallmark characteristic of mitochondrial disease is fatigue, which worsens as the day progresses. Knowing this about the diagnosis can help you to make better decisions about daily energy management and energy conservation. For example, can you schedule your days so that activities that require mental and physical effort (i.e., shopping, attending school, doctor's appointments, work hours, physical therapy) take place in the morning or early afternoon, before fatigue begins to set in? Can there be more or longer opportunities for rest as the day progresses? Controlling our schedule isn't always realistic or possible; however, it is important to make adjustments accordingly. For example, if a clinic visit is pending that afternoon at 4 pm, don't try to also fit in some errands while on your way. Instead, recognize the energy demand that will be necessary for the important (later) activity, and plan for it by pac-

ing yourself and resting or taking care of less strenuous business in the morning. Adult patients and parents alike have trouble getting the hang of this as it is often counterintuitive to stop and rest when everyone around us is working, playing, socializing, etc. However, the benefit of pacing is that you will require less recovery time and ultimately be able to manage your or your child's energy levels better so that you **can** do more of what you desire.

6. **Recognize the drain of emotional stress.** Emotional stress can have as much negative impact on a person's well-being as an illness. Emotional stress and anxiety are often overlooked, especially for children and teens, but they can take a very physical toll on someone with Mito, and can dramatically impact his energy levels. Recognizing this and working hard to create a supportive environment is critical.

7. **Oxygen hunger is also a potential pitfall for people with Mito**, due to the failure of dysfunctional OX-PHOS and mitochondria to fully utilize all circulating oxygen. You may also notice that people with Mito breathe faster with minimal exertion, just as a runner will gulp air and breathe faster to fuel the muscles. **Be aware of this**, and look for it as a cue that you or your child may need to slow down and take a break.

Nutrition

"Eat right to stay healthy" should be the daily motto for kids and adults with Mito. In fact, perhaps the jingle for Mito patients should be "Eat right and eat often!" Nutrition, like hydration and rest, is another area that is often overlooked as part of a comprehensive approach to managing Mito symptoms. For people with Mito, eating small, nutritious meals throughout the day is akin to fueling a fire with kindling to keep it burning. We need to continue to feed the body with the proper fuel in order to keep the energy output at optimum levels.

Most people with Mito should avoid excessive amounts of foods that are high in simple sugars. Simple sugar carbohydrates (white rice, plain bagel, granola bar) can help kids and adults get an energy rebound during a time when energy is really depleted (some people call this a "crash" but it actually looks more like a "slump"). However, a steady diet of simple carbohydrates causes the mitochondria to potentially have more free radical by-products, so opt for a balance of fruits, vegetables, whole grains, healthy fats (like peanut butter and olive oil), and easily digested protein (like yogurt, eggs, and fish) instead. Talk to your physician about recommendations for your diet or that of your child, and seek the advice of a nutritionist in a hospital as well.

Nutrition for kids and adults with Mito is all about balance—and striking that perfect balance takes some trial and error for most people. You can, however, follow some general guidelines in regard to nutrition and mitochondrial disease:

- Follow the "3+3" diet—three small meals and three snacks a day (so, you or your child will be eating about every two and a half hours).
- If you have slow digestive motility, try foods with high nutrition value and higher liquid content/softer texture, such as yogurt and fruit smoothies, chocolate milk, and creamed/pureed soups which are easier to digest.
- Keep a food log. As important as it is to track hydration, getting an idea of one's actual diet is useful as well. In addition, if you are able to seek the counsel of a nutritionist, your first assignment will be to keep a food diary!
- Watch out for "empty" calories from sugary drinks (beware also of long-term use of IV solutions containing dextrose if weight gain is a problem for you).
- Eat slowly. Some patients find that sipping liquids between meals is easier than drinking a lot with a meal.
- Eat a complex carbohydrate (anything whole wheat or whole grain, most fruits and vegetables, beans, nuts, and legumes) with a protein at every meal and snack. For example, try peanut butter and apple slices, eggs and toast, cheese and crackers, or celery with cream cheese and almonds.
- Avoid large servings of simple carbohydrates, such as plain pasta, white rice, white bread, cookies, etc. A large serving of these foods is broken down into more glucose than the body can metabolize for energy at once. However, a small serving of simple carbohydrates can make a child or adult with Mito feel better quickly when depleted.
- **Avoid fasting.** This is a very important rule. Do not go for long periods of time without food or drink. In some cases, especially before surgery, a period of fasting (called NPO) is required. However, even in these cases, discuss this with your or your child's doctor to determine the minimum amount of fasting time allowed. This can prevent an energy deficit and negative metabolic consequences.

Part 2: Specific Symptoms, Explanations, and Suggestions

It can be said that the symptoms that children and adults with Mito are feeling and experiencing are not necessarily the focus of mitochondrial medicine and research. For example, the almost universally reported symptom, pain, is not well defined in research papers or thoroughly addressed in the clinical textbooks of mitochondrial medicine. Why not? Let's use the analogy of an onion, where what we see on the outside layer is the patient and his symptoms. Underneath that layer there are many layers that lead to the core of the problem. At the very center of our onion are the molecules that define the disease. In today's understanding of mitochondrial disease, we are looking at the onion from the inside out—we are learning as much or more about the molecules than we are about the corresponding patient symptoms! As patients, parents, and clinicians, we feel the knowledge gap when trying to interpret and manage multitudes of symptoms. As of yet, no standards of care for patients exist, although trends are emerging and patients themselves are helping to bridge the gap between the molecular science and the patient symptom experience.

What Is a Symptom?

People are often confused about the difference between signs and symptoms. Symptoms are subjective and are felt by the child or adult with mitochondrial disease, while signs are found during clinical exams or via diagnostic testing. There are both signs and symptoms associated with mitochondrial disorders. Symptoms include muscle weakness, headache, fatigue, pain, dizziness, nausea, etc. Signs include lactic acidosis, ataxia, low blood pressure, exercise intolerance, strokes, and fever. Signs help definitively define the disease and/or classify the root cause of symptoms. Symptoms are typically a person's chief complaint; for example, you wouldn't say "I have a lactic acidosis today," but you would say "I have a headache and feel tired." We will focus primarily on the symptoms in our discussion here, but understanding the difference between these terms can help you to better "speak the language" when communicating with your healthcare providers.

How can there be so many possible symptoms associated with one disorder? If we approach our understanding of this by remembering the underlying energy deficit inherent to Mito, then the long list of potential symptoms makes more sense. After all, if the body's energy factories are not working as they should, how can anything in the body work effectively? Imagine that the mitochondria are like the power stations in a city. Suppose a dozen power stations supply the energy needed for one area of the city. One of the power stations fails, so now the energy currency is decreased. The lights will go out on a couple of blocks in that city. Do the lightbulbs need to be replaced? No, the energy source needs to be turned back on. When there is an ineffective or insufficient energy supply due to a defect in the body's powerhouse, then *any* system of the body can be affected. As we have discussed before, the organs and functions of our bodies that require the most energy to function will be affected most dramatically.

Understanding mitochondrial disease symptoms is helpful for parents, patients, and caregivers because it helps us to a) identify new symptoms, b) know better how to treat them, and c) feel confident about actively managing those symptoms as part of the healthcare team. Not all potential symptoms are discussed in this chapter; rather, we'll take a closer look at some of the more common issues and discuss practical options for improving the way that you or your child feel.

Typically, clinicians are trained to view the body (and symptoms therein) by a review of systems—heart, digestive, central nervous system, skeletal, etc. As a result, when your physician or nurse is working with you or your child to understand your symptoms, he is reviewing them through that "systems" lens. However, because so many patients with mitochondrial disease experience so many unrelated symptoms (in multiple organs or systems), a segmented review of systems can be less helpful for patients who are struggling to make sense of the "big picture." Therefore, I have chosen to write this section by focusing on "chief complaints" instead, i.e., what would you or your child be feeling, bothered by, essentially complaining of. My hope is that approaching the most common symptoms in this manner will diffuse the medical complexity and allow you, as patients, parents, and family members, to get straight to the most practical and relevant information about each symptom. Finally, there are many symptoms that affect children, teens, and adults with Mito that are not listed here; rather, the partial list below illuminates the most universal issues for our Mito community.

Fatigue

Probably the most common and most pervasive of all Mito symptoms is fatigue. Children and adults with mitochondrial disease wear out easily, especially as the day progresses, during periods of illness or stress, and with physical exertion or excessive activity. Adults and teens who can verbalize their fatigue describe feeling "flu-like," "worn-out," "fuzzy," "unable to focus," "weak," or "heavy and clumsy." Not all patients who have mitochondrial disease and fatigue feel drowsy or sleepy as their energy is depleted. In fact, some children and adults with Mito may become increasingly agitated, unfocused, irritable, and uncontrolled as their fatigue worsens. In these cases, their bodies are still fatigued, but the low energy state results in worsening of symptoms and loss of control.

In addition, Mito patients may find that subtle symptoms, such as shakiness, tremors, dizziness, slurred speech, drooping eyelids, difficulty focusing, and impaired concentration become much more pronounced when fatigued. Likewise, some parents report that they can recognize when their child with Mito has become overtired because he will "zone out," avoid eye contact, regress in speech and behavior, be emotionally "flat," become hyper-agitated, or act floppy and listless. Adult patients frequently describe a "brownout" when they become fatigued, where they are awake but feel unable to focus and have difficulty with short-term memory and concentration (even to carry out a simple conversation or complete simple tasks). Both adults and kids share profound weakness and feelings of exhaustion after exercise. Adults, teens, and parents of affected kids also universally agree that there is an inevitable "payback" if they do too much and become overtired, causing them to need two to three times longer to recuperate than they would have required otherwise. This is especially apparent during busy holiday seasons, vacations, and when children go back to school and are expending more energy than usual. Illness, physical stress, and emotional stress can also zap a Mito patient's energy reserve almost instantly, leaving them profoundly fatigued and often unable to do much more than rest in bed.

Obviously, all people—with and without mitochondrial disease—get tired. Further, we know from the research that people get more tired as they get older as a result of reduced mitochondrial function that occurs naturally to some degree with aging. However, pronounced, frequent, persistent fatigue and exercise/activity intolerance are uniquely characteristic of people who suffer from mitochondrial dysfunction, and are directly related to impaired oxidative phosphorylation and diminished ATP production. While resting does help, it is important to recognize that supportive management of fatigue involves much more than relaxation. Fatigue is the underlying common denominator for many of the symptoms that trouble children and adults with mitochondrial disease and therefore should always be considered when planning activities, both in the short- and long-term. As mentioned before, an approach that prioritizes rest, hydration, nutrition, supplementation with the Mito cocktail, and careful symptom management is likely to offer the most relief and give kids and adults with Mito improved energy and a higher overall baseline.

On the other hand, one of the most perplexing characteristics of mitochondrial disease is variability in energy levels and symptom presentation. Parents of young children are often baffled by day-to-day, moment-to-moment fluctuations in energy, symptoms, and ability that seem to ebb and flow without rhyme or reason. They find it difficult to explain to therapists and school professionals why their child was unable to speak on Monday but can play on the playground on Tuesday. (Unfortunately, they may even become the subject of suspicion by inexperienced providers.) Likewise, adults who are working, caring for a family, and caring for themselves are frustrated by their inability to plan for fatigue or predict the onset of other troubling symptoms. Most eventually begin to recognize the individualized triggers that cause fatigue and worsening of symptoms in themselves or their children, such as poor liquid intake, poor calorie intake or hypoglycemia, overexertion, overheating, or overstimulation. However, even for intuitive parents, patients, and families, living with mitochondrial disease and dealing with the fluctuating levels of fatigue can be a constant balancing act.

Like a laptop that is running on a battery that cannot hold a charge, running multiple programs simultaneously becomes problematic when the battery is almost empty. For Mito patients, a "low-battery state" and subsequent fatigue is frequently inevitable and occurs alongside worsening of other unrelated symptoms. Children, teens, and adults with Mito tire easily, become weak after minimal effort, and are likely to notice an effect in many areas of the body when tired. Improving energy production and implementing energy conservation strategies are essential cornerstones to reducing fatigue and providing the opportunity for plenty of meaningful and therapeutic activities.

Heat Intolerance

A great majority of children and adults who have mitochondrial disease suffer from heat intolerance. Heat intolerance is a marked inability to handle humid and/or warm environments. Heat intolerance may be associated with lack of or inefficient sweating, elevated body temperature, redness or mottling of the skin, dramatic loss of energy and stamina, or sudden decrease in muscle tone (looking or feeling "floppy" or "heavy").

Heat intolerance can occur both indoors and out. Naturally, very hot and humid climates are difficult for most Mito patients and dramatically impact their energy level and stamina. Consequently, many families learn to plan vacations or trips during cooler months in order to be able to enjoy more time outside while away (i.e., choosing not to visit Disney World in July). However, indoor environments that are too warm, especially if compounded by poor air circulation, are just as difficult for kids and adults with Mito. In particular, parents should be thoughtful about recognizing environments away from home where kids may find themselves overheated, such as the school bus, a hot car or vehicle without air conditioning, classrooms with large windows facing the sun, classrooms with poor ventilation, heated swimming pools, and outdoor areas without shade.

There are some strategies that can help improve heat intolerance for kids and adults with mitochondrial disease. Primarily, aggressive hydration and use of cooling vests or special cooling clothing will not change the Mito patient's ability to tolerate heat, but can reduce the lethargy and irritability that occurs. There is a theory that heat intolerance occurs in people with mitochondrial dysfunction because the body's autonomic nervous system, which controls body temperature, is affected by the dysfunctional energy metabolism. When the body is overheated, from a fever or from the environment, the enzymes in the mitochondrial electron transport chain are less effective, thereby decreasing ATP production and consequently resulting in worsening of symptoms. Kids and adults with mitochondrial disease may not realize that they are becoming overheated until a dramatic drop in energy occurs, at which time they may develop an inability to focus, slur speech, have difficulty standing or sitting upright, and obvious fatigue. Therefore, it is extremely important to plan ahead in anticipation of heat intolerance occurring. The following are some basic suggestions for staving off the effects of heat intolerance:

- When going outdoors in warm climates wear lightweight, breathable clothing.
- Dress in layers that can be easily shed as the temperature rises.
- Avoid overdressing during the winter months.
- Drink plenty of fluids, more than usual, in the few hours before going out and continue to aggressively hydrate while outside.
- Use cooling vests with ice packs that fit inside of a fitted undershirt-style vest, or that rely on a special fabric that, when wet, evaporates and cools the skin much like sweating would do.
- Carry wet washcloths packed in a cooler or Ziploc bag with ice that can be used on a person's face, neck, head, and chest during a hot day to help keep the body temperature closer to normal.
- Plan ahead by seeking out shady areas or planning occasional rest periods inside when enjoying warm weather activities.
- Swimming is also a great way to stay cool, as the water creates a natural cooling effect on the body.

Very cold temperatures are also difficult for people who have mitochondrial disease, although the primary symptom reported by patients when they are cold is deep muscle pain and fatigue. When we are cold, our mitochondria help generate heat, so it makes sense that moderate temperatures are easiest to tolerate and provide the greatest opportunity for kids and adults with Mito to feel their best. Finally, it should be noted that some people with mitochondrial disease are able to endure extreme temperatures (hot or cold) at the time, but later suffer from a "hangover" characterized by the fatigue, muscle pain, etc. described above. In either case, anticipating the additional energy demand required by the body to keep a constant body temp in very warm or cold environments is essential.

Nausea, Vomiting, Constipation, Reflux, Abdominal Pain, and Poor Appetite

Vomiting, abdominal pain, constipation, chronic nausea, cyclic vomiting, dysmotility (slow digestion when muscles of the digestive tract do not work normally), anorexia (loss of appetite), and reflux are just a few of the gastrointestinal (GI) symptoms that plague some children and adults with mitochondrial disease. For Mito patients who have these and other GI symptoms, manifestation of these symptoms tends to be dramatic and can significantly impact the child or adult patient's everyday life. For many years, mitochondrial disease was considered a neuromuscular disease and GI symptoms were disregarded or overlooked. However, as the spectrum of mitochondrial disorders broadens, more and more patients—of all ages—are reporting significant digestion problems as a primary symptom of their diagnosis.

The gastrointestinal system is highly metabolically active, meaning that the cells are rapidly renewing and are consequently highly energy dependent. It is not completely understood why the gastrointestinal system is so significantly affected by some mitochondrial disorders, although research suggests that bacterial overgrowth in the gut, smooth muscle dysfunction (see the section entitled "Muscular Issues" below), as well as autonomic nervous system dysfunction play a large part. Your autonomic nervous system is responsible for "automatic" functions in your body, including digestion, respiration, heart rate, and perspiration. All of these autonomic nervous system tasks can be disrupted by poor energy metabolism. When this happens, patients can feel terrible, "flu-like" symptoms that come on suddenly and are difficult to treat. Dysfunction of the autonomic nervous system is called dysautonomia, and is another hallmark feature of mitochondrial disease. The part of the autonomic nervous system that controls organ function involved with digestion is called the enteric nervous system. Sometimes the enteric nervous system is called "the second brain" because it can operate independently but also communicates intricately with the nervous system and the brain. Research hypothesizes that the dysautonomia, which occurs as a result of mitochondrial dysfunction, has an impact on the enteric nervous system. Gastrointestinal dysfunction results, which contributes to very slow (or stopped) peristalsis that normally occurs to move food through the digestive tract. Patients, accordingly, may have abdominal pain, nausea, vomiting, bloating, constipation, reflux, and poor appetites. Anorexia and lack of appetite caused by the distressing GI symptoms worsens the overall motility, causing more nausea and dysmotility, resulting in a cycle that is difficult to break and that leaves children and adults feeling rotten. In addition, lactic acidosis and dehydration can induce nausea, which also contributes to gastrointestinal distress and dysmotility. Some patients are even diagnosed with pseudo-obstruction, a condition where the normal function of the gut is completely stopped without obvious cause (as if there were something blocking the intestinal tract and preventing the normal movement of food through the digestive system).

Because mitochondrial function and energy production are so dependent on good nutrition and hydration, many children and adults ultimately require supportive nutritional interventions (beyond what they're taking in by mouth) in order to get enough calories and fluids. For example, it is common for Mito patients with disabling GI symptoms to use a "g-tube" (gastrostomy tube) or "j-tube" (jejunostomy tube) as an opportunity to increase overall calorie and fluid intake as well as relieve uncomfortable pressure that can build up in the stomach or upper intestine. Especially useful for those who are at risk for malnutrition or dehydration, g-tubes and j-tubes are feeding tubes that are surgically placed into the gastrointestinal tract. A g-tube is placed directly into the stomach, whereas a j-tube is placed into the jejunum, which is the upper part of the small intestine. In both cases, many physicians who care for children and adults with chronic GI distress and mitochondrial disease would agree that the benefits of g-tubes and j-tubes typically outweigh the risks of surgical placement. First, use of a g-tube or j-tube allows the enzymes present in the digestive system to continue to be excreted and used. Second, even for patients who have extreme dysmotility, continued use of the gut (even minimally) is better than not using it at all. Gastrostomy tubes (g-tubes) require normal stomach function and emptying, therefore patients with slow emptying (gastroparesis) may benefit from a j-tube. In either case, after placement of the tube, a "button" (with one or more capped opening called a "port") is placed right onto the skin that allows special nutritional formula, fluids, water, or medication to be administered via a tube. In the case of j-tubes, an electric pump controls the infusion rate. Patients who require g-tubes or j-tubes can benefit from the advice of specialized home infusion companies as well as gastroenterologists who have experience with dysmotility.

Nausea and vomiting are symptoms that frequently affect mitochondrial disease patients and obviously can make patients feel miserable and dramatically impact their quality of life. A percentage of people with mitochondrial disorders actually suffer from cyclic vomiting syndrome (CVS), which is characterized by persistent, chronic nausea and repeated vomiting (several times within an hour). Some researchers believe that CVS is a type of mitochondrial disorder and can be improved when overall nervous system function and energy metabolism is improved. In addition, slow gastric emptying (food doesn't empty from the stomach properly) also contributes to terrible and persistent nausea, and can also cause vomiting, bloating, abdominal pain, and lack of appetite. Children may become afraid to eat or drink if they suffer from persistent nausea or vomiting for fear that eating will trigger the symptoms. In these cases, it is extremely important to recognize the increased energy demands of children who are growing and to take measures (g-tube, j-tube, medications) to help them to feel better and get enough calories and fluids.

Many adults and children find that tube feeds of water, electrolyte solutions, or special formulas that are administered slowly at night are game-changers because they stop the nausea/vomiting cycle. Patients and parents who live with chronic GI symptoms, nausea, and pseudo-obstruction report that frequent, small meals that include soft foods like yogurt, noodle soups, and whole vegetable/fruit juices are helpful. Two medications commonly used for nausea include Zofran® (ondansetron) and Benadryl® (diphenhydramine). In addition, some patients and parents have reported long-term successful control of GI symptoms by following a "pseudo-obstruction diet" composed of six small meals per day of low-fat, low-fiber, lactose-free foods.

For patients with chronic GI symptoms as part of their mitochondrial disease presentation, it is critical to have a trustworthy and active team involved in managing their nutrition/hydration status. Ideally, the team should include a gastroenterologist, primary care physician, and a nutritionist. While every medical center may not offer these specific resources, many hospitals for children and academic centers offer a complex care service for people with chronic illnesses. It is worth doing the research to seek out centers in your area, as managing these symptoms can not only be overwhelming but are potentially able to improve quality of life and the affected person's health when optimally managed.

Constipation has been related to autonomic and enteric nervous system dysfunction as well, and may be related to poor nerve communication as well as low muscle tone in the intestines. Constipation can cause abdominal pain and discomfort in children and adults with Mito, especially when peristalsis (muscular contractions that move food through the gut) is extremely slow or stopped. Increasing fluids along with regular use of maintenance, low-dose stool softeners and osmotic laxatives such as MiraLax® (polyethylene glycol) are commonly prescribed. However, as with use of any laxatives, be careful of dehydration and diarrhea, and increase fluid intake appropriately. The ultimate goal for children and adults who suffer from GI symptoms and dysautonomia is to feel better while never compromising excellent nutrition and hydration status.

Pain

Pain and the experience of coping with pain is one of the greater challenges facing children and adults with Mito, as acute or chronic pain can literally consume one's energy both physically and emotionally. Some adult patients have confided that pain is the most difficult of all of the symptoms that they face, as it makes them feel cornered, helpless, isolated, hopeless, and despondent. Further, pain is extremely individualized, and is difficult to quantify and difficult to treat. Moreover, chronic pain is often less effectively managed than acute pain, and may contribute to depression and feelings of hopelessness, especially when family members, friends, and healthcare providers dismiss the patient's pain. The affected person's *perceived* level of pain is important to recognize on an ongoing basis, as the experience of pain is not only physical, it is mental, spiritual, and cultural as well. Pain, and the anxiety that often occurs alongside it, is also a tremendous energy drain, and should be taken seriously, frequently evaluated, and managed as part of an ongoing symptom management plan.

There are several different types of pain that can manifest in people with mitochondrial disease, although the most common kinds of pain are abdominal pain, migraine/headache, nerve pain in the arms, hands, legs, and feet (also called neuropathy), and muscle pain.

Abdominal pain can be mild or severe, and may feel like cramping, burning, or deep pressure caused by persistent reflux, distention of the stomach or intestines due to slow emptying, or other autonomic dysfunction. It is important to note that some pain medications, particularly those classified as narcotics, have known effects on gut motility and can potentially relieve symptoms but worsen the underlying problem. Chronic abdominal pain may be better treated by a combined approach of medications, such as Elavil ® (amitriptyline), along with medications that improve the GI symptoms (motility, nausea, reflux, etc.). This is best managed by a primary care physician or GI specialist who can follow you or your child closely.

Many people with Mito also experience frequent, disabling headaches and/or complex migraines. Headaches can be caused by a variety of factors, some of which are not different for kids and adults with Mito than would be for the general population. Common triggers include sinusitis, anxiety, exhaustion, hormone fluctuations, dehydration, and hypoglycemia. Unique to Mito patient are headaches that are potentially caused by autonomic nervous system dysfunction (dysautonomia) as a result of impaired regulation of the blood flow in the vessels (lined by smooth muscle cells rich in mitochondria) that provide blood supply to the brain.

Despite the variety of causes, the approach to treating headaches should include prevention as well as acute pain relief. Prevention is critical, and begins by identifying headache triggers in the environment. Parents or patients should keep a careful log of the headaches, noting the time of day they occur, foods eaten prior, activity level, environmental factors and stressors, and a rating (scale of 1-10) of the headache for at least a couple of weeks in order to get a snapshot of the headaches and better identify factors that can be controlled in an effort to minimize the painful headaches. For children who get headaches at school, consider their food and fluid intake, energy expenditure, classroom lighting and temperature, as well as stimulus level. Identifying these possible triggers and attempting to prevent the headaches by practicing good nutrition, hydration, and energy conservation can significantly reduce the number of headaches in some people.

Further, during the time of an acute headache, there should be a plan already in place for acute pain relief. Consider having the conversation in advance with your child's pediatrician or with your nurse practitioner or physician to determine what medications should be taken and how often. Can a dose be repeated if the painful headache persists? What if the migraine is accompanied by vomiting and poses a potential risk of dehydration? Interestingly, there is some research that suggests that Coenzyme Q10 can help with some types of migraine headaches, potentially improving the vascular issues caused by mitochondrial dysfunction in the smooth muscle of the blood vessels. B vitamins and L-Carnitine are often reported to be helpful as well. Many adults and children who suffer from chronic, painful headaches have reported success with alternative therapies, such as acupressure/acupuncture, biofeedback, and meditation/relaxation techniques.

Neuropathies describe painful, tingling nerve sensations in the arms, legs, hands, and feet that are caused by a disorder or dysfunction of the nerves in the peripheral nervous system (the nerves that connect to the brain and spinal cord). Many neurologic disorders feature symptoms of neuropathic pain, which can be very painful or mildly uncomfortable. Continuous neuropathic pain is deep, burning, and aching; paroxysmal neuropathies feel like sudden, sharp stabbing shocks; paresthesias may be described as tingling, prickling, or numbness in the hands and feet that may be mild or severe. Children and adults alike can develop neuropathic pain, and may also feel numbness or total loss of sensation in the arms, legs, hands, and feet along with pain. Peripheral neuropathies may be helped by supplements in the Mito cocktail, including Coenzyme Q10, L-Carnitine, and alpha lipoic acid. Physical therapy, hydration, and the medication Neurontin® (gabapentin) are also frequently prescribed. Patients may notice worsening of neuropathic pain (e.g., many symptoms) during periods of illness, stress, or dehydration.

Muscle pain is also very common in children and adults with mitochondrial disease and is likely a result of impaired energy production in the highly energy-dependent, mitochondria-rich muscle cells. Muscle pain can manifest as deep, aching pain in the legs, arms, or back and may be worse when lactic acid levels are high. TENS therapy (transcutaneous electrical nerve stimulation) has been used safely in some patients, although generally treatment through use of vitamins and supplements to improve energy production is most helpful, along with frequent low-intensity exercise to improve overall muscle strength.

Treatment of all types of pain is important and can be greatly improved if made a priority of a patient's healthcare team. Often, specialists may be distracted by abnormal laboratory findings and acute symptoms and overlook pain. However, recognizing that pain is a significant energy drain on the body motivates us to better manage the pain, as a child or adult who is pain-free will likely be able to manage other symptoms better as well. Of interest is recent research that suggests that cellular signaling mechanisms that are mediated within the mitochondria may play a role in chronic pain. When treating pain, it is important to "stay ahead of the pain" and not allow a window of opportunity to open where the pain gets out of control and much more difficult to manage. In real terms, this means keeping on top of regular dosing, taking advantage of alternative therapies like acupressure, and tracking pain using a log to help determine and control the pain triggers as much as possible. In addition, palliative care programs (focused on helping patients with quality of life) are frequently established at large hospitals and medical centers and often include a pain specialist on the team who can help be your advocate and help with big-picture approaches to pain management.

Developmental Delay, Autism, and Difficulty with Concentration and Memory

Almost half of all children diagnosed with mitochondrial disease have some neurological issues, including developmental delay, autistic features, cognitive delay, and seizures. Approximately 20 percent of children with Mito have global developmental delay, and of those, it is estimated that another 4 to 20 percent have features of autism, PDD-NOS, or other cognitive delays (including speech and motor delays.) (See Chapter 8 for more information on the ASD/Mito connection.) In addition, a number of adult patients suffer from memory loss and/or thought processing issues, which may be worse during periods of stress, when fatigued, or can progress over time.

Developmental delays are classified by functional development in areas where children typically reach milestones that are predictable by age and stage. Children may have developmental delays in speech, physical, social, emotional, or cognitive development; children with mitochondrial disease, especially children who present with symptoms in infancy or young childhood, often have developmental delays in multiple areas. Physical developmental delays can be misinterpreted as cerebral palsy in very young children, and communication delays in combination with social/emotional delays may be mislabeled as autism in children who are later determined to have a mitochondrial disorder.

Regardless of the cause, dealing with a child's developmental delay can be upsetting and frustrating for parents. Children with developmental delay frequently are unable to clearly communicate discomfort, which is difficult for parents trying to interpret pain, crying, and classify symptoms. Parents of kids with Mito who have developmental delays also face additional responsibilities of working with their children to foster their physical, speech, and cognitive development on top of managing their classic Mito symptoms. Some children with mitochondrial disease have symptoms of developmental delay that, while persistent, do improve over time. In some circumstances, seizure disorders arising from mitochondrial disease may interfere with normal cognitive development; in others, characteristic lesions in the brain's white matter are thought to contribute to the delays.

The good news is that there are many services now available to children with developmental delays, especially for young children and children under the age of three. Early intervention services are available for children who meet state-dictated criteria and include physical therapy, speech therapy, and occupational therapy, as well as vision therapy and therapy for children who are hearing impaired. Your pediatrician is the gatekeeper to a referral to early intervention—if he forgets to mention it to you, don't be afraid to ask. These services can significantly help improve children's baselines, adaptive abilities, and give parents a team of support during critical years.

The majority of older kids, teens, and young adults have fewer issues with developmental delay but struggle with cognitive processing issues, including simple and complex problem solving, memory, and executive function. Skills such as planning, organizing, transitioning, and completing tasks can be very challenging for some teens and adults affected by Mito. In addition, social/emotional thought processes, such as self-monitoring, goal setting, and self-awareness, can be affected (and potentially more difficult to identify). In these circumstances, neuropsychological testing offers the opportunity for a person's abilities and weaknesses in specific cognitive function areas to be assessed. Behavioral aspects are assessed as well, and the results of the testing can be an invaluable tool to use in shaping specific therapies, recommending services (in school and/or in the community), and helping target areas that can help the affected person function better. It is very frustrating for teens and adults with Mito to have "fuzzy thinking," and it can affect their jobs, their ability to care for their families, and to keep important medical information organized. The combination of fatigue, autonomic nervous system dysfunction, and a slew of other symptoms can cause a person's cognitive ability to fluctuate in severity as well. As there is not a specific treatment for cognitive degeneration in mitochondrial disease, other than neuropsychological therapy, improving symptoms in other areas (dysautonomia, for example) and maintaining optimal baseline through nutrition, hydration, rest, and supplementation is considered the best approach.

Muscular Issues

The word "myopathy" is taken from the Greek words "muscle" and "disease," and is a fitting term used for mitochondrial disorders, which are also sometimes called mitochondrial myopathies. A hallmark characteristic of mitochondrial disease is weakness that affects the muscles. Muscle weakness can vary in severity—for some children and adults, the weakness is mild and is most apparent during illness or after significant physical exertion. For others, muscle weakness is more profound and more generalized, causing issues not only with walking, but also with standing, sitting, breathing, talking, and chewing. When we think about a disorder that causes weakness in potentially all of the muscles in our body, we can really understand how Mito can dramatically impact a person's everyday quality of life and overall ability.

There are several different types of muscle in our body, including skeletal, smooth, and cardiac muscle. Muscles are an integral part of our body's skeletal system, not only allowing our body to move but also providing the tone and structure for our bones to grow and function properly. Layers of skeletal muscle protect our bones and internal organs, and skeletal muscles allow our eyes to move, help us to breathe, allow us to walk, give us expression in our face, and allow us to chew and swallow. Moreover, some organs, such as the stomach and intestines, are lined with smooth muscle, which contracts and helps regulate digestion. Likewise, the vessels and arteries that regulate blood flow to our heart, brain, gut, and important organs are lined with smooth muscle. Finally, our heart is a muscle, composed of cardiac muscle cells that activate the heart's motion, circulating blood to our lungs and the rest of our body. Each of these muscle groups is rich in mitochondria and needs abundant energy to function properly.

Can a defect in the mitochondria's electron transport chain (energy producing mechanism) impact these muscle cells' ability to function as they should? Absolutely! In fact, the degree to which these cells, and the subsequent muscle function, can be affected is often under-recognized by patients as well as healthcare providers inexperienced about mitochondrial disorders. From a "big picture" perspective, the mitochondria-dependent muscles do much more than give us mobility; muscles are essential to healthy organ function and can be at the root of many of the symptoms that children and adults with Mito dysfunction feel. For example, some research suggests that cardiomyopathies (heart defects), migraine headaches (caused by dilation of the blood vessels that supply blood to the brain), stroke (also related to blood flow in the major vessels), and slow intestinal motility all have a mitochondrial component.

Exercise intolerance and low stamina are also hallmark features of mitochondrial disease and affect both adults and children. Many patients and parents find that they don't have the energy to walk long distances (walking around a mall, for example) and that they become easily and quickly fatigued with minimal activity. Some people suffer from muscle cramping, pain, or feelings of heaviness in their arms and legs, which is worse after physical exertion. In addition, a majority of children and adults with mitochondrial disease complain of muscle weakness, which is most evident by measuring how quickly the muscle fatigues and becomes weak, floppy, or simply cannot perform as before. As a result of these symptoms, many families with mitochondrial disease shy away from activities that require physical effort, including physical therapy and exercise. However, research is increasingly supportive of moderate, low resistance aerobic exercise in order to actually improve mitochondrial function. Exercise can help slowly improve a person's baseline as well as actually increase the number of mitochondria in the cell. Consequently, physical and occupational therapy should be considered a therapeutic approach to improve muscle pain, weakness, and fatigue, and should be practiced at least twice a week, if possible. Like most therapeutic approaches to mitochondrial disease management, the key in this circumstance is moderation and careful attention to find the perfect balance of "how much is too much." Further, weakness, cramping, and muscle fatigue typically worsens as the day progresses, so therapies or exercise programs should be adjusted appropriately.

Hypotonia is also a characteristic that is very common, especially in children with Mito. Hypotonia, or "low tone," refers to a decrease in the tension normally found in a muscle. Hypotonia is not the same as muscle weakness, although both may occur in the same person. A person with low muscle tone appears "floppy," and may seem to have trouble sitting up, holding up his head, walking, holding objects in his hands, and balancing. Hypotonia also can cause swallowing issues, difficulty talking, and drooling because the facial muscles are not supportive enough to perform adequately. Hypotonia in mitochondrial disease can be caused by motor nerve impairment in the brain or by poor muscle strength and the severity can fluctuate (improve or worsen) over time. Again, physical therapy, occupational therapy, pool therapy, and speech therapy are wonderful therapeutic approaches to improving hypotonia and improving functional use of a person's arms and legs despite the low tone.

Low muscle tone can additionally manifest in the digestive system as constipation or very slow digestive motility, and can be a problem for babies and children who do not have the strength to suck or swallow properly and consequently are unable to take in enough nutrition and fluids by mouth. In this case, support through early intervention programs and local feeding professionals should be sought.

Happily, a majority of both children and adults report improvements in muscle tone as well as muscle strength and overall stamina with ongoing use of the Mito cocktail, particularly L-carnitine, creatine, and Coenzyme Q10. Great nutrition and attention to hydration (plenty of fluids) are also important considerations.

Seizures/Epilepsy and Stroke

The medical literature suggests that more than 60 percent of mitochondrial disease patients have seizures or will develop seizures or epilepsy during the course of their disease. In addition, most children and adults with mitochondrial disease have seizures that are difficult or unresponsive to typical treatment recommendations (this is also called "refractory to treatment"). Researchers suggest that mitochondrial dysfunction contributes to seizures and stroke-like episodes in Mito patients, and may also play a role in epileptic seizures in the general population as well.

Epilepsy is also called seizure disorder, and both are terms used to describe a condition in the brain where recurring seizures have the potential to occur. A seizure occurs due to a burst of abnormal electrical discharges of neurons in the brain. Many seizures are characterized by a period (a few seconds to a few minutes) of lost consciousness along with confusion and/or memory loss (called "absence" or "petit mal" seizures; some also involve jerking or involuntary spasms of the muscles (called "tonic-clonic" seizures). Sometimes people experience clues (called an aura) that indicate to them that a seizure may be about to occur, such as a sensation of a strong smell, a sensation of a flashing light, headache, mood changes, a dreamy feeling, nausea, or an unusual taste. If you or your child experience seizures, you may hear your physician refer to epilepsy as a secondary diagnosis. In this case, that means that mitochondrial disease is your primary (main) diagnosis and epilepsy is the secondary diagnosis. While related, each can also stand alone for insurance and eligibility purposes, as well as for treatment.

In many cases, the occurrence of seizures is unpredictable and unrelated to activities, although some patients and parents feel that stressful circumstances, such as lack of sleep, illness, or emotional distress, can bring about a seizure. Research suggests that low blood sugar (hypoglycemia) can trigger seizures; therefore children and adults with Mito and seizure disorders need to snack frequently and stay hydrated.

There are several different types of seizures, and children and adults with mitochondrial disease typically experience more than one type (although at different times). Generally, seizures can be classified as partial or generalized. These terms don't describe how the patient acts during the seizure but instead describe the area of the brain where the seizure begins. Partial seizures arise from a localized area in the brain, whereas generalized seizures cause a more widespread electrical abnormality within the brain. The symptoms for each type of seizure are slightly different. Myoclonic seizures are common for children and adults with Mito; this type of generalized seizure is characterized by brief, involuntary jerks of the body (especially the legs and arms) along with a brief loss of consciousness. Myoclonic seizure disorder is also called myoclonic epilepsy, and like most seizure disorders, is primarily treated by medications used to control (limit) the seizure activity in the brain. Other types of seizures common in children and adults with mitochondrial disease are atypical absence (also called petit mal), primary generalized, and atonic seizures. Children and adults who experience seizures should have precautions in place (such as constant support and supervision by a personal care assistant and a medical alert bracelet) as there is the opportunity to fall and be injured during a seizure or have difficulty breathing.

As mentioned before, seizure disorders in children and adults with mitochondrial disease tend to be resistant to treatment. The ketogenic diet, a very strict low-carbohydrate, high-fat diet, is sometimes recommended and is only implemented under careful medical supervision. Likewise, vagal nerve stimulation (VNS) is also considered safe for Mito patients, although there is mixed opinion on both of these methods' rate of successful seizure control in this population. Drug therapy is also used, although valproic acid (also called Depakote®) is contraindicated in some types of mitochondrial disease (especially Alpers disease and POLG1 mutations) and should be used with caution.

Stroke-like episodes also can occur in children and adults with certain types of mitochondrial disorders, and are different from seizures. These strokes and stroke-like episodes occur as a result of mitochondrial dysfunction that affects the central nervous system. This subsequent inflammation or impact on the brain is called encephalopathy and is associated with several types of mitochondrial disease including MELAS and Leigh syndrome. A person having a stroke or stroke-like episode may be confused, have numbness and/or weakness, speech difficulties, and difficulty with vision during the episode. Some stroke-like episodes may be preceded by migraine or seizure, but it's important to note that these migraines or seizures are not actual strokes or stroke-like events.

Seizures and stroke-like events in people with mitochondrial disease occur when the energy demand of the brain is unable to be met due to defective energy metabolism. Remember that mitochondrial dysfunction is associated with "mitochondrial oxidative stress," wherein free radical molecules are produced in large numbers and cause damage to nearby cells. Mitochondrial dysfunction and subsequent increased free radical damage has been associated with seizures not only in people with Mito, but also in the elderly and people with other types of seizure disorders. Recent research suggests that chronic oxidative stress and subsequent mitochondrial dysfunction may make the brain more susceptible to seizures. Hence, we can recognize what an important role the mitochondria play in the stability of the brain, and how mitochondrial dysfunction and oxidative stress can be both a consequence as well as a cause of epileptic seizures.

What to Do During a Seizure

- Help the person to a lying position, loosen tight clothing, and place something soft like a pillow or jacket under his head.

- If able, assist by placing a soft folded cloth (like a washcloth) between the person's teeth. Do not force anything into the person's mouth if his teeth are clenched and do not put anything hard into his mouth.

- Gently turn the person's head to the side to help him continue to be able to breathe.

- Stay with the person and reassure him after the seizure, telling him that he is all right, reorienting him, and gently informing him to relax because he has had a seizure. People are often sleepy and disoriented after a seizure, with no memory of what happened.

- Many physicians ask parents and patients to keep a seizure log and to document when seizures occur.

Perhaps you know what to do during a seizure, but do your child's teachers or those who work with you also know what to do? Teach them! It is also important to point out to those who are unfamiliar with seizure disorders that children and adults who suffer from seizures may have multiple seizures a day. Under those circumstances, a seizure is not an emergency, but a protocol should be in place for everyone's safety.

Depression

It is unfortunate that depression and other psychiatric issues that affect adults, teens, and children with mitochondrial disease are often overlooked or attributed to "personality," "stress," "hypochondria," and even "fictitious symptom disorder." Many adults and teens in particular *are* struggling to cope with the challenges and symptoms of mitochondrial disease, but are also susceptible to depression as a consequence of their mitochondrial dysfunction. Despite the regrettable neglect of these symptoms by a patient's family or physicians, there is growing research evidence that many mental health conditions, including depression, schizophrenia, and bipolar disorder, are associated with mitochondrial dysfunction. In fact, impaired energy metabolism and inadequate or ineffective energy production in the brain have been observed in patients with these conditions (who do not necessarily also have a concurrent diagnosis of mitochondrial disease).

Let's begin by objectively defining depression. Depression (clinically known as major depression) is characterized by persistent sad mood, disrupted sleep and appetite, and inability to experience pleasure. While disruptions in sleep, appetite, and mood may be present or even "normal" for many children, teens, and adult patients who have Mito, they should not also have persistent feelings of hopelessness and sadness. It is important to recognize that many patients and family members who live with the challenges of Mito may have bad days and feel sad or depressed;

however, overwhelming feelings that do not improve after a few days or weeks and that interfere with sleep, self-care, care of another person, or daily activities is concerning. Family members, spouses, and even parents of kids and teens may be afraid to approach the affected person about depression; however, it is actually a gift to be able to help advocate for another person who is suffering from depression by finding appropriate counseling and psychiatric care that will help him feel better. There are medical and cognitive-behavioral therapies that can help, and the first step is to approach your primary care physician about referral to a psychologist or psychiatrist. While some would argue that psychiatrists are better equipped to help people with mitochondrial disease since psychiatry is medically-based, other patients report success with counselors, therapists, or psychologists who are willing to learn about mitochondrial disease, and who may also be more available, accessible, and motivated by long-term therapy.

For children and adults with mitochondrial disease, coping with fear, grief, sadness, stress, anger, etc. can cause feelings of depression. All patients, parents, and caregivers who struggle with depression should seek professional support, for there are effective therapies available to help with depression. Depression is normal in these circumstances, and is more common in people who live with or care for someone with a chronic illness than in the general population.

There is still controversy over the exact cause of depression, as the condition is likely due to a variety of physical, genetic, psychological, biochemical, and environmental factors. However, periods of depression may occur in people with known mitochondrial disorders that are not situational but rather are directly related to their mitochondrial dysfunction. Researchers have proposed that defective energy metabolism due to mitochondrial disorders plays a part in the cause, development, and effects of some psychiatric diseases, mainly depression, bipolar disorder (also called manic-depressive disorder), and schizophrenia.

The brain contains a large number of mitochondria and has a very high energy demand. As a result, it makes sense that the brain is more susceptible to inadequate energy production caused by a defect in the mitochondria. In fact, some animal research has even shown that chronic stress-induced depression alters metabolism and impairs the ATP production in the electron transport chain's enzyme complexes (Complex I-IV). In other words, our brain metabolism is coupled to our psychiatric well-being, and our physical well-being is coupled to well-functioning metabolism.

Treatment for depression in people with Mito should be two-pronged and include cognitive-behavioral therapy as well as use of medications, when necessary. Psychiatric medications are commonly used to treat depression, including antidepressants like the drugs classified as SSRIs (selective serotonin reuptake inhibitors). Celexa®, Zoloft®, Paxil®, and Prozac® are examples of SSRIs that are often used to help patients who have depression and mitochondrial disease. However, because of potential side effects, psychiatrists familiar with mitochondrial disease recommend that a slow, cautious approach be used when prescribing medications to treat depression (even SSRIs, which are generally considered safe for most people in this population). Generally, patients should try one medication at a time at the lowest recommended dose and pay careful attention to side effects, impact on other Mito-related symptoms, as well as potential benefits. Because mitochondrial disease is a metabolic disease that also affects many other organs and body symptoms, it is possible that the intended dosage or therapeutic benefit of psychiatric medications could be different for kids and adults with Mito. Finally, there are some preliminary studies that suggest that supplemental creatine can improve the symptoms of major depression in some people, both with Mito and in the general population.

Emergency Situations

For the most part, clinicians who are leaders in the field of mitochondrial medicine agree that the majority of symptoms that trouble Mito patients should be treated as they would in any person experiencing those symptoms. While there are exceptions to this rule of thumb (avoiding use of valproic acid to treat seizures, for example), in many cases, kids and adults with Mito find that ongoing trial and error and careful attention to symptoms can keep them under control. In addition, successful patients and families also learn to prioritize symptoms in order to effectively treat them. In other words, although you or your child may suffer from fatigue, nausea, pain, muscle weakness, headache, constipation, and processing/concentration issues, it is not realistic to expect that ALL of these can be addressed at every appointment. Further, is it realistic or worthwhile pursuing specialists for every symptom? Doing so may result in weekly visits to the clinic, multiple sub-specialists, multiple tests, frequent follow-up appointments, and a litany of individual treatment plans that could be prevented by prioritizing. Which symptoms are the most troublesome? Which are most threatening, long-term, to your own or your child's health? Knowing this and feeling confident in making these decisions takes time and experience.

However, there are some situations when symptoms and related issues become potentially life-threatening or otherwise devastating and require immediate medical attention. Examples of these are outlined briefly below. Parents and family members should have a plan in place before these situations arise so that appropriate medical support can be implemented with as little additional stress and subsequent energy drain as possible (see Appendix C).

In addition to emergency protocols, every patient with mitochondrial disease should have a basic medical letter that can be used in the event of an emergency and that includes essential information about you or your child, such as: name, diagnosis, attending (primary) physician, allergies/contraindications, current medications and doses (including vitamins, supplements, and special formulas), and contact information for physician sub-specialists involved in your care. Having this letter handy for travel, unexpected emergency room visits, school, etc. can help streamline the process of getting immediate and appropriate help for you or your child during a crisis. Patients, parents, or caregivers can actually draft this letter as described above **for** their physician and ask him to approve it, sign, and copy on their practice letterhead for your safekeeping. Ideally, of course, this would be done during a follow-up visit, not during an emergency.

Above all, please remember that even minor illnesses such as a fever or the stomach flu can be devastating for a person with mitochondria disease. When in doubt, seek medical advice!

Surgery or Procedures Requiring Anesthesia

Many children require sedation for routine surgeries such as placement of ear tubes, and many adults may be sedated for routine procedures as well. There is a growing body of research surrounding the negative effects of anesthesia on the mitochondria, and the relationship between the administration of certain types of anesthesia and mitochondrial myopathy. As a result, physician leaders have created anesthesia protocols, which can be found online at both www.MitoAction.org and www.UMDF. org. These protocols should, ideally, be "on file" in your medical record or your child's, as well as in place at your local hospital emergency room. These protocols were designed for patients to share with primary care physicians as well as specialists prior to surgery (and other times anesthetics are used) as a precaution against unwanted side effects. A number of Mito patients report difficulty waking up after surgery, and most report a subsequent regression in skills, which may or may not be completely related to the anesthesia but can certainly be attributed to the increased energy demands of the body during the healing and recovery process.

Key points to remember related to use of anesthesia during surgery or emergency situations are:

- Avoid use of lactated ringers IV solution; D10 or D5 with electrolytes at one and a half times normal maintenance is recommended before, during, and after surgery, as well as in emergency situations. Hypoglycemia and prolonged fasting should be avoided;
- Propofol should be avoided or used only for short periods (less than sixty minutes);
- Patients with mitochondrial disease may be at higher risk of malignant hyperthermia (MH); therefore, anesthesiologists should follow standard MH precautions;
- Avoid any anesthesia, elective procedures, and elective surgery if possible during times of illness or infection;
- Expect a longer recovery period and increase metabolic support postoperatively or in an emergency, including use of fluids, parenteral nutrition, electrolytes, and IV L-Carnitine.

Again, share these recommendations with your physician and ask for the advice of anesthesiologists and other specialists prior to the event if possible.

Fever

Fever dramatically increases the body's energy demand and can be devastating to mitochondrial disease patients. Patients, parents, and research reports that fever is associated with marked lethargy, temporary or prolonged loss of skills/regression, weakness, and metabolic crisis (manifested by increased lactic acidosis, etc.). Impaired energy production is impaired even further during illness, especially illness that occurs with fever. Body temperatures greater than 101 degrees Fahrenheit cause greatest concern, although it should be noted that many patients with mitochondrial disease have lower than normal baseline temperatures and therefore elevated temperatures should be adjusted accordingly.

Not only is the body temperature and degree of fever important but clinical signs and symptoms of how the affected person is doing are also critical. Very young children and babies have a very low threshold for managing fever, as do teens and adults who are ill, recovering from surgery, or otherwise already compensating for increased energy demands. Fever should be treated aggressively with fluids and medications such as ibuprofen and acetaminophen. Both ibuprofen and acetaminophen have a degree of mitochondrial toxicity that is concerning to parents and patients; however, controlling the fever and lowering body temperature is typically more important than the potential associated toxicity, especially during acute periods where the medication is used for a short period of a few days. Aggressively increasing hydration is also critically important in children and adults with Mito who are suffering from a fever. Seek immediate medical attention if during an illness with a fever (called a febrile illness) the affected person is unable to increase and maintain adequate fluid intake.

Finally, it is always a good idea to have a conversation with your primary care doctor or pediatrician before a febrile illness about the risks associated with fever, so that, when needed, a call to the physician begins a discussion about the immediate plan of action. Expect a longer recovery as well as regression of skills (especially in children) after a febrile illness; depending on the severity, some children and adults may take weeks to months to return to baseline.

Dehydration Due to Vomiting or Diarrhea

Any situation that causes potential dehydration, including vomiting and diarrhea, is cause for serious concern and medical attention for a person with mitochondrial disease. Positive hydration status tends to be fragile in those who have a mitochondrial disorder, and therefore the propensity to become dehydrated is much greater. Dehydration is very, very serious. Even minor dehydration contributes to overall worsening of fatigue and other symptoms, and may also result in lethargy, seizures, and even unconsciousness. Like fever, it is important that patients, parents, and their healthcare team all understand the seriousness of potential dehydration so that a plan is in place to administer IV fluids in the event of such an illness.

Medications and Toxins

Certain medications are known to worsen mitochondrial function or have the potential to cause organ failure (kidney and liver dysfunction usually). In general, people with mitochondrial disease should use caution with:

- valproic acid
- statins (cholesterol-lowering drugs in this class)
- aminoglycoside antibiotics
- erythromycin

In addition, some drugs and environmental substances are considered mitochondrial toxins, including:

- cigarettes
- antiretrovirals (HIV medications)
- aspirin
- aminoglycoside and platinum chemotherapies
- acetaminophen
- metformin (Glucophage®)
- beta-blockers

Symptoms are such a challenge for families who are trying to make sense of the diagnosis of mitochondrial disease. Struggling with a variety of symptoms while dealing with multiple specialists, school, work, finances, and stress is overwhelming. The glossary provided in the back of this book is a great resource to use when you are trying to make sense of new symptoms, laboratory findings, and recommendations from your physician. It seems simple, but all symptoms for people with mitochondrial disease are aggravated by illness, dehydration, and "overdoing it." Your role as parent, patient, or caregiver can be much more meaningful if you are able to accurately identify and describe symptoms, prioritize, and do your part in keeping up your baseline or that of your child's as much as possible.

Key Points from This Chapter

■ No two patients with mitochondrial disease "look" exactly alike; however, "classic" Mito signs and symptoms may include fatigue, muscle pain and weakness, seizures/stroke, slow digestive motility, and developmental delay in children.

■ Nutrition, hydration, rest (energy management), and use of the Mito cocktail are the cornerstones to managing mitochondrial disease.

■ Mitochondrial disease is better "managed" than "treated." Much like auto maintenance, daily routines are just as important as major therapies and medications.

■ Hydration is probably the most frequently overlooked area that can have an immediate positive impact for the well-being of people with Mito.

■ People with Mito should avoid fasting (going without food or drink). Eating small, frequent meals is a more effective means of making and regulating energy than consuming large meals. Think of keeping a small fire burning with kindling—it needs constant attention.

■ Be vigilant about prevention of infections through frequent hand washing, preventive disinfection of homes and classrooms, avoiding crowded indoor places, and so on. Infections and illnesses are very difficult to overcome if you have Mito. Fever can be especially devastating and should be treated aggressively.

■ Mito symptoms affect many different organ systems in our bodies. The neurologic system, digestive system, musculoskeletal system, and cardiovascular system are the areas that are most commonly affected.

■ Clinical depression is often misinterpreted as "situational" depression in children and adults with Mito. In truth, there is a correlation between adequate energy metabolism and psychiatric well-being.

■ Anesthesia and emergency situations propose certain risks to individuals with Mito; anesthesia and emergency management protocols (available online, see Appendix C) should be followed.

6

Children & Teens with Mitochondrial Disease

If there were a "help wanted" advertisement for a Mito parent, it would include the following requirements: flexible, able to work well with others, able to handle stress well, organized, strong advocate, has pseudo-medical degree, willing to work long hours without breaks, must be prepared to change expectations, have courage, and, most importantly, must have a strong sense of hope.

—Evelyn, mom to Sabrina (five years old with unspecified mitochondrial disease)

You're a parent. Not just any parent, however, you're the primary guardian of a child with mitochondrial disease. That means you are the voice for your child, the primary advocate, the caregiver, the care coordinator, the therapist, and, most importantly, the expert. **You** know your child better than anyone else, and YOU are her best advocate.

Having said that, you probably didn't ask for this degree of responsibility! Many parents feel out of their comfort zone on a daily basis, and are asked to comprehend and manage more than a high-paid executive with a comfortable salary. Many of you have the same skill and hands-on medical knowledge as a critical care nurse, but have no formal education or training. You navigate and organize reams of data as part of the ongoing process of keeping medical records and school education plans up to date. You know how to get a live person on the phone at the insurance company and you can haggle for medical equipment or supplies while throwing together a pizza dinner.

Despite feeling completely overwhelmed most of the time, you are actually incredibly talented, resilient, and loving. You are not expected to be perfect, although you do expect it from yourself and get very frustrated by setbacks. It's hard to ask for help, even though you might recognize that you need it. Your biggest wish is that others—doctors, family members, teachers—would be as committed to your child's care as you are. And of course, every day you wake up hoping that today is a *good day* for your child.

Parents react very differently to their child's diagnosis of mitochondrial disease. For some, they feel that Mito is the enemy, and struggle with resentment and anger. Others feel emotionally overwhelmed and have a hard time knowing what to do day-to-day. Many feel confused, and disappointed by the lack of support that is offered to them by their community and their medical system. Some embrace the diagnosis and are passionate about helping others. Whatever emotions and feelings you may have about your child's diagnosis, you still have something very important in common with other parents who have children with Mito (or arguably, any degree of special needs). You want the best for your kids; you want them to be happy and you want them to be surrounded by supportive people who love them.

In medicine, kids are known to be incredibly "resilient," and compensate much better than adults facing similar conditions. Nonetheless, as the parent of a child with mitochondrial disease, you have the very important job of being the "GPS" for your child on your family's Mito journey. You are there to offer guidance along every step of the way—at school, at home, at the clinic, at the hospital, in the community, and in the family. Understanding the symptoms and preparing for the road blocks along your journey will help you to feel empowered, give you clarity, and help you to make important decisions along the way.

Common Mito Symptoms in Children

Not all children with Mito have the same set of symptoms. Even more importantly, no two children with a diagnosis of mitochondrial disease look, behave, or feel alike! The spectrum and degree of delay, symptoms, organ involvement, and severity of the disease can be mild to very severe, and can fluctuate from month to month and year to year. The "hallmark characteristics" listed below are so broad that it makes it very difficult for parents and children to find other families whose children are in the exact same boat. However, from a big picture perspective, children with mitochondrial disease all have one thing in common: an energy shortage, which can result in any or all of the issues in the following list. Having mitochondrial disease is like operating with a "low battery," but this doesn't mean that a child is just tired; it means that many areas of her body will suffer from the lack of energy or power that they need. We can better understand mitochondrial disease by using this analogy: A house has lights, air conditioning, a dishwasher, electrical outlets, a microwave, a dryer, a television, etc. All of these things require power to run. Not only do they require power, they require AMPLE power in order to work properly. If your house was being run on a generator, there wouldn't be ample power for all of the appliances and lights in the house to work at once. The lights might dim if you turned on the microwave; running the hair dryer while the televisions and computers were on would break the circuit and cause a power outage. In this same way, the body's organs have a need for ample power. The major organs with the most work to do require the most power to run properly: the brain, central nervous system, the digestive system, and the muscles. Any or all of these organ systems can "short out" or not function as they should because the body just isn't able to generate enough power or energy (from the mitochondria). Depending on the demand, symptoms can vary too.

The unpredictability of mitochondrial disease is very prevalent in and very challenging for children. Day to day, moment to moment, it is not uncommon for children to be feeling great, then awful. Parents can feel crazy and exhausted trying to predict the next challenge and handle the fluctuation of symptoms. The most challenging symptoms for children and teens with mitochondrial disease are as follows:

Hallmark Characteristics of Mitochondrial Disease in Children

- **Developmental delay** (including delays in some or all areas of speech, physical, and cognitive development)
- Loss of skills or **regression**, for example, a child develops difficulty walking or remembering words when she had not had trouble before
- **Slow digestive system** (called gastric dysmotility or gastroparesis) that causes constipation, reflux, vomiting, and stomach pain
- **Feeding issues**, potentially related to a number of factors including fatigue, lack of strength, nausea, difficulty sucking or swallowing, and lack of interest in food
- **Hypotonia** (low muscle tone), such that the muscles make the child's arms, legs, and trunk more "floppy" and weak
- **Lethargy**, lack of reflexes, and weakened levels of alertness (specifically in infants)
- **Muscle weakness** and lack of strength, so sitting up unsupported, walking, climbing, or picking up heavy things is challenging or impossible
- **Fatigue** and complaints or signs of being tired when other children are not, especially after any episodes of stress (including crying) or physical exertion
- Issues with **eyesight**, including vision loss, drooping eyelids (ptosis), sleepy eyes, or difficulty focusing
- **Hearing loss**
- Frequent "**meltdowns**," irritability, and/or behavior issues that are often actually related to low energy but that can result in a diagnosis

of autism spectrum disorder (ASD) or pervasive developmental disorder (PDD) (More information on Mito and autism in Chapter 8.)

- **Heart problems**
- **Headaches**
- **Seizures**
- **Kidney problems**

LIBBY

My name is Libby and I am fourteen years old. I have had mitochondrial disease my whole life. There are times when living with mitochondrial disease can be really taxing. Whenever a basic cold or virus comes along, I know that I am in for a long rehabilitative period. It's hard to do daily things, and really hard to maintain friendships, not because friends don't care, but at times they really don't understand the level of energy expenditures it takes just to "be."

You miss out on a lot of social things, but overall the biggest concern for me is worrying that I am going to have something happen to me that I won't be able to bounce back from. Still, I don't live waiting for the next crisis—I just adapt and try to keep moving forward. You really never know how you're going to feel the next day after resting. You could have done everything right and your body just says, "not doing that today," which means that there can be a lot of disappointments.

I also hate it when people say, "You look too good to be sick!" That drives me nuts. I have learned, though, that just because you have a name for your disease, you can't let it rule you. When people hear you have mitochondrial disease, they don't understand the magnitude of how it impacts every minute of every day of your life. You do learn to adjust but it's hard.

In my family, we joke a lot and we think about people who have been through worse things and come out on the other side. I like to escape in books, and do silly things like play video games. Most of all, I count on my family to help me when I am sick, and I do the same for them. We also pretend that my brother and I don't have it, and that we just have a bug or something, and this way we don't focus as much on the Mito but just the symptoms and ways to relieve them.

I wish everyone knew that with proper supports and management you can do a lot. I play the guitar, I do fencing, and I go to school when I can. I want to be a pastry chef one day. I've learned that you always have to look to the future or you get caught up in how hard everyday life is.

Special Issues by Age

Infants & Children: Birth to Age Three

Not all children with mitochondrial disease are symptomatic from birth, but many are. Some babies are born struggling, and a diagnosis is often found within their first eighteen months of life. Looking back, parents of children who have Mito describe their babies as sleepy, relatively content, having had to be wakened to be fed, or who would not eat at all. Sometimes these little ones have marked impairments and multiple health problems that manifest right away. They are frail, failure-to-thrive and have trouble acclimating outside of the womb. They just don't seem to have enough strength to "get better." They fight periods of breathlessness (apnea), kidney and heart problems, and require feeding tubes or central lines for nutrition and for medication. Babies who are born with mitochondrial disease seem to have the most difficult time remaining stable during the first three years of their lives, and can be very small, very sick, and a source of great distress for parents, brothers, and sisters.

It is very overwhelming to be a mother or father of a small child who is going through the diagnosis of mitochondrial disease. It is difficult to know how to devote your time and attention when bombarded with so much new information. The following are suggestions of areas that should be prioritized during this stage.

Fluids and Nutrition

Because babies and very young children are so small and often very weak, the simple act of getting enough fluid and nutrition into their bodies can be very challenging. However, fluid management and adequate nutrition (both calories and protein) is absolutely crucial during this stage. Many children benefit from use of a g-tube (a gastric feeding tube that is placed through the skin directly into the stomach as an alternate way to ingest formula or medicines) in order to get enough nutrition without the additional exhaustion of feeding by mouth.

In addition, speech and language pathologists (SLP) that specialize in oral motor therapy techniques can be of great assistance by using "Beckman Oral Motor Techniques" to help strengthen and activate the muscles of the face and mouth that are needed for effective chewing and swallowing. Speech and language pathologists in a hospital setting can also assist by evaluating your child's ability to swallow effectively through a noninvasive procedure called a swallow study. The goal of speech therapy for very young children with Mito is primarily to develop muscle, and improve strength and coordination, which can in turn improve both speech and feeding.

Helping babies and very young children with Mito to remain metabolically supported through good hydration and nutrition should be a daily priority—for parents as well as the child's medical team. Many parents keep a feeding log or track daily calories and fluid intake. (Smart phone apps are a great way to do this; although some apps may be designed for weight loss, any app that tracks calories from a food database and allows you to enter the volume of liquids consumed will be helpful.) A consult with a nutritionist can be very useful in helping you determine the minimum number of calories required for your baby based on weight, age, and metabolic needs. Every baby benefits from breastfeeding, even if the breast milk is only used as a supplement

ROSE

Rose appeared healthy at birth, although, in retrospect, there were soft signs of trouble even then. She was a sleepy, placid newborn who sometimes had to be wakened to be fed. I began to be concerned when she was two months of age, and we took an infant massage class. All of the babies were approximately the same age, but Rose was much less active than the others.

By her four-month well-child visit, I was concerned enough to mention it to her physician. Fortunately or not, she rolled over for the first time during that appointment, so he brushed my concerns aside. Still, Rose did not show any interest in solid food. It was as if she didn't know what to do with it. As the months went by, Rose fell on the weight chart from the 50th percentile between birth to six months to the 5-10th percentile by twelve months. She was sitting by the second half of her first year, but not crawling or pulling herself up to stand. I was by this point full of anxiety and sadness, which no one else seemed to share. She was such an alert, interactive baby that everyone was content to "watch and wait" for a little while longer. We were thrilled when she said her first word at nine months, but a shaking episode around this time sent us to a pediatric neurologist. He determined that it was not a seizure.

Finally, at thirteen months of age, Rose was evaluated at a children's hospital. She had serious developmental delays in all areas. My husband and I were heartbroken. And we began the journey that is so common to families with children with disabilities, making the rounds of sub-specialists, searching for a reason why. Our daughter was evaluated by geneticists, neurologists, metabolic specialists, developmental pediatricians, psychologists, speech pathologists, physical and occupational therapists, and there were no answers. Except that she had developmental delays in all areas.

We began to see the feeding team, as her growth had become a serious concern, and Rose was still unable to eat solid food. I was told that she wasn't eating because she was being breastfed and wasn't being "allowed to develop an appetite for mealtimes." Appointments with the feeding team finally became so humiliating and of so little use to us that we stopped going. By sixteen months of age, Rose was a delightful child and sitting well but hardly eating at all and keeping multiple appointments every week with an army of developmental experts. Although we still didn't have a Mito diagnosis, we had entered the world of early intervention in earnest.

to a high caloric, high protein formula. Babies and toddlers with mitochondrial disease tend to be very small and are often "not on the chart" for growth by height and weight. A better measurement for these children is to track the child's weight weekly, monitoring closely to ensure that the child is continuing to gain weight. Some parents are able to request home health services (weight checks weekly by a nurse beyond the initial postpartum period) or a home baby scale (digital) once their child's weight gain pattern is established.

Wellness

A fever (body temperature greater than 101 degrees) puts enormous physiologic stress on a young child's body, and for the child who suffers from mitochondrial dysfunction, an infection or virus with fever can truly be disastrous. Be very cautious about exposure to other children who are not well, or who even may have common childhood colds or illnesses like the flu or strep throat. Become vigilant about hand washing and be smart about exposure to crowds, indoor public places, or groups of young children (like a preschool or daycare center). An infection or virus and fever is so energy demanding it can wipe out an infant or young child's reserves, leaving her very weak and physically struggling. Even for children with suspected mitochondrial disease whose diagnosis is not yet confirmed, parents are encouraged to be extremely cautious and to be aggressive about treating fevers and even minor illnesses. Pediatricians need to be aware of the risk of metabolic crisis to your baby or young child, and parents and physicians should have a plan that includes careful observation and potential hospitalization for supplemental IV fluids, increased dosages of supplements (see Chapter 4 on treatment), and metabolic support when your little one is battling an illness.

Therapies & Early Intervention

In the United States, eligible children under the age of three are entitled to free early intervention (EI) services (implemented via an Individual Family Service Plan or IFSP) through the US Department of Education's 2004 Disabilities Education Act (Part C). Under the umbrella of "inborn errors of metabolism," children with Mito (or suspected Mito) qualify for these services. In fact, any child who *has* or is *at risk* to have a developmental or physical delay qualifies, and this is great news for your family!

An IFSP is part of the federal law in the United States that protects children under the age of three who have disabilities. It is a process in which a document as well as a family-centered team is created in order to create appropriate goals for a child, and to implement services (i.e., speech therapy) to help the child attain those goals. Recognizing the importance of family-focused services for very young children with special needs, the intention of the IFSP is to meet the developmental needs of the child via a "multi-disciplinary" approach that includes the parents as well as community professionals. While federal special education law mandates use of an IFSP, each state manages their IFSP process and related services differently. Each state has at least one parent-to-parent network (part of a federal grant program) that can provide specific information for parents about the available services, processes, and providers in your state. A complete listing of these parent-to-parent networks is available online at http://www.parentcenternetwork.org/parentcenterlisting.html.

Typically, when your child begins missing important developmental milestones (such as talking, rolling over, standing, walking, feeding herself, etc.), your pediatrician will refer you to your local IFSP community leader (often a nurse or social worker, who has a background in special education and may also be a special needs parent) and the process begins. However, for kids with mitochondrial disease and Mito-autism (see Chapter 8) it is not uncommon for the child's medical issues to overshadow her developmental needs. In this case, parents who are concerned about their child's development can initiate the early intervention process by contacting local providers, such as their community's or county's Department of Public Health (DPH), their state's Department of Developmental Services (DDS, previously DMR), the special education superintendent of schools in their community, or their pediatrician.

The process of developing the IFSP begins with a meeting and an assessment of your child. Federal law (again, under the 2004 IDEA) clearly dictates the criteria that should be met for a child to qualify for early intervention services and development of an IFSP. Usually the initial meeting and assessment will take place in your home, and includes a period of observation by the IFSP coordinator as well as a series of questions about your child and her development. Following the initial meeting, the IFSP begins to be developed, and is a collaborative effort that includes your opinion and concerns as the parent.

While the process of the IFSP described in Figure 6.1 is clearly defined by federal law, options for families in regard to therapies and services vary dramatically state-to-state. Each state has its own laws that determine (often based on funding and available resources) the level of services that your child is eligible for, and how they will be offered. For example, in some states, early intervention (EI) services (occupational therapy, physical therapy) are offered through home health agencies, local community hospitals, or rehabilitative centers. In other states, a local agency or organization, such as the ARC, may provide all EI services for your community. Once connected to a local IFSP coordinator, you can ask for specifics about your state. Your IFSP coordinator will also make recommendations about the community resources available to your child, including speech therapy, developmental groups for parents, parent information services, case management, etc. Again, the extent of services offered and structure of reimbursement varies by state; in most cases, children receive a variety of services, most of which take place in the child's home, and payment is arranged through a combination of private insurance, state health benefits, and early intervention community benefits.

What services and therapies would offer a benefit to the child with mitochondrial disease? Depending on your child's symptoms and specific presentation, there may be many opportunities for benefit. Most children with Mito should receive physical therapy (PT), occupational therapy (OT), and speech/oral motor therapy at least twice each week. Specialists who offer vision and hearing therapy should be included as well, if appropriate. Early intervention programs vary by state, and can include group sessions as

Figure 6.1   IFSP Guidelines & Benefits

Early intervention is the term for special education for children from birth to age three. The IFSP is the document and the process that governs your child's "education" and services (a.k.a. therapies) during her early childhood years.

According to the IDEA, the IFSP specifically must address:

- the family's resources priorities and concerns related to enhancing the development of their child;
- information about a child's developmental status across the five domains (physical [including vision and hearing], communication, cognition, social-emotional, and adaptive);
- statement of outcomes for the child and family including pre-literacy skills when developmentally appropriate;
- criteria, procedures, and timelines for child and family outcomes;
- identified early intervention services to meet the child and family's needs. These services should be based on peer-reviewed research;
- statement regarding natural environments in which services are delivered and an explanation as to why services may not occur in the child's natural environment;
- dates and duration of planned services;
- the identification of a service coordinator; and
- transition plan from part C, and other services as needed.

Benefits to the Family

In addition, there are benefits for both families and professionals that are accomplished through the IFSP.

The IFSP assures families:

- a predictable process for discussing and documenting the child's and family's changing needs;
- "family-centered services" in which both the child's needs and needs of the larger family will be considered;
- a focus on outcomes deemed most important to the family;
- a "living" document that changes and grows as the needs of the child and family change;
- a written plan of who will do what, when, and where for a six to twelve month period of time;
- both family and professional input to the development and implementation of plans;
- access to available educational, medical, and social services in a community to help the family and their child;
- the expertise of professionals from many disciplines including: physical, occupational and speech therapy, social work, nursing, nutrition, audiology, psychology, child development and education; and
- coordination of those special services across agencies and professionals in a manner attractive and useful to the individual family.

Benefits to the Professionals

The IFSP allows professionals from different agencies and different professions to:

- engage family members as colleagues in a team effort to help the child develop;
- access family expertise and knowledge about the child's preferences and needs;
- share their expertise with the family and with each other;
- reduce redundancy of information and service and prioritize efforts;
- discuss shared interests for the child and family; and
- understand the context of the family in which the child is living and growing.

Reprinted with permission. Source: www.ifspweb.org

well as individualized therapy sessions. Parents can request that their pediatrician write a prescription for home health services so that therapies can take place in the child's home. This is recommended in order to maximize the child's energy and opportunity to benefit from the sessions, as well as to decrease potential exposure to communicable illnesses.

Early intervention teams work together with your family to develop a comprehensive plan (the IFSP) as well as goals in many areas of development, including physical, cognitive, communication, social/emotional, and adaptive development. While the process varies by state, IFSP meetings are typically held at least once every six weeks and require written documentation by all of your child's service providers (therapists) about your child's development and progress toward meeting your child's IFSP goals. As your child makes progress, those goals are adjusted. Likewise, if your child should have a period of illness and experience some regression, the goals will be adjusted. These meetings take place in your home, as the emphasis of early intervention across the country is to support the child and family in their natural environment.

You might find it difficult to set goals during these meetings, especially if you are in the midst of the diagnosis process and are unsure of what the months ahead will look like for your child. Frequent hospitalizations or low-energy days can also make this process frustrating. It's important to keep the big picture in mind during the development of your child's IFSP, and to try to set realistic goals that can be reached. Active participation in your child's therapy sessions is a great way to get to know your child and begin to understand—sometimes through trial and error—her limitations and how she responds to exercise, stimulation, etc. Help your therapists understand that mitochondrial disease is an energy metabolism disorder (i.e. goal is to maximize battery) and work diligently together to learn how to help your child make progress by pushing her just a tiny bit beyond what she can comfortably do without causing exhaustion.

Your therapists are your allies and your advocates, and having a long-term relationship with the same therapists can really help you as a family to build a foundation for your child's future growth. By participating in your child's therapy sessions with the therapist whenever possible, you can also learn to identify subtle cues that may indicate that your child is getting tired or needs a break. Recognizing these cues becomes very important as your child grows and gets ready to transition to public school-based services at the age of three.

Getting Support for You

It can be so difficult facing a world where a disaster seems to lurk around every corner, and it is very painful as a mom or dad to watch your baby or toddler miss milestones, endure frequent appointments and hospitalizations, and fail to grow in comparison to the other children around them. Not only is the stress of caring for a baby with mitochondrial disease exhausting because of the baby's physical needs, but the emotional stress of seeking (and receiving) a diagnosis compounds a parent's fear and emotional devastation. Parents in this stage are frequently too exhausted, too overwhelmed, or too nervous to ask for help. "Reaching out" and asking for support can be particularly tricky for dads, who often would rather "do something" or "fix it"

JESSICA

Our beautiful daughter, Jessica, came by induction two weeks early because of lack of fetal movement in the womb. As new parents, we were worried, but you just never think anything bad would really happen to you. Two days after we brought her home from the hospital, Jessica became listless, lethargic, and would not eat. We rushed her to the hospital to learn that she was having her first metabolic "crash." Since then, she has had too many hospital stays to count, and visits the hospital frequently for labs, pain, and to see her specialists. She was diagnosed through a fresh muscle biopsy at one year of age. Five years later, physicians have yet to be able to identify the exact type of mitochondrial disease that she has, but almost all of her organ systems are affected.

On a daily basis, Jessica fights severe hypotonia (low muscle tone) that prevents her from being able to sit, crawl, stand, walk, or move independently. She also has swallow dysfunction and is fed through a feeding tube that bypasses her stomach and goes directly into her intestines. Her most serious symptoms are lactic acidosis and renal tubular acidosis, neutropenia, pancreatic enzyme deficiency, and obstruction of her digestive system. Each and every day is a struggle for Jessica and all of us.

Jessica will light up the room with her smile and laughter. She loves people, especially little children. She cannot speak, but adores books. Jessica has taught us so much about courage. She has taught us to appreciate the simple things in life—a hug, a smile, the innocence of a child. We have discovered family in unexpected friends, and have been disappointed by family who were supposed to be our support system. We have learned to trust our own instincts and advocate for her in moments when her life was in jeopardy. We have adjusted our life expectations and ultimately have found a stronger love than we could have ever imagined before Jessica came into our lives. We are thankful for each day that we can share with our little angel.

and have a hard time coping when they can't. Physicians often are primarily focused on their role of diagnostician during a child with Mito's infancy and early childhood, remaining focused on ordering and interpreting tests. Tests are important, but consequently physicians are often less aware of the family's need for support.

Because having a baby or very young child with Mito can be stressful, sad, scary, and isolating, it is particularly important to prioritize and to keep perspective as much as possible. Do not go into this journey alone. If you're married or have a partner in all this, take the time to listen to each other as much as you can, and recognize that you may not be able to offer one another what each of you really needs right now because you are BOTH living in your own emotional crisis. Many parents are very focused on looking for answers during this time as their young child struggles, yet it is paramount to turn your focus inward to your child and to your family's immediate needs. Your child doesn't know about mitochondrial disease, they just know how comforting your touch can be. If you are a single parent, it is even more important for you to make an effort to reach out to the mitochondrial disease community and find support in other parents. You have every reason to ask (and receive!) help!

Find others who have children with chronic illnesses through your hospital or online. Yahoo! Health groups (see Appendix C for specific group names) and community support groups or online forums (such as www.MitoAction.org/forum) can be a tremendous resource and place to vent, ask questions, find hope, and feel less alone. Many parents share that finding one or two "Internet friends" who have children with similar issues is like a lifeline for them during the first year or two of their child's life. No one can understand your feelings of confusion or anxiety like another parent who is going through the same thing.

Your family can really benefit from the support of others in your community as well; however, it will serve you well to recognize early on the important difference between support and understanding. "They don't understand what we are going through" is a true and common protest by parents of children with Mito. Furthermore, it can be extraordinarily difficult to trust anyone else to care for your child who has mitochondrial disease. The symptoms are erratic and often serious. Children at this age with Mito are typically nonverbal, so understanding their needs is often based on parents' instinct. While family might not understand these needs, they can still offer support through this stage, especially if you are dealing with the needs of your other children, multiple visits to the doctor, hospitalizations, etc. Try to take the assistance of others from your neighborhood, your family, your church, etc. with the recognition that many people *cannot understand* what your family is dealing with, but they can give you dinner, walk the dog, take your other children to their activities, or run some errands that can help you nonetheless.

In this way, support can be defined in two different ways—emotional, and practical. Focus on the practical support at this time from the people in your community so that you and your spouse can do your best to be rested, well-fed, and focused on helping your child. Seek emotional support from new friends and from people who can be objective, such as counselors or therapists. While this journey may feel rocky and scary today, there *is* hope for tomorrow and there are real joys and opportunities that you and your family will find once you have weathered this difficult time. No doctor can predict the future and no one has the right to put a limit on your children's lives or their potential because of their diagnosis. One nugget of advice for parents of young children is to keep your faith and keep your perspective by focusing on what you and your children CAN do. This is a difficult but precious lesson that will carry you forward for many years to come.

Your role as advocate begins now, and it will be a tenure position with lifetime benefits! Keep your perspective! Take the time to step back and step away from the overwhelming situation at home with your child. Take a walk, find and use family and babysitters for short periods of time, go out to dinner, take an exercise class. You can become exhausted and unable to see the big picture when you don't have perspective.

Pre-school (Ages Three through Six) and School-age Children (Ages Six through Twelve)
Transition Services and Educational Plans

School is an important part of your child's life socially, emotionally, and physically. If you feel overwhelmed by the "alphabet soup" that was thrust upon you in early intervention (IFSP, OT, PT, ABA, etc.), then you are probably further confused when your child becomes eligible for services through public school. In addition, it is not uncommon for parents to share that school is a "low priority" for their child from their perspective. After all, some children who are between the ages of six and twelve may be in the process of getting a Mito diagnosis, dealing with health issues, hospitalizations, troubling daily symptoms, behavior issues, developmental delays, changes in family support and services, and so on. Furthermore, school-aged children who are physically delayed or disabled due to Mito are heavier, require new and more specialized equipment, and have different needs than they did when they were younger. On the other hand, children whose Mito is an "invisible" disability may struggle during these years because it is difficult for others (teachers, friends, coaches, family) to understand their illness and fatigue if they "look so good." It is a challenge to look great on the outside, yet physically feel awful most of the time.

Special education services for children change when your child turns three. About three months before your child's third birthday, your child begins the transition from early intervention to public school-based special education. Under the 2004 Individuals with Disabilities Education Act (IDEA), your school-age child may be eligible for an Individualized Education Program (IEP) if she meets the criteria, which are determined by your state and commonly include ten to fourteen broad impairment categories such as developmental delay, physical, intellectual, neurological, communication, or emotional impairment, and other health impairment (OHI). In addition, it must be determined that your child cannot "progress effectively" in the regular curriculum because of her disability. In other words, due to your child's unique issues and disabilities from mitochondrial disease, your child cannot meet the required standard of the curriculum and cannot meet her potential, including cognitive and social/emotional growth potential.

This can be a confusing transition for parents of preschool age children, since you are accustomed to having services out in the community and in your home. Now, your child's therapies will be primarily offered by the public school, and in some cases, supplemented by outpatient providers through your private insurance or state Medicare benefits. There are many new changes to address and understand during this transition period, including the IEP, the best program and school placement for your child, structure of your child's day, transportation to and from school, and so on. In addition, the change in structure and orientation to new people (teachers and therapists) as well as the new environment is potentially stressful for parents and their children. Be patient with yourself and the people on your child's new team during this transition, and take the opportunity early-on to request a meeting with your child's new teachers and therapists. Be prepared to share your specific concerns, information about mitochondrial disease, and tips on how the new people in your child's life can recognize her subtle cues when she is becoming depleted. It is very common for preschool children with Mito to have a shorter day and for the focus of school to be on therapies and group interactions. While many parents are hesitant to put their children in school when they are still very young and, in many cases, very fragile, school can be a successful opportunity for kids to make progress and parents to work or rest.

Many children with mitochondrial disease who are school age and who had EI services will qualify for an IEP. Likewise, kids with a later onset of symptoms during elementary school years can also find the necessary support through an IEP. An IEP requires that certain modifications **and** accommodations be made in order to provide access to the curriculum for your child. Your child is required to have an IEP that is updated at least once annually in order to receive special education and related services. The IEP is truly a unique plan for your child and should reflect appropriate and attainable goals as developed by your child's IEP team: teachers, school administrators, related service providers (such as therapists), and you—the parent(s)! Even those children who are developmentally on target for their age can have a voice about what is included in their IEP.

BETTY AND HER SON ALEX

Betty's son, Alex, is six years old and has Mito. Alex has been home most of his life because he has many food allergies and because he frequently got colds when he attended preschool. Betty has grown accustomed to being Alex's advocate. She is vigilant about teaching others about his allergies and his needs. She had a special book made for Alex that tells others all about his special needs so that his therapists, babysitters, teachers, etc. will know how to best take care of him.

Alex, however, doesn't look sick. He is playful, he is a chatterbox although his speech is slurred, and when he is tired he becomes more hyper instead of sleepy. Alex's teachers initially describe him as "unfocused and hyper." It seems incongruent to them that Alex has a mitochondrial disease that is characterized by fatigue when he appears to have so much energy, and it also seems suspicious that Alex's mom has gone to such great lengths to be his advocate when he seems "normal."

Alex is ready for kindergarten now, but his mom isn't sure if he should go. She is worried that he will get sick and that he won't be able to eat the special foods that she is accustomed to preparing for him because he has many food allergies. She has trouble trusting anyone else to take care of Alex as she has become very aware of his needs and his nonverbal cues that help her to know how he is doing. Alex has his blood sugar checked daily and uses a nebulizer treatment if he has trouble breathing.

When the time comes for Alex's first IEP meeting, Betty comes prepared with a long list of requirements for Alex. She has trouble identifying what the school can offer Alex other than making it "just like home." Betty requests that some specific measures be put in place for Alex such as an air conditioning unit in his classroom and a microwave for his special foods. She would like Alex to be able to call her throughout the day to let her know how he is feeling. Betty is very worried that by allowing Alex to go to kindergarten, he will "get worse," and will end up in the hospital. Some of Betty's friends have children with mitochondrial disease who are very fragile and who are frequently hospitalized in the intensive care unit. Betty wants to be sure that she protects Alex from this fate.

Unfortunately, Betty and Alex live in a school district that has never encountered a child with mitochondrial disease before and that has experienced drastic budget cuts in the last few years. The school is unsure how and is unwilling to meet Betty's requests for several reasons. Primarily, they don't "see" Alex's needs in the way that his mother describes them. Most of the symptoms that Betty describes are not obvious to them. They have not seen Alex "crash" in the way that Betty describes. No other parent has ever made so many requests of the school before and the school really has no idea how to provide these accommodations for Alex. Rather than address each request separately on her list, as well as offer some additional modifications of their own, they dismiss the entire list as "unreasonable and unnecessary."

After meeting with the team, Betty feels that the school is being difficult and that the teachers don't care about Alex. Conversely, the teachers and school administrators feel that Betty is overreacting and being overprotective of Alex. How can both parties move forward in this situation and determine what is best for Alex?

First, the school requests Betty's permission for Alex to have a neuropsychological evaluation so that they can better identify Alex's needs and to establish a baseline for his school performance and abilities. For Betty's part, she asks her pediatrician to work with her to modify a template of an individualized healthcare plan that specifically outlines priority health needs for Alex. Betty seeks the support of a special education consultant who acts as a mediator between Betty and the school and successfully gets a one-on-one aide to help him throughout the day. A year later, at Alex's annual IEP meeting, Betty asks again for an air conditioner for Alex's classroom. Now that the staff has gotten to know Alex, they can recognize his subtle cues when he is overheated and becoming overtired. Interested in seeing Alex continue to stay healthy and make progress, one teacher suggests that the school reach out to a local heating and air company to install the AC at a reduced cost.

Things are coming together now that Betty and Alex's school are cooperating. Even though he missed many days of school each month, Alex was excited to go to his first birthday party when invited by a classmate and says he "likes school a lot!"

For kids with Mito, finding the appropriate modifications and accommodations in school may be more challenging. Parents share that they are surprised at how involved they need to become in order to educate teachers and school staff about Mito and about the importance of preventing a metabolic crisis. It becomes your responsibility to help your child's teachers, therapists, and school or community team really understand how Mito specifically affects your child. Just as important as understanding, however, is prioritizing. There are limitations to what schools and school staff can do, and progress often comes slowly. This can be really frustrating to parents. The

Common IEP Modifications and Accommodations for a Child with Mito

- Shorter school day
- Extended school year
- Transportation in an air-conditioned vehicle
- Temperature-regulated classroom
- Sink in the classroom for hand washing and/or easy access to hand sanitizer for all students
- One-on-one aide (consistent)
- Physical therapy, speech therapy, and occupational therapy at least two times per week, thirty minute sessions, in the morning (when energy is highest)
- Alternative or shorter physical education (gym) period
- Use of a stroller or wheelchair to go to the gym, playground, cafeteria, and on field trips
- Use of technology such as Skype and a home tutor to interact with the classroom during prolonged absences
- Opportunity to have access to a snack and water at all times
- Opportunity to take breaks in a quiet place (such as a reading corner or the nurse's office) as needed or regularly
- Modified curriculum based on the child's developmental and cognitive abilities
- Use of assistive technology
- First floor classroom
- Provide positioning support such as special seating, cushions, foot or back support, etc.
- Provide daily or weekly progress reports and symptom checklists (both from home to school and from school to home)
- See samples of IEPs, symptom checklists, and healthcare plans at www.mitoaction.org/education and in Appendix D.

adage "pick your battles" couldn't be more relevant in this situation—you must help the team see how BEST to meet the needs of your child by prioritizing those needs. The most successful parent/teacher teams approach the child's plan from each other's point of view, working hard to keep the needs of the child and the goal of progress and health center stage, despite budget limitations, lack of awareness amongst teachers and staff, and stressed or overwhelmed parents. If you can't have everything that you want for your child, what are the most important requests that will ensure her health, safety, and best opportunity for a great school experience?

An IEP is a safeguard and in many ways is a tremendous opportunity for success when developed appropriately. Further, while many children do not have *obvious* physical or cognitive disabilities as part of their Mito diagnosis, they *do* qualify for an IEP under the other health impairment (OHI) umbrella. OHI criteria are also determined by the state and typically include children who have an inability to attend school or learn due to prolonged absences, fatigue, or lack of alertness due to a chronic or acute health problem. In many cases, mitochondrial disease certainly fits that description!

Kirsten Casale, an educational consultant for children and families with mitochondrial disease, offers this fundamental advice to parents going through the IEP

Universal IEP Goals for a Child with Mito

IEP goals are very specific to your child's development, ability, and unique needs. In addition, IEP goals change at least once each year, and are adjusted to your child's health, growth, development, physical, social, and academic needs. However, there are some universal goals for the team to keep in mind when developing your child's IEP and/or healthcare plan:

• To aid and educate (Child's name) school district about the medical complexities of her mitochondrial disease and other medical conditions as it pertains to how her body utilizes energy in beneficial and nonbeneficial ways;

• To ensure proper accommodations and modifications in her developing IEP are aiding her in using her energy expenditures appropriately;

• To ensure that (Child's name) remains safe and educationally challenged, while also managing her energy expenditures;

• To better her chances in reaching her grade level expectations/academic goals, while not exacerbating her chronic illness symptoms, which could lead to progression of her mitochondrial disease and other medical conditions;

• To have this document implemented through the school district so that (Child's name) has **"the highest level of expectation"** academically as described under IDEA; while being properly supported in the **"least restrictive environment"** while accessing her legal right to **"free access to public education,"** as is guaranteed her under the Federal laws listed in IDEA/2004.

Source: Kirsten Casale, Educational advocate for MitoAction, from a "Sample Health Care Plan"

process: "Know the law, and know your rights. However, it is your responsibility to be a part of the team, not a source of opposition. When you can prioritize your child's needs and give tangible, real-life examples of how the modifications and accommodations that you request will actually help keep your child safe, healthy, and able to learn, it is my experience that teachers and schools are willing to do what it takes to help your child." Kirsten also suggests developing an educational health plan with your child's doctor, and has found tremendous benefit in bringing pediatricians into the discussion early in the process of developing a child's IEP. Samples of IEPs and educational health plans for kids with Mito are available online at www.MitoAction.org/education.

Some children with Mito may NOT qualify for an IEP but can benefit from a Section 504 plan. First implemented as part of the American Disabilities Act (ADA), a 504 plan provides accommodations for your child but does not provide modifications. What's the difference? Accommodations alter the environment or the tools available to the student in order to more effectively access the curriculum. Accommodations include seating your child more comfortably or closer to the teacher, allowing use of a tape recorder, voice recognition software, or a scribe in the classroom, breaking assignments into shorter segments with breaks in between, untimed tests, reading assignments or test questions out loud, moving the classroom location to the first floor, using a stroller or wheelchair to get around the school, using an air conditioner to counter heat intolerance, and use of a sign language interpreter for the child who is hearing impaired. Modifications, as allowed in an IEP, include actual changes to the curriculum so that the content is simplified or the requirements are changed based on your child's unique disability. One important distinction between the two is that, unlike an IEP, a Section 504 plan does NOT require an individualized program designed to meet your child's needs. In addition, a team meeting (and consensus) is required before a child's IEP can be modified; however, this is not the case with a 504 plan. An IEP is usually more rigorous, more expensive (for the school district), and more detailed than a 504 plan. Children who have cognitive *and* developmental delays more frequently have an IEP. However, both are used, and used successfully to allow children with Mito to attend school!

Homeschooling—An Option for Kids with Mito?

Some parents choose to homeschool their children. For you, as the parent of a child with Mito, this is a very individual choice. Some parents are overwhelmed by their child's medical needs and can really benefit from the team approach offered by school. Others find that meeting the schools' requirements in light of their children's medical needs is too overwhelming and creates more chaos. Here are some words of wisdom from parents who homeschool their children with Mito (*Source:* Parent contributors on www.MitoAction.org):

Benefits to Homeschooling for Kids with Mito.
- You get to monitor the health of your child, without having to rely on the teachers or classroom aides to provide care or report how your child is doing.

- There is less exposure to viruses and infectious germs that could exacerbate a chronic condition.
- You, as the parent, can determine how much "work" your child can handle before she becomes overly fatigued. You can adjust your program accordingly, and provide education in smaller, more manageable chunks, especially if your child fatigues easily.
- It is MUCH easier to get a doctor's appointment, and you can go during "off" hours. This also leads to lower germ exposure, since you can be in and out of the doctor's office long before the other kids get out of school.
- You can visit museums, stores, and other public places during school hours (school field trips to museums are usually done by 1:00 pm or so) while they are less crowded, thereby reducing your child's risk of virus/germ exposure.
- You can make sure your heat-intolerant child has an air-conditioned vehicle for transportation and an air-conditioned room at home that she can comfortably study in.
- The variety of approaches, methods, environments, and materials for homeschooling is endless. With homeschooling, you can choose whatever you find most appealing for you and your child, unlike the school system where teachers are limited to specific topics, textbooks, and materials. Remember even though your child has mitochondrial disease there are always options available for her to succeed academically!

Disadvantages to Homeschooling for Kids with Mito.
- Parents who homeschool have a tremendous level of responsibility as advocates for everything from medical care to academic benchmarks. This can be overwhelming and exhausting.
- Without excellent organization skills, a homeschooling family can fall behind and become overwhelmed.
- Requires personal investment of money in most cases for textbooks, supplies, etc.
- Requires space in the home conducive to "school time," which can be difficult in large families or smaller spaces where distractions abound.
- May be difficult to get community support or access to expert resources in areas where few kids with chronic medical conditions are homeschooled.
- Potential for both children and parents to become isolated.
- Children may miss the opportunity to learn from others and to interact with other kids their age.

To Learn More.
- Join a homeschooling support network in your area. Search the Internet. Check out Yahoo groups. You will most likely have no difficulty finding such a group in your area.

- Join online support groups. There are online homeschooling curriculum support groups for just about everything you can think of.
- Search general homeschooling sites on the Internet.
- Read books about homeschooling.
- Go to your State Education Department's website. They usually list their curriculum standards for each grade. Another great resource is www.Homeschool.com.

Germs and Illness at School

Germs, germs, germs! What is an annoying cold or virus and a day in bed to one family is a potential crisis for the family who has a child with mitochondrial disease. Difficulty overcoming even minor illnesses is a common occurrence for children with Mito. For some children, immunity issues brought on by mitochondrial disease make them more susceptible to infections and illnesses. Most children with mitochondrial disease, however, are not more susceptible but simply do not have the energy reserves to overcome common childhood illnesses.

Being sick is extremely difficult for children with mitochondrial disease and often causes them to experience increased fatigue, lethargy, muscle pain and cramping, nausea, headache, and an overall aggravation of all of their symptoms. Children with Mito often require prolonged absence from school when sick, as recovery takes longer, and rest, fluids, and nutrition are more paramount. School-age children also frequently regress or lose some skills after an illness. It is critically important to tackle and pro-actively plan for exposure to germs and illnesses in school for your child at the beginning of the school year, and to address and adjust the plan as the seasons change.

Tips for Preventing and Managing Illness during the School Year.

- Consider incorporating the potential for prolonged or frequent absences into your child's IEP in anticipation of unforeseen illnesses that may take weeks of recovery.
- Ask your child's teacher and/or school nurse for permission to send a letter home to children in your child's classroom that explains a little bit about Mito and kindly requests that parents remember to let the teacher know when their child has a fever or contagious illness.
- You may find that your child is sick every year right after the school year begins and right after every holiday vacation, so you may keep your child home or interact with the classroom using Skype or other technology during those high-risk periods.
- In winter months, your child's physician might recommend increasing vitamin C and fluid intake in order to improve the body's ability to fight an infection or illness.
- Preventive measures such as flu vaccines are highly recommended, again, as part of a plan for keeping your child as healthy as possible during the school year.

- You may have to make some tough decisions for your child, and require them to stay home when the class is going on a field trip to a busy museum during cold and flu season. Your role as your child's advocate is to constantly and realistically weigh the risks against the benefit for every situation.
- Most teachers are willing to encourage use of hand sanitizer in their classroom, and will cooperate with your request to frequently disinfect common surfaces such as toys, desks, pencil sharpeners, markers, etc. Although the approach may seem simple, writing a checklist of all the ways that your child's teachers can help minimize germ exposure can actually be very helpful. The checklist makes a great back-to-school gift along with a canister of disinfecting wipes and a bottle of hand sanitizer!

If your child does become ill, be vigilant about alerting your pediatrician and teachers, and increase your child's fluid intake immediately. Illnesses that cause a fever are extremely difficult for children with Mito and should be diligently managed by using acetaminophen and ibuprofen (alternating) every four hours. (Discuss with your doctor the appropriate protocol for your child.) Some illnesses, such as the flu or a stomach virus, may be better managed in the hospital. Intervention and metabolic support (fluids, rest, supplements, good nutrition) early in an illness can help prevent regression and a cascade of additional symptoms. Again, as much as possible, prevention is key.

Red Light, Green Light...Yellow Light

Even in elementary school, children can and should be able to recognize their body's need for rest. In fact, Dr. Irina Anselm of Children's Hospital in Boston says that helping a child with mitochondrial disease to verbalize or otherwise communicate fatigue and pain can significantly help improve her overall health and success in school. How can young children understand the complicated concept of energy management? Children at this age respond very well to concrete analogies. With your help, children can develop a visual and interactive activity that serves as a reminder to check-in with their body and to rest, drink, and eat as needed. To illustrate, some elementary school-aged kids love trains and understand that trains need to make stops to refuel. While it may be difficult for children to express that they are tired and need to "refuel," they are able to move the train around the tracks and dock the train in the station for rest and refueling. Similarly, you could use a car (a toy car or a picture of a car) and something that depicts a road. You can talk about the fact that the car needs to slow down or stop at the gas station. Teachers and aides can use concrete analogies like this to help children be cooperative about pacing themselves, and to teach them how important it is to check-in with themselves to assess their need for a break.

- Some children with more advanced thought processes can understand a "stoplight" analogy and can use colored circles (green, yellow, and red) on a blank traffic light to indicate how they are feeling. Teachers can also enforce and guide periods of rest using these tools by telling children, "Yellow light—we have to slow down and take deep breaths and have a break" or "Your gas tank is empty so your car needs to stop and refuel." When children are told what to do without their involvement, not only are they more likely to be resistant but they are also failing to read and understand their own body's cues. Even children with developmental disabilities can learn to participate in this important process. An insightful one-on-one aide in the classroom can be a child's greatest ally by learning to recognize subtle cues of fatigue, hunger, or illness.

- Effective metabolism is dependent on oxygen (keyword: OXIDATIVE phosphorylation). Therefore, children with mitochondrial disease need oxygen! While deep breathing exercises are useful for all people, Mito patients especially benefit from taking full, deep breaths. Unobstructed breathing is likewise important; ensure that there is never an obstruction to the airway (sometimes this happens during sleep or when a child is slumped in a chair) that would impair oxygen flow.

- Children with mitochondrial disease may need regular "refueling" and often benefit from frequent high protein, high carbohydrate snacks and plenty of fluids spread throughout the day. Coupled with breaks (including the opportunity to lay down flat on occasion), we can help our kids conserve energy so that they can get the most out of the most essential activities of their day.

Teens

Puberty

Puberty and infancy are probably the two most challenging periods in the life span of a person who has mitochondrial disease. Your teen's body already has a lot to overcome and compensate for from Mito, and now we add hormones! Emotional stress and hormone fluctuations can cause many teens to experience an increase in or exacerbation of symptoms. Some teens find that all of their "old" symptoms come back while other teens are presented a brand new set of challenges and confusing symptoms to figure out. Physicians and parents agree that for teens with Mito, puberty consistently makes symptoms more erratic and therefore more confusing to interpret and treat. As teens' bodies are changing, so is their awareness of the world and of their life with a diagnosis of mitochondrial disease.

As is true in other stages of childhood, no two teens with Mito are alike. Some children are not diagnosed with Mito until their teen years when they become more symptomatic. Other teens with Mito are more profoundly developmentally delayed and may suffer from multiple symptoms involving multiple organs. Some teens with Mito can suffer from profound setbacks during this period after years of a plateau, while others become more independent and have an intense desire to live and to express themselves. Some teens have outlived their prognosis by ten years or more, such that every day and every year is a new beginning and a new opportunity. No one knows the future for any of our children with mitochondrial disease, and it is vital that teens

Top Ten Back-to-School Survival Tips

1. Pack **extra snacks and fluids** that can be kept with the child at all times. Drinks and snacks are energy saving measures, and help to maintain a healthy energy baseline.

2. Buy your child a **backpack with wheels** to lessen muscle fatigue.

3. Buy the classroom teacher a **giant bottle of antibacterial gel** and request that it be kept by the door where students can use it every time they go in and out of the room. Good handwashing is a must! Many school nurses will offer a handwashing campaign in your child's classroom if you ask.

4. Request a free copy of MitoAction's **ENERGY 4 EDUCATION DVD**—a great way to get teachers and therapists up to speed on mitochondrial disease in less than ten minutes!

5. Provide your IEP team with a sample IEP that outlines suggested modifications and accommodations for kids with Mito, including protocols and daily health symptom checklists. Share these materials at least two weeks before your child's annual IEP meeting. A sample IEP can be found in Appendix D.

6. **Schedule a meeting with your child's school nurse** to share any changes that took place over the summer. This is a great plan right after holiday breaks too.

7. **Advocate that your child's schedule be adjusted** to suit her "better times of the day." For example, can physical therapy take place in the morning?

8. Give your child's teachers and nurses a small card with **all of your contact information**, reminding them that you are only a phone call away if they have ANY questions or concerns during the day. It helps to gently remind the people who care for our children at school that with mitochondrial disease, things shift quickly!

9. While maintaining every student's right to privacy, ask that your child's teacher and school nurse **let you know if there is a known contagious illness in the classroom**. Children with mitochondrial disease aren't always more susceptible to infection (some are), but almost all have difficulty recovering from even a minor illness.

10. Share a copy of this list with your child's teachers and therapists and encourage them to learn more about mitochondrial disease!

are encouraged to live full, bountiful lives and to have dreams that are meaningful to them. Puberty feels scary, overwhelming, and isolating for ANY teenager, and these feelings can be amplified in a teen with Mito. Families who have the mantra "We will not *survive* Mito, we will *live* it" are frequently the most successful at finding balance between living each day and juggling symptoms during the teen years.

Puberty and the changes that take place in a boy or girl's body during puberty devour a huge amount of energy. It is very common for teens with Mito of all abilities to be exhausted or irritable. New and unexplainable symptoms may emerge and may go away as suddenly as they arrived. Body temperature regulation often becomes more challenging during puberty, and teens may have unexplained fevers or spikes in temperature that are not related to illness. They may be too cold or overheat easily, and shiver or be unable to sweat. Teens with Mito complain of body aches, joint aches, and muscle pain, especially in their arms, legs, hands, and feet. Helping teens find ways to preserve their energy by lying down, using text-to-speech software, and other assistive technology or accommodations can help but may not alleviate the pain as it did in earlier years.

For some teens, puberty coincides with increased expectations in school, and vision issues (primarily related to eye fatigue) may become apparent as reading and computer use increases. Growth spurts between the ages of twelve and sixteen can be a source of incredible fatigue in teens with Mito and may result in a dramatic increase in the amount of sleep needed per day. More frequent breaks or rest periods can help as well. Puberty is difficult for girls as they suffer from hormone highs and lows associated with their period, as well as pain from menstrual cramping. Some physicians recommend chemically stopping or controlling a girl's menstrual cycle with low-dose birth control pills in order to stabilize the hormone swings (the patch is not recommended).

Puberty can bring about unexpected blood pressure changes that were never a problem before, and parents should seek advice from a cardiologist if their teen complains of dizziness, a pounding heart, or a feeling of being "drained of all energy." Often these symptoms, which are related to autonomic nervous system dysfunction, are more apparent and more unpredictable during puberty. Teens may complain of heartburn or feel nauseous as hormones can cause their sense of taste to change and the stomach increases more acid. Eating a couple of salty crackers before every meal, and changing to small, frequent meals (five to seven meals per day) can help your teen reduce acid reflux, conserve energy, and feel more stable.

LUCY

I hated being younger because I would always worry about what other people thought. Like when I was in my wheelchair, I didn't want people to think I was faking because I could get out and walk around. I just used it for energy saving mostly. One time, a woman in a store came up to my mother and said she should be ashamed of allowing me to play around in a wheelchair when I could walk. I had gotten out and held up a pair of pants to see if they would fit, so I turned to her and said, "When YOU have a life-long challenging disease with no cure, then you can say something like that, but I bet you don't!" My mom said that was the day she knew that I was going to have a strong voice and be a good advocate for myself.

Mood swings are normal during puberty; however, the energy demand of emotional stress should not be underestimated. Many teens are worried about school, their health, fitting in, their family, and have a lot to deal with every day. These worries, on top of more intense schoolwork and social pressure, can be invisible energy drains that leave your teen exhausted and susceptible to setbacks. Teens need more support—physically and emotionally—than they did before puberty set in. On a brighter note, after a roller coaster ride of erratic symptoms and hospitalizations, most teens settle back into a new baseline that carries them through their young adult years after puberty.

Some teens with mitochondrial disease may have shown "soft signs" of their disease prior to reaching puberty, such as fatigue or difficulty recovering from an illness, but experience a major setback during adolescence. This can be emotionally devastating for a family and for the teen. As your teen's parent, you must recognize that you and your child's doctor become the beacons of hope for your teen. If you and the physician want to have a conversation about progression of symptoms, consider doing this over the telephone instead of in front of your teen. Teens with Mito share that they are scared and worried about the medical aspects of their disease, and that they feel out of control. Some teens have resigned themselves to fate with an almost callous attitude like, "Well, I might die anyway."

High School Survival Tips

- Request an extra set of all textbooks (one for home and one for school). Not carrying books to and from school saves physical energy.
- Ensure that all medications (including medicines used only occasionally) are current and available at school, along with detailed directions, emergency protocols, and letters from the prescribing doctors. High schools do not allow students to carry medicines of any kind with them during school, and school nurses as well as county paramedics need to know that emergency protocols are in place.
- Have a plan to allow scheduled access to snacks and water throughout the day. Nutrition and hydration makes a big difference in keeping energy levels consistent.
- If there are dietary restrictions, communicate them to the school in writing before school starts each year. It helps to share this information with your teen's teacher and the school nurse as well.
- Insist that your child have the opportunity to have one-on-one meetings with a guidance counselor throughout the year.
- Use lightweight notebooks, pens, pencils, and a calculator. A tablet like the Apple iPad is a wonderful tool for high school students who have Mito and shouldn't carry more than they absolutely need to.
- All assistive technology used at home to ease unnecessary energy expenditure should also be made available at school, including: laptop/e-tablet, calculator, voice dictation software, and a handheld digital recorder.

You can help be a source of encouragement for your teen and can keep her on track by listening more than providing solutions. Helping your teen learn to manage her disease and listen to her body will help your teen more than trying to "fix" her problems (both social and physical). Teens with Mito may have a tendency to become pessimistic if they don't feel supported by friends and family or if they feel that their symptoms and feelings aren't validated. Help your teen find a hobby that is realistic and enjoyable and that is unique to her. Some teens with Mito are great singers, guitar players, hold record scores in video games, are avid readers, do crossword puzzles, study ancient cultures, learn all about the computer, and can be truly inspirational. Relationships with other teens who have Mito or chronic illness can help teens feel connected and less isolated. Many states offer camps for kids with chronic illnesses that provide leadership and camper opportunities—experiences like those found at camp can be life-changing and can really help teens find their voice and independence.

Helping Your Teen Achieve Independence

"I have Mito."
"Hey everybody, I have MITO!!!"
"I don't have Mito—what are you talking about?"

Do you announce it over the PA system or do you act as if nothing is wrong? This is such a personal matter, but in talking with parents and teens who have survived middle and high school with Mito, there is consensus on a few things. One, people will notice if something changes. If your teen needs to begin using a wheelchair because of fatigue or limited/lost mobility, it's difficult to act as if nothing has changed (even if the person inside is the same). If your teen is absent for three weeks, other students will get worried and curious and eager to ask and know "What happened to you?" Being evasive can unfortunately cause more issues than being upfront. Some teens with Mito are worried about what others will think of them and adamantly deny that they have the disease because "I don't want people to feel sorry for me." However, teens thrive on drama and are known to spread rumors, especially when they don't understand their peer's situation. Unfortunately, some teens with Mito are victims of bullying and may feel extremely isolated or depressed as they are faced with the daily reality and limitations of their disease. They may even feel that school is a battleground and complain that they don't have the energy to go to school or do their work.

Being a teen is difficult, and being a teen with Mito can be grueling. Parents and teens who have "survived" agree: It is important to keep perspective—middle school and high school are not forever. Are there alternatives? How can you achieve a high school degree with as little physical and emotional stress as possible? Is a home tutor an option? Can a neuropsychological evaluation help establish appropriate resources for your teen? Is a GED and early college admission an alternative for a homebound high schooler? Can your middle schooler have a Mito awareness campaign or fundraiser that the students in the class help to organize? Is there a speaker who could educate your child's class about Mito? Can your child show a movie or multimedia presentation about mitochondrial disease? Can your child write (remember voice dictation software!) a piece to be published in the school newspaper about her life and challenges with Mito?

Your family must also be open to discussing your teen's feelings and validating her experiences and fears at her level. Even teens with physical and cognitive delays are often more aware, more frustrated, and yearn for more independence or self-expression during their teen years. While they may have the desire, most teens need a lot of support to be able to feel important and to learn how to be themselves despite the daily reality of their diagnosis. Having family discussions in which everyone in the family has to share their feelings and wishes is one way to help your teen learn ways to express herself and her needs.

In addition to finding ways to help engage teens so that they feel important and included, parents can really help their teens with Mito by being careful to *empower* them rather than *enable* them. Teens are on the cusp of becoming young adults. Young adults wish to have more independence and to have purpose in their daily life. Your support and guidance now can help your teen have realistic and satisfying goals and plans for the next phase of her life. Throughout your child's life, you may have become accustomed to making sacrifices or accommodations because of your child's illness. It is very challenging but very important that parents of teens with Mito give their kids the opportunity to test out their own decisions (and make their own mistakes) whenever possible.

For example, Danny is sixteen and has struggled with the symptoms of Mito since he was twelve years old. He has lost some of his vision and he has missed a lot of school over the last few years because of frequent illnesses and health problems. Nonetheless, Danny is really bright and is in many ways more mature because of his diagnosis. Danny knows that if he has an assignment for school, it will take him three times longer to do it because of his disabilities. However, because Danny is *capable* of doing it without risk to his health, his parents (and therefore his teachers) expect him to complete the assignment. Danny also knows that if he complains to his mom that he is too tired to go to school after staying up late to work on the assignment (that he should have been working on earlier), his Mom is not going to budge. Danny will be tired—in fact, it might take him days to really recover from staying up too late. But Danny's mom wants him to learn to pace himself, so she enforces their plan (do the assignment over time beginning as soon as you get it) and enforces the consequences (go to school, even if you are really tired) as long as Danny's health and safety are not threatened. This is really tough as a parent: knowing when to protect your child and when to let him experience the natural consequences. However, Danny's mom believes that if she always protects Danny and lets him skip assignments or stay home from school when he feels tired, he may perceive himself as a victim of the disease, and this perception can haunt Danny and potentially disable him more as an adult than his actual medical diagnosis.

What Does Fatigue in Children Look Like?

Fatigue not only looks different in every child but also is much more complex than just being "sleepy." Children with mitochondrial disease are frequently suffering from fatigue on some level, although their expression of fatigue may vary from hyperactivity to depression. It is important to lay a foundation with everyone who helps teach or care for your child about what she looks like when tired. Let's look at several different scenarios:

1. Some children become more agitated and irritable when fatigued. They may act out, yell, or become obtrusive. Although others may describe these children as "hyper" or "defiant," they will note that these children are not happy or smiling when exhibiting these behaviors. Perhaps these children lose self-control when they are fatigued because they simply do not have the energy to "keep it together" any longer. If your child is this way, perhaps she is so exhausted that she becomes very anxious. She cannot express herself and may have loud outbursts of yelling, throwing things, or crying without being able to explain why or respond to direction. Help your child's teachers look at your child's behavior from a different point of view and realize that it is often misinterpreted. Gently remind them of the research on sleep deprivation and how, for some children with Mito, a bad day can be equal to a day or more without sleep. Help these children slow down and get into a quiet, safe, and comfortable place to rest. A shorter school day, a cooler classroom, or less stimulation can help right away.

2. Some children with Mito may become distracted and unable to focus when fatigued. They retreat into themselves in order to cope with the fatigue. They are not good at expressing their feelings by the time they are this tired. They cannot learn or focus. Their speech may be slurred and they avoid eye contact or cannot seem to hold eye contact with others. They become very quiet, don't want to talk or respond, and become upset when pushed to participate. Help these children before they get so tired that they need to retreat. They will feel much happier when they are recharged frequently!

3. The most obvious sign of fatigue in children with Mito is sleepiness. There are times when a child is overtired or has gone too long without food and drink and looks like a wilted flower. She is droopy, her eyes are half-closed, and she may want to lay her head down or lean on someone or something and doze off. When a child is this tired, she may seem listless and not be able to participate in normal activities.

EVA

For six months we had been fighting with our insurance company in order to get our daughter Eva a wheelchair. She was turning four and all of a sudden we had to leave the world of overgrown baby items and cross over into the land of special needs and durable medical equipment. Eva has Leigh's disease, a form of mitochondrial disease, that affects her muscles and neurologic system such that she cannot walk or talk. Sounds terrible, right? In reality, since we've gotten over the diagnosis, we find so much joy in Eva. For a little one who doesn't walk or talk, she has more personality and charisma than many adults that we know.

Dealing with insurance for basics like formula or durable medical equipment (i.e., wheelchair, feeding seat, way to take a bath) for a parent who already has her hands full working, running a family, and caring for her dependent child with special needs is the definition of stress. I have a Pavlovian response when I see an envelope in the mailbox from the insurance carrier.

Meanwhile, in January we finally got Eva's wheelchair and it's fantastic! The degree of support and size are perfect for her. At the time of delivery, the vendor commented, "This must be so hard for you...putting your daughter in a wheelchair." Are you kidding? I'm ecstatic. She weighs forty pounds, and finally she feels comfortable. We've come a long way from the earlier days when Eva was so frail we couldn't go out of the house unless medically necessary. So, right away I pack up my kids and away we go to the mall (early, before the crowds). Eva's siblings have a blast pushing her all over the mall at race-walk speed. Eva is loving it. We are having more fun here than we would at Disneyland. We even have ice cream and hot dogs!

However, I can't help but notice that people are giving me sympathetic looks or sad smiles. One woman even stuck out her bottom lip—really! We zoomed into the Disney store (Eva loves princesses) and well-meaning mothers sheltered their children and cleared the aisle. Keep in mind Eva looks pretty normal. While we were happy, jubilant, in fact, to be out with Eva and her new wheels, I was taken aback by the sympathy and assumption that our daughter was somehow less fortunate because of her situation. I sensed that people were afraid to interact with us.

As I mulled this over, I started to think about how much we depend on appearance in order to estimate one's ability. That's probably the Achilles heel of mitochondrial disease. When someone "looks normal," how can she really be dealing with a disease or disability? I've been out with Eva plenty of times in a stroller and we never got a second glance, even during the times when I really needed extra help (boarding an airplane, for example). Putting her in a wheelchair changed everything.

Many adults and kids with Mito can walk...some of the time. Or they can talk... until they run out of energy. Have we moved beyond discriminating against people with disabilities to a point now where we, as a society, have adopted a hands-off approach instead? For fear of showing prejudice, the aisles will clear when the wheelchair enters. How do we, the community of people with all kinds of abilities and special needs—visible and invisible—teach our neighbors to embrace us instead?

Even though she might feel better with a drink or a snack, the child may have no interest or energy to even try. This type of fatigue isn't temporary, rather it is a symptom of mitochondrial disease that can be prevented by helping the child to have plenty of breaks, as well as plenty of nighttime sleep (or daytime naps if needed).

Helping children recognize their fatigue signals when they *begin* to get tired is the most effective way that adults can help them. Once a child with Mito becomes so tired that she acts like one of these examples, it takes much longer for that child to recharge and come back to her "normal."

Key Points from This Chapter

■ Children with mitochondrial disease can look very different from each other, and symptoms and abilities vary greatly.

■ Many children with Mito experience developmental delay, muscle weakness and fatigue, heat intolerance, difficulty with attention and memory, and issues with coordination. Many children with Mito also have underlying medical issues that fluctuate in severity, such as digestive disorders, seizures, and kidney or heart problems.

■ Children with mitochondrial disease under the age of three qualify for early intervention services, which include development of an IFSP, physical therapy, occupational therapy, speech therapy and developmental assessments and support.

■ Children who are preschool and school-age with mitochondrial disease may have an IEP, a 504 plan, or an OHI. Your child's specific needs and abilities will determine which is best for her. Most kids with Mito have an IEP and receive PT, OT, and speech at least once per week in school, especially between the ages of three and twelve.

■ Teens with Mito have an especially difficult time because of hormone fluctuations and "normal" fatigue associated with puberty. Additionally, these kids often struggle with identity and independence during their adolescent years.

■ Fatigue for kids with Mito means many things. Children who fatigue as a consequence of over-expenditure of energy don't always act "sleepy," but can also manifest their fatigue by being irritable, unfocused, nonverbal, and agitated.

■ Goals for helping kids manage their mitochondrial disease should be focused on energy conservation and prioritizing the needs for the child so she can have the best quality of life possible and opportunity to meet her potential.

■ An abundance of information about kids with Mito exists online at www.MitoAction.org/education.

■ Don't go it alone. Make the effort to connect with other parents of kids with Mito or with similar special needs. Additionally, take a stand as a team player with your child's teachers, doctors, nurses, and community. You know your child best. When you have concerns, speak up!

7

Adults with Mitochondrial Disease

If you, your spouse, or your adult child has mitochondrial disease, chances are that you feel as if you are a needle in a haystack. Life as an adult living with Mito can be lonely and isolating since many of your friends and family members will have never heard of the disease, and because your symptoms are often not visible to others.

The mental battle against mitochondrial disease is also exhausting. Everything emotional and physical about mitochondrial disease for you as an adult patient leads back to fatigue and very likely a feeling of hopelessness. Unlike your friends or family who may have faced a battle against cancer and won, there is no "end" for which we can rally. Fighting for a cure, a period of remission, a chance at survival gives us strength and encourages our optimism that there is light at the end of the tunnel. This hope gives survivors of terrible diseases incredible resolve to endure periods of horrible nausea, hospitalizations, pain, alopecia, etc. But if you have mitochondrial disease, or if your spouse is affected, it may feel like there is no hope. There is no end-point in sight, no light at the end of the tunnel, and life can become a blur of days that are generally no good.

Unfortunately, there is no team around to cheer for you if you have mitochondrial disease, especially if you're an adult. The lack of coordinated care is a result of Mito's complexity and variety of symptoms, and a general lack of awareness. This makes Mito a disease that is difficult to diagnose, difficult to treat, and difficult for the medical system to support. Today's medical system uses a compartmental approach based on

BEN

I'm Ben, and I was diagnosed with Kearns Sayre Syndrome in my forties. I was slightly asthmatic, uncoordinated, and rather weak in my childhood and teens, which my family attributed to lack of effort. Around age sixteen, I developed ptosis (drooping eyelid) in my left eye. Looking back, those were my first real symptoms of mitochondrial disease.

In my thirties, I underwent surgery to address the ptosis in my left eye, which was now disabling. I battled months of eye infections, depression, and general lack of interest and good health. At the time I thought that my problems were my own fault, and everyone around me told me that I just needed to try harder. In hindsight, most of those problems were also symptoms of my mitochondrial disease.

When my father developed Myasthenia Gravis in my forties, I arranged a consultation with a neurologist. The neurologist took a biopsy from my left shoulder and diagnosed me with Kearns Sayre Syndrome (KSS). He sent me to the hospital library for information on the condition. There was none.

Within two years, I couldn't work. I'd had a major metabolic "crash" after moving some furniture and carpets one weekend and was laid up for days. My symptoms have progressed quite a bit since diagnosis and I am considerably weaker and certainly feel more fragile than I ever did before.

diagnostic tests, diagnostic and descriptive codes, and treatment endpoints. For the adult Mito patient who is self-advocating through the medical maze, nothing fits. The diagnosis is complex, difficult to obtain, and, in a shocking majority of cases, remains "suspected" or "probable." Yes, that means more than 50 percent, so if you're in this category don't let anyone tell you that you're hard to categorize. Diagnostic and descriptive codes for mitochondrial disease are obscure; in fact, insurance companies didn't create billable codes for the diagnosis until the 1990s. Beyond the initial testing in order to obtain a diagnosis, additional tests (MRI, blood tests, exercise tolerance tests, CT scans, EEG, sleep study, etc.) may be desirable but the benefit isn't always a) clear, or b) easy to justify for a disease with no endpoint or treatment plan. To the medical system, there is not a plan for patients with mitochondrial disease, and this is especially messy for adults who have complex and varied symptoms that are tiresome for the medical community to interpret. It's human nature, especially in our society in the United States, to focus on the goal, the cure, the victory, and the moment we can get back to the way things used to be…or better. But, what do we do, how do we cope, if this isn't a realistic scenario? We redefine what it means to live. We make an energy budget and learn to savor the moments worth recognizing rather than struggling for maximum gain.

This is your goal: LIVE. Mitochondrial disease is a diagnosis, not a death sentence. It is a lifelong condition that will force you to decide where you want and need to spend your energy. You and your partner are your best advocates. You can be happy and you can learn to make the most of the energy that you have so that you can do the things that you enjoy.

ASMA

*A*sma is a volunteer advocate and has two teen children who are both affected by mitochondrial disease. After years of navigating the healthcare system and teaching dozens of doctors, teachers, therapists, and nurses about her children's needs due to their condition, she was recently diagnosed with cancer, a devastating setback for her family, but one that ultimately she was well prepared to take on.

Asma was awed and surprised at the outpouring of structured support she received. She said of a three-day hospital stay, "They were offering me free nutrition advice, counseling, support groups, home visits, medical supplies...heck, they even offered me free massage in my home! I looked the social worker in the eye and I said, "I have been trying to get just one of these things to be offered, much less paid for, for years for my kids with Mito!" For Mito patients, the challenges of their diagnoses are complicated by the lack of awareness and treatment regimen that some other diseases may have. The exhausted patient has to be her own cheering squad.

Much of what you knew before your diagnosis may need to be redefined. It won't be easy, but it is possible. I can tell you that with confidence because I am privileged to know many, many adults with mitochondrial disease that have meaningful lives, relationships with their families and friends, and find purpose and strength in sharing their story with others.

Three Types of Adult Mito Patients

In my work educating physicians, patients, and families about managing mitochondrial disease, I have found that there are generally three types of adult Mito patients. While many of your daily challenges are the same, the process by which you came to a diagnosis of mitochondrial disease as an adult greatly influences your point of view as well as your resources.

1. The young adult who has outgrown their pediatrician—and their prognosis.

Twenty years ago there were a handful of pediatric geneticists who understood and were able to clinically diagnose mitochondrial disease. Parents of these children were often told, "Your child is the only person in the world with this form of mitochondrial disease." The first case of mitochondrial disease was described in the medical literature in the late 1960s and, in those early case studies, broad statements about the condition were made. Pediatricians and geneticists of this era held a few beliefs about mitochondrial disease that have since been debunked—by the patients if not the scientists. These beliefs include:

- that mitochondrial disease is a genetic condition, always inherited from the mother,
- that the hallmark characteristic of a mitochondrial defect is neurological devastation that is apparent clinically (the patient has extraordinary physical and mental disabilities) and on MRI (the brain appears patchy or has classic lesions in the gray matter and the basal ganglia),
- that children with a mitochondrial defect cannot live to be more than ten years old.

These beliefs are based on a crucial fact: *Only the most clinically severe and interesting cases are described when a disease is first discovered.* It takes years—fifty or more—for the epidemiology (the descriptive evidence about who has a disease, how often it shows up, and why people get it) to evolve. In the case of mitochondrial disease, the disorder is so complex that this process is still not where it should be, as the mitochondria are in many ways a mystery that has a potential impact on every element of disease and aging yet to be discovered.

Teens and young adults with mitochondrial disease have disproven the medical explanations of the 1960s, '70s, and '80s. I can joyfully report that I have encountered dozens of teens and young adults who have lived longer than their parents ever dreamed. They are going to college, they are artists, they are hopeful that they can pursue a degree in medicine, and all of them face incredible challenges and an ongoing battle with their Mito symptoms. But they are *alive* nonetheless, and they are the heroes who offer hope to the parents of babies and children struggling to make sense of the diagnosis.

However, if you are one of this group of patients, you face your own crisis. The vast majority of metabolic, neurology, and genetic specialists who sub-specialize in mitochondrial disease were trained as pediatricians. They have tiny exam tables, jungle animals on the walls of their clinics, and coloring books and cartoons in their waiting rooms. Their offices are not equipped to handle adult patients, and more and more hospitals are not allowing the over-eighteen population to be seen by their pediatric doctors, even if those doctors have been following the patients for eighteen years! A group of displaced young adult patients with complex medical histories and special needs have been "released" by their pediatricians only to be unable to find another physician who will take them as a new patient. The end of this chapter suggests strategies that help young adult patients and their parents advocate for the opportunity for ongoing support and medical care.

2. The middle-aged patient, usually female, with a maternal mitochondrial DNA mutation inheritance (mtDNA) that her children exhibit also.

Often, this type of patient can look back and recognize symptoms or issues that were never severe enough to warrant a diagnosis earlier in her life. Sometimes these women are diagnosed during or after a pregnancy when the stress of childbearing worsens their health and exacerbates their symptoms, creating an environment where the healthy mitochondria are no longer able to compensate for the lack of energy produced by their dysfunctional counterparts. Common symptoms during this type of adult onset may include extreme fatigue, muscle weakness, extremely frequent vomiting, difficulty maintaining normal blood pressure or heart rate, dizziness, and mental fog that is worse than even the most troublesome "normal" pregnancy. In other situations, Mom may require bed rest during pregnancy, and it is only after the birth of her baby (often a second or third child, when fatigue is truly inescapable) that advanced mitochondrial disease progression begins. It is not uncommon for these women to share in retrospect that they have been "dealing" with these symptoms for a long time, sometimes for years, and that only when their baby began the diagnostic process did they too get a diagnosis.

In this situation, help from social services and your community is critical to your health. This is one of the most difficult aspects of maternally inherited mitochondrial disease. How can you take care of your children when you are also affected by the same disease? As a mom living with Mito and caring for a potentially sick child, the parenting advice to "apply your own oxygen mask before assisting others" couldn't be more relevant. It is often easier to get state funded nursing hours for your child than it is for yourself, and you should plan to take advantage of every offer from organizations, church, friends, and family to help you with your children. For many families, this situation requires a serious reality adjustment about what you and your family can or cannot do. You will probably find it most helpful to be upfront and honest with your community about the challenges that you and your children face; others are more likely to help if they understand tangible ways that they can make your life easier and why something as simple as grocery shopping can be exhausting for you.

3. The otherwise healthy man or woman (frequently, but not always, in his or her forties or fifties) who is shocked when devastating neuromuscular symptoms don't get better.

What a challenge you face if this is the path by which you have arrived at the land of mitochondrial disease! Imagine a slow but steady onset of confusing symptoms that are seemingly unrelated. This group of patients often suffers from cognitive function or memory loss in addition to fatigue and muscle pain. It can be speculated that the frustrating *"now where did I leave my keys?"* that happens naturally with aging can be blamed on tired and aging mitochondria, which cannot fuel the synapses or connections of the brain as well as they used to. When you look at this group of adult patients, their symptoms are often difficult to describe as they seem to affect just about every body system, *but these folks don't always* <u>look</u> *sick*. As the primary care physician is listening to you describing mental fog, extreme fatigue, muscle pain, ringing in the ears, dizziness, nausea, reflux, inability to exercise without near collapse, unexplained weight gain or weight loss, vision loss, hearing loss, etc. it is not too difficult to imagine that you could be unfairly judged a hypochondriac, depressed, attention-seeking, or, well, crazy. After all, no disease can affect every part of the body, right?

If we step back and think about energy production and the role that the mitochondria play in converting food into fuel for the body's organs to function, then the array of symptoms makes sense. Every light in your house goes dim when there is not enough power. There may be more lights in the office of the house, so the office seems the darkest, but it is as equally affected as the laundry room, which is tiny and has one light bulb. The brain, muscles, and digestive system require the most "power" for proper functioning (imagine all that goes into play just for every organ to do its job to digest a banana!) and are frequently the most visibly affected by declining mitochondrial function.

It is important to note that an overwhelming number of adult patients report a "tipping point" that they identify as the trigger for the onset of the mitochondrial dis-

CECILIA

My name is Cecilia and I suffer from Complex IV, COX, with Leukodystrophy. In 2001 I had a year of seemingly unrelated symptoms that escalated into complete atrophy after a bout of pneumonia. After that, I cycled between bouts of complete atrophy to moderate quadrepresis. I took short-term disability from my job as a physical therapist until I began suffering severe dementia a few months later.

The more I did, the worse I got, and I was only thirty-seven years old. I was the director of a physical therapy clinic with twenty-seven employees, and had always been athletic and very healthy. Prior to that year, I ran marathons, competed in triathlons, and cycled fifteen miles every day. My onset was very sudden and catastrophic; I was never able to return to work, and I am currently on disability and social security. My life is completely different than it used to be.

After two months in the hospital, an MRI determined I had bilateral symmetrical leukodystrophy and I was airlifted to Cleveland Clinic in Ohio, twelve hours away from my hometown. A month later, I was discharged and sent home to the care of my family with complete amnesia and severe dementia. By Christmas my amnesia lifted and I gradually improved, although I was not expected to recover or live.

For the next two years, I spent most of my time in rehabilitation, which included speech therapy, neuropsychology, physical therapy, general conditioning, and being studied for a diagnosis. I made very, very slow progress. My symptoms were very severe.

Finally, in 2006 I had a muscle biopsy and I was officially diagnosed with Mitochondrial Disease COX complex IV deficiency. I have two teenagers and a husband that are learning to understand the complexity of Mito and its lifelong impact on individuals and their families. I'm very passionate about advocacy and what people like me can do now to help improve the lives of people with Mito, their families, and those seeking diagnosis.

ease. There is really no research to support or describe this phenomenon, but having worked with hundreds of adult patients over the last several years, I believe that there is a remarkably similar trend that emerges from their stories. A period of stress, heat stroke, a surgery (especially one that required general anesthesia), an illness (especially one that resulted in a prolonged fever or period of dehydration), menopause, or an injury can, upon careful reflection, be pinpointed as the "beginning of the end" for many middle-age patients. During a support group that I run for newly diagnosed adult Mito patients, I took an informal poll in which thirty-six out of forty of the participants noted a particular period of illness or a physiologically stressful event that seemed to precipitate the slow but unmistakable onset of symptoms that ultimately led them to a diagnosis of mitochondrial disease (often after years of testing and declining health). Perhaps in the future this will change the way we look at "routine" illness or surgery, especially if we know that a percentage of the normal population in our country is predisposed to mitochondrial myopathy.

Four Myths about Adult Mito Patients— and How to Set the Record Straight

Myth #1: "Mitochondrial disease is a childhood disorder."

Physicians of yesteryear were taught that mitochondrial disease was a childhood disorder. As a result, mitochondrial disease often doesn't even make it on the "differential," or the list of possible diagnoses, when an adult is being evaluated by his physician. Now before we blame anyone, let's figure out why this myth exists in the first place.

Doctors and nurses only know what they are taught, and until recently, mitochondrial diseases were often not included in the textbooks or curriculum for medical students unless they decided to sub-specialize in biochemistry and genetics. If they were addressed, it was always in the realm of pediatric genetics.

The literature is lacking. There are publications in professional journals that describe the genetic inheritance patterns of mitochondrial disease, describe devastating childhood cases, or that describe discoveries made about oxidative phosphorylation (see the Glossary and Chapters 2 and 10 for explanation of these terms) in mice, yeast, and other nonhuman things. Yet, there is a distinctive lack of large or population-based studies that describe cohorts, or groups, of real patients who are living and dealing with mitochondrial disease.

We need better advertising campaigns. Think about the commercials you might see when watching evening TV that advertises drugs that help patients with everything from Alzheimer's to asthma. There are few federally approved drugs and consequently a lack of pharmaceutical companies interested in marketing their drugs to medical professionals as well as the general public, and, sadly, no commercials (yet) for Mito.

The truth is that over half of *diagnosed* mitochondrial disease patients are children, and that many more children are being diagnosed each year as testing and awareness improves. However, there are thousands of adults who have mitochondrial disease, and there are likely many more adults that have been misdiagnosed or have conditions related to dysfunctional mitochondria.

Finding a specialist who is willing to see adult patients with mitochondrial disease can be challenging. I recommend a strategic approach, and that you find someone—your spouse, a friend, a parent, a sibling—who will be your ally and your advocate. This person should be able to make a commitment to attend medical appointments with you and be able to act on your behalf if you are ever unable to make your own decisions. Your advocate doesn't need to know all about mitochondrial disease but should be willing to learn with you along your journey, and most importantly, should really get to know what triggers your most devastating symptoms so that he can offer you the perspective and support needed to manage the daily challenges and help you make important decisions.

You, the adult living with Mito, are not alone, and it's important that you connect with other adult patients so you have a lifeline to people who understand what it means to be in your position. Use of the support section in Appendix C in this book should be a priority for you. Don't rule out the opportunity for support or friendship with parents of affected children as well, as you can learn so much from one another. Many children with mitochondrial disease are unable to talk, and you can help verbalize the symptoms that they may be feeling—a tremendous help to the parents. Likewise, parents can share with you strategies for treatment or support that may be more readily suggested in the pediatric world but that are helpful for you as well. A great example of this took place during an educational seminar that I was leading on the topic of pain in mitochondrial disease. Adult patients, spouses, and parents of affected children were all present. During our discussion, a very outgoing woman in her forties began to talk about her muscle pain, and that she had discovered that the pain in her legs was worse at night if she was even the least bit dehydrated. The parents there were eager to ask her questions like, "What does the pain feel like? Does it get better with massage, or with over-the-counter pain relievers? How long does the pain last? Does position make a difference?" Their children, unable to communicate effectively, were having the same nighttime pain but couldn't convey details helpful to their parents. Subsequently, a mother of a young child whose muscles were severely weak due to his mitochondrial disease began to talk about warm water swimming, and shared that she was able to get insurance coverage for "pool therapy" from her occupational therapist since the therapist was able to cite an orthopedic reason for the therapy. The adults patients in the group could benefit from warm water swimming too, and could use the same approach from their own therapeutic facility. It had never been offered to them by their doctor but there was no reason why there couldn't be a similar benefit. Mitochondrial disease is not just a childhood disease anymore.

SYDNEY

*H*i, my name is Sydney and I am twenty years old. I live in Nevada with my very supportive family. I have complex I, II, and probably V abnormalities. This currently manifests itself in general fatigue, muscle weakness, fairly poor food absorption, extreme temperature intolerance, and most likely I'm forgetting something.

In hindsight, I recognize there were a few signs of the disease even when I was little. I've always had trouble with hot and cold weather, and I would feel sick if I didn't get a full night of sleep at a sleepover. When I was thirteen, I started struggling with feeling really tired even with lots of sleep each night. A couple different doctors told me I was fine, so I figured everyone must feel this way. At the end of my junior year of high school I started really struggling with the orchestra rehearsals that I had been able to handle for years. That summer, I started going to many, many doctors. I thought that if I took care of my back pain, everything else would go away. After seeing the usual medley of doctors, I went to a doctor who said that my back pain was caused by insulin resistance and whipped my diet into shape. While the back pain did eventually go away, none of the other symptoms did.

Already homeschooled, I limped through my senior year. I went to college; it was a struggle to play cello and take eighteen credit hours my first semester. Halfway through second semester, I had a bout of not being able to move at all. In the nine months since then I've been doctor hopping and relearning how to live. I have been told that playing cello will not work with my body. My favorite thing about music has always been teaching private lessons, so I hope to one day become a tutor of something else.

Myth #2: "Exercise is impossible when you have Mito."

In fact, exercise intolerance is a hallmark characteristic of mitochondrial disease. Adult patients and children with Mito typically are unable to withstand intense physical activity, and often require more rest, oxygen, carbohydrates, and fluids following any physical activity. In other words, even VERY low-impact or small amounts of exercise can leave you feeling "wiped out," complaining of fatigue, shortness of breath, weakness, and an increased heart rate (tachycardia). As a result, for years doctors have recommended maintaining a low activity level to their Mito patients.

So, you think you get to be a couch potato because you have Mito? Not so fast. Turns out, a sedentary lifestyle may actually NOT be keeping your mitochondria functioning at their best. Recent studies published in the BioScience Reports (a publication of the Biochemical Society) in 2007 found that the mitochondrial function in muscle cells of people who were exercising was both more effective and more efficient. The idea of exercise training as a treatment for mitochondrial disease began after numerous research studies found beneficial effects of exercise on healthy mitochondria. However, the question remained: How will exercise impact patients with mtDNA defects?

The results are encouraging and should especially motivate adult patients to try to incorporate an exercise regimen into their weekly routines. Groups of mitochondrial disease patients who participated in twelve to fourteen weeks of regular exercise experienced an overall benefit as a result of their increased activity. The benefits were similar for patients participating in various types of exercise, including endurance training, aerobic conditioning, and resistance training. As a result, exercise is now being considered a possible therapeutic approach for people with mitochondrial defects. According to the published studies, exercising patients demonstrated a higher baseline activity tolerance, less deconditioning (loss of muscle tone and aerobic ability), and a better overall quality of life. Even more convincing, the beneficial effects experienced during the exercise training subsided when the exercise training was stopped. Mitochondrial function improves as a result of exercise, as shown by a better use of oxygen, nutrients, and efficient energy production.

However, if you have mitochondrial disease, it's still hard work. The theoretical and proven benefits of exercise don't change the hallmark characteristic of mitochondrial disease—fatigue. In fact, a benchmark variable of many clinical trials for patients with mitochondrial disease is improvement in exercise tolerance—and "exercise" for adults with Mito is NOT the same "exercise" that other gym-going adults engage in. Exercise here means consistent activity that helps to improve your overall baseline (i.e., the amount of activity that can be typically tolerated without experiencing negative symptoms, such as extreme fatigue, pain, shortness of breath, etc.), and includes walking, paddling around in a pool, stretching, and light resistance exercises.

Nonetheless, the idea of exercising as well as the exercise itself is really tough for many mitochondrial disease patients. Margaret Klehm, a nurse practitioner in a metabolic clinic in New England gives the following advice about exercise training: "Start slow, and be prepared to build up your tolerance very, very slowly," she says. "Endurance exercises, like swimming, walking, or stationary bicycling are best." Always stop the activity before you experience pain. Resistance exercises, like leg lifts or using resistance bands, are also useful and can be done in small amounts. Always HYDRATE! The mitochondria cannot work effectively without enough fluid and oxygen in the cell, so drinking plenty of low-sugar fluids before, during, and after any physical activity is critically important for an adult with Mito.

Be smart, but don't give up. The key to exercise if you have mitochondrial disease is to start slowly and be realistic about how much you can tolerate while slowly increasing the intensity and duration of the activity. For mitochondrial disease patients, doing this over time (months to years) can actually improve their baseline performance.

More research is needed, but the proven benefit of exercise to both mitochondrial function as well as ability to increasingly tolerate activity is encouraging to anyone who suffers from mitochondrial disease. Several publications have directly addressed the benefit of exercise for mitochondrial disease patients. Consult with your doctor and request physical therapy (more likely to be covered by your insurance) to create an exercise plan that makes sense, and plan to literally take it one step at a time.

Myth #3: "Keeping your job is the most important thing you can do for yourself."

You may be facing a difficult decision about how to financially support yourself or your family while balancing the energy demands and potential health toll of having a job. Working gives many people more than just a paycheck; it can be a way to find gratification, and may be an important part of their identity. When faced with the challenging symptoms of mitochondrial disease, many things, including if and how to keep a job, come into question.

Lee Rachel Jurman is a private disability advocate and case manager with Personal Disability Consulting, Inc. She helps adults living with disabilities and their families navigate the maze of public and private systems, and make informed decisions about living and working with disabilities, and I think she has great advice about the implications of deciding to work or not to work. She says that the decision to transition from full-time work to part-time work or to no work is highly charged. The common assumption among most professionals and patients alike is that work is good and that people want to work and need to work in order to get benefits. She suggests that adult patients facing difficult decisions about disability make the transition slowly. Begin by asking for workplace accommodations, then leave work in stages if it becomes necessary. This approach follows the advice of "planning for the worst but living the best," and hopefully gives you as much control as possible.

Though we cannot predict the future, we can prepare for it. Lee recommends some basic but important questions to ask when considering whether or not to work: *What has changed for me? What can I do? What can I no longer do? What do I know about the future?* To answer these questions, you must take an honest look at your personal situation. Because we are often not as objective as we should be, get help with this "taking stock" exercise. Family, friends, and professionals are all able to help in this task. Further, ask yourself: *Can I make myself sicker by working?* If yes, then you should make a change. *Have I put my job in jeopardy?* If yes, then again, a change is needed. Do not wait for others to make this choice for you (ahem, others such as your boss); you need to make the decision yourself. Give yourself a pop quiz:

- What is the price of working?
- Where have I been and where am I now?
- What is coming in the future?
- How many hours/day, days/week can I sustain?
- How much physical exertion does work require from me?
- How much mental exertion/stress is a result of my job?

Think about your own individual stamina and pain level as well as how much physical, mental, and emotional stress you can handle or *want* to handle. *What happens when you do too much? Can you pace yourself in your current job? Do you need to travel and does this add stress? Do you need breaks during the day or do you need a day off each week or several days each month?* Consider all of these as you decide whether or not to work. I recommend that you make a chart with the answers to your "taking stock" exercise and keep it so that you and your self-appointed advocate can dust it off periodically and assess what has changed. *Is working giving you energy, or depleting you?* For you, the adult with mitochondrial disease, this is a very important question.

There are obviously huge benefits of staying at work—self esteem, income, insurance, professional identity, etc. And likewise, there are consequences if you cannot work—isolation, loss of self worth, loss of income, and change in family role. But consider the fact that *not* working may give you an opportunity to do new things within the limits of your chronic illness.

Myth #4: "Your doctor knows more about your diagnosis than you do."

How we wish that were true! But alas, we're not in Oz and your doctor is not the wizard. In reality, even if you are one of the lucky few who has an outstanding doctor who is very experienced with mitochondrial disease, the reality is that your doctor is not your best advocate. YOU are.

One of the most challenging aspects of mitochondrial disease is that every patient's symptoms are a little different, and, to compound the confusion, your Mito symptoms likely fluctuate day to day and week to week, based on a whole host of factors. Your doctor cannot possibly keep track of this degree of detail for you and every other patient that he has, no matter how great of a physician he may be. You know yourself best, and you live with your disease every day. Become a "Mito meteorologist" and track your symptoms every day just like professionals track the weather. You can learn your own forecast and adjust accordingly. Looks like rain? Pack an umbrella. Spent Monday too busy with work, family, doctor's appointments, etc. and missed the opportunity to rest? Be prepared to have plenty of fluids and bed rest on Tuesday to give your mitochondria a chance to regenerate. Predictability can help us to cope.

We know by now that there is the likelihood that multiple organ systems may be affected as a result of your mitochondrial disease. To compound that fundamental complexity, we all agree that there is a lack of awareness about Mito. One might even go so far as to say that there are misconceptions about mitochondrial disorders (i.e., the disease only affects children, or that a patient must be neurologically devastated in order to have Mito). At best, the healthcare system is not very supportive of patients who live with chronic diseases, and at worst, it may be destructive. The responsibility of coordinating multiple specialists becomes a challenge and frequently is delegated to the patient or caregiver himself.

Know Your Priorities: Special Thoughts Just for Adult Patients

Why is it so difficult for adult patients with mitochondrial disease to feel supported? In part, I believe that this is related to the burden of care which, if you are an adult patient, often falls on your own shoulders. Many adult patients are struggling with grief at a very deep, emotional level while simultaneously dealing with not feeling well. The grief that you may feel (this is true for spouses as well) is very much justified. You may feel as if your future has vanished and that there is nothing but uncertainty ahead. In addition, adult patients are often accustomed to being able to make their own decisions. However, when you have Mito, you are often forced to substantially rely on other people. You may no longer be able to "do it all" or to even take care of your own basic needs. This can be incredibly frustrating. Adults with Mito are also grieving the loss of their dreams and their identity, especially when their disease takes away their ability to work and earn an income or career recognition. Some adult patients confess that they feel cornered and are very resentful of all that the disease has taken away from them. They feel that children get more support, and don't feel validated by the medical community or even by their own family.

First and foremost, your feelings are valid. It *is* hard to be an adult patient with mitochondrial disease, and to not acknowledge that would be dishonorable. Give the freedom to yourself to grieve. Give yourself permission as well to let go. When you are dealing with so much, it can feel like a slap to encounter people who seem not to care or understand your suffering. Give yourself the power to choose to forgive.

Dare to ask yourself: What will mitochondrial disease give me? It will give you incredible strength. It will teach you to fight for yourself. It will teach you to step back and think critically. It will teach you that some people are not worth your energy, and it will teach you to get comfortable with yourself. You will learn to read your own body, and to trust yourself and your instincts. You will learn to find value in people and things that others overlook. You will learn to say "no" and to say "thank you." You will become your own best advocate. It is my hope that one day you will be able to say that you learned more about yourself by having mitochondrial disease than if you had not.

You are not alone in this journey. Further, no one can predict your future. Those who are coping the most successfully with their mitochondrial disease diagnosis have this to say: *"A diagnosis of mitochondrial disease forced me to make choices. It immediately eliminated all the silly stuff because I simply don't have and can't afford wasting my energy on it. I conserve my energy so that I can do the things that I want to do, that I must do, or that my family needs me to do so that I feel whole as a person. It was only when I accepted that I had a limited amount of energy and that it was my choice how I could use it, did I begin to live with Mito."*

Key Points from This Chapter

■ Adults get mitochondrial disease too, although for many years Mito was thought to be a "childhood" disorder. Some adults may have had "soft signs" of Mito their entire lives, while others may experience a sudden onset. Sometimes adult patients can identify an event that seemed to trigger the onset of their symptoms, such as a major illness, surgery, or pregnancy.

■ Adults with Mito face some unique challenges that are different from those of children and parents.

■ Dealing with symptoms and being your own advocate can be overwhelming—get a partner to accompany you to appointments and who would be able to speak on your behalf if necessary.

■ Mito is not just a childhood disease, and can affect adults of all ages, races, and genders.

■ Connecting with others who have Mito or similar chronic conditions is very important for your emotional well-being.

■ Exercise is a very important aspect of improving quality of life for adults with Mito. Although very difficult, even a very low-impact and consistent exercise regimen can dramatically improve a person's baseline, and help him feel better.

■ Taking care of a family, working, and taking care of yourself is all very overwhelming for most adult Mito patients. Consequently, adults with Mito have some tough decisions to make about work, sharing responsibilities, and managing symptoms.

■ Give yourself freedom to grieve, forgive, and let go of other's expectations so you can focus on what really makes you happy.

8

Autism and Mitochondrial Disease: Special Challenges and the Diagnosis Debate

"Who in the world am I? Ah, that's the great puzzle."
—Lewis Carroll

Autism spectrum disorder (ASD, or "autism" as it is sometimes referred to in this book) is a developmental disorder characterized by speech delays and difficulties with social interactions and communication skills. The Autism Society of America estimates that 1 to 1.5 million children and adults are autistic in the United States, and that the number affected grows exponentially each year. There are many debates about what causes autism, but there is growing evidence that there are a percentage of children with autism who have a mitochondrial defect at the root of their developmental and behavioral disability.

Doctors, like Dr. Marvin Natowitcz of the Cleveland Clinic, are beginning to speculate that there are triggers that act as the catalyst for the onset of autistic symptoms in children who have been labeled autistic but have an undetected energy metabolism defect. This interaction may explain many parents' persistent sense that vaccines caused their children's autism, as well as science's widely accepted conclusion that the evidence for causality is lacking. The administration of multiple simultaneous vaccines does not *cause* autism directly, but it may trigger symptoms by destroying the body's ability to compensate for an underlying mitochondrial defect. Organs, like the brain, require significant amounts of energy (in the form of ATP) and are vulnerable targets to the effects of dysfunctional energy metabolism, such as Mito causes. As a result, many Mito sufferers can experience atypical neurological functioning. Any physiologic stress such as illness or a routine childhood surgery has the potential to reveal an underlying mitochondrial defect; vaccines are only the most talked about possibility. A group, or cohort, of children is being identified with a primary mitochondrial disorder with features of autism. (Primary mitochondrial disease implies that the ASD features are secondary to or can be considered a symptom of a primary mitochondrial defect.) Studies published over the last decade estimate that anywhere from 4 to 20 percent of children with autism or an autism spectrum disorder can attribute their symptoms to an energy metabolism defect. However, estimates are difficult, given that the actual incidence for both ASD and Mito are not well-defined.

These findings are just beginning to infiltrate the community of parents of autistic children and are not even fully recognized by the medical community despite a flurry of recent research and related publications. Ultimately, if you are a parent of a child who is on the autism spectrum and you are dealing with additional unexplained medical issues, you should learn more about mitochondrial disease.

The vaccine debate is contentious and very emotional for angry parents and for doctors who rightly feel that vaccines are one of the most astounding achievements of medicine. Children with Mito are very delicate, and no parent or doctor can be expected to protect them from every potential stressor. The most important point is that sudden onset of autistic symptoms following a physiologic stressor is one indicator of an underlying mitochondrial susceptibility. The approach to diagnosis and treatment path that you decide to follow may be different if your child has a mitochondrial disease *and* autistic symptoms. Dealing with either of these diagnoses is a struggle, and to deal with both can be exceptionally stressful for everyone involved.

The Chicken or the Egg?

For years, parents of some children with confirmed mitochondrial disorders have described features of autism as part of their child's clinical "Mito" presentation. Now, parents of children with a primary autism diagnosis are being evaluated for mitochondrial disease. Parents long to know whether Mito might be a potential cause of autism or whether the conditions might be related in some other complex way.

No one has a definitive answer, and speculation and disagreement on the subject abounds. However, a few points emerge:

1. There is a relationship between the two conditions in some children. Some children with autism spectrum disorders have a mitochondrial defect known as impaired oxidative phosphorylation. It causes ineffective energy production. Other types of mitochondrial disorders (such as those that are inherited from mtDNA) are considered rare in children with autistic disorders.

2. Not all children with autism have mitochondrial disease, and not all children with Mito have autism. Clinicians and researchers disagree on the percentage of individuals who have a coexisting diagnosis.

3. The majority of physicians and public health clinicians strongly refute any relationship between vaccines and autism, yet there is an undercurrent of concern and disagreement in the parent population that must be acknowledged. All the physicians that I consult in my work emphatically agree that vaccination is imperative, because the illnesses they prevent would be disastrous, potentially fatal, for children with Mito. However, the fever and immune system stress that are potential consequences of vaccines can exacerbate an underlying (unknown) mitochondrial disorder. A key point is that the fever or the immune response—not the vaccine—is the trigger, and children with an underlying Mito disorder may develop symptoms in response to *any* fever, illness, or stress.

4. More research, large population studies, and discussion are needed. (Of course, everyone agrees about that!) Unfortunately, there are substantial obstacles—a research trial involving deprivation of vaccines to a control group of children would be unethical, and unwise!

There are many reasons why there have not been sufficient studies at this point to help parents definitively understand the relationship between autism and mitochondrial disease. Diagnosis of mitochondrial disease is complex, and in order to be accurate must include a combination of specific clinical features, laboratory findings, and defective "enzymology" determined by DNA sequencing (more about diagnosing Mito in Chapter 2). Diagnosis of autism is also complex; in fact, autism is being described by parent advocacy groups as "a puzzle." Even to simply compare the brains of children with autism to those with mitochondrial disease, researchers need permission to anesthetize children for brain scans (a risk for any child, and a heightened risk for the child with mitochondrial disease).

Despite the urgency felt by both the autism and mitochondrial disease communities, there are complex yet subtle relationships that must be teased out over a long period of time through rigorous and careful studies. While we recognize that there is a relationship between the two conditions, many of the specifics and the current recommendations are fuzzy. As a result, the path that each family chooses remains very individualized, and is often based quite a bit on parents' ability to interpret information, navigate the healthcare system, pay for additional testing, the relationship they may have with their child's doctor, and the recommendations of friends or teachers.

Research and studies of groups of patients are providing the community with descriptive data about autism and mitochondrial disease, but the answers are still not as clear as we hope they will be in the future. In the words of a mother struggling to make sense of her son's symptoms, "When it is your child who is affected, you don't like the pace of science." In the meantime, I will focus in this chapter and throughout the book on managing daily challenges and finding quality of life with mitochondrial disease.

How Do I Know If My Child with Autism Also Has Mitochondrial Disease?

The response to this question is all too often, "Talk to your child's doctor." Obviously, if you are a parent of a child who has multiple behavioral, developmental, and health issues, you are most likely already in regular contact with your child's doctor; now might be the time to ask about Mito. Unfortunately, the number of patients in need of a specialist who understands mitochondrial disease outnumbers the number of physicians who are equipped to manage these patients. This becomes even further complicated if you are seeking a physician who understands mitochondrial disease *and* autism! Despite these obstacles, I have found that the passion and determination that YOU, the parents of these special kids, possess is extraordinary. You are amazing champions for your children.

Markers of Mitochondrial Disease in Children with Autism as a Primary Diagnosis

The possible relationship between metabolic disorders, elevated lactic acid levels, and features of autism spectrum disorder has been described in the medical literature since the early 1990s. In fact, much research exploring the correlation between ASD (autism spectrum disorder) and mitochondrial dysfunction has been published throughout the last decade.

A 2008 cooperative cohort study from the Cleveland Clinic, the Kennedy Krieger Institute, and Massachusetts General Hospital sought to describe the most common features that coexist in children who have both autism and documented mitochondrial dysfunction. A cohort study takes a small sample (i.e., twenty-five children) that could be considered "representative" of the population in question and investigates each study participant in great detail. The results of a cohort study are often generalized to the broader population. This is especially common in the early phases of a disease's research, when larger groups of patients are not readily identified or available to participate in a trial. This study has been instrumental in helping parents and healthcare providers to identify "red flags," or reasons to suspect mitochondrial disease in a child who also has ASD or PDD-NOS.

Let's take a look at some key findings from the study that are relatively easy to identify and that make these children, who have **both** diagnoses, different than children who "only" have autism:

1. Children in the study who had a primary diagnosis of autism and a subsequent diagnosis of an electron transport chain defect (a.k.a. mitochondri-

al disorder) had one or more major clinical abnormalities <u>atypical</u> for autism. *Plain English: The first red flag is the presence of additional, atypical, unrelated "chronic medical issues" in kids who are autistic. Sometimes we refer to kids in this category as having "atypical autism" or "autism plus."*

2. Children in the study who had autism and a history of nonneurological medical problems were more likely to have an underlying metabolic defect. *Plain English: If your child with ASD is sick, has an unusually difficult time recovering from common childhood illnesses, has had a chronic or acute medical condition, or has other "unrelated" medical problems such as severe gastric dysmotility, this is a red flag.*

3. Constitutional symptoms, such as excessive fatigability, were present in 75 percent of the children studied who had autism <u>and</u> a mitochondrial defect. *Plain English: Kids who are tired all the time, have difficulty recovering from an activity, decline during the course of a day, or resist activity or communication with others more often when tired should be investigated further for mitochondrial disease. Fatigue is a hallmark characteristic of Mito, not of autism.*

4. Marked delay in early gross and fine motor milestones and unusual patterns of regression occurred in over one-third of children studied. *Plain English: Loss of skills, including speech, ability to walk or perform fine motor tasks like tying shoes or fastening a button, especially following any fever, illness, or period of unusual stress is a red flag. In addition, babies who missed early milestones, such as crawling, sitting, eating solid foods, talking, and walking, could be experiencing that delay as a result of an energy metabolism defect.*

5. Laboratory findings that were consistently abnormal in the children studied who had autism and subsequently confirmed mitochondrial disease include elevated blood lactate, elevated plasma alanine, and elevated serum ALT/AST. *Plain English: Before taking your child to a specialist or pursuing a muscle biopsy, some additional information can be obtained through simple blood tests. Lactic acid levels are elevated in the majority of all patients who have mitochondrial disease, therefore this is a big indication that there could be an underlying metabolic issue beyond a child's autism.*

Markers of Mito-Autism

A small number of population studies describe a surprisingly large number of patients with a diagnosis of ASD who were also found to have abnormalities in lactic acid or pyruvic acid levels. While elevated lactic acid is a marker of mitochondrial disease in the general population, it is not considered a *definitive* finding for diagnosis. Some people with certain types of mitochondrial disease, particularly the mtDNA mutations, may or may not have elevated lactic acid levels. However, the studies looking specifically at children with ASD and suspected mitochondrial disease show that abnormal lactic acid, pyruvic acid, or lactate/pyruvate ratios were relatively common and are considered a "red flag" warranting further testing. The simplest explanation behind the frequent elevation of lactic acid in the blood for all people with mitochondrial defects is that lactic acid is a by-product of the breakdown of glucose in the cell. Abnormal mitochondria aren't effectively breaking down and using all the "parts" from the glucose once broken down, so lactic acid accumulates in the blood. These abnormalities (high levels of metabolic by-products such as lactate and alanine) are markers of a disorder of energetics (energy metabolism), which is a mitochondrial function.

So, how can we translate a patient's lab findings, such as lactic acid levels, to the presence of mitochondrial disease? We must recognize that such findings do not *independently* correlate with mitochondrial disease. In fact, there continues to be debate about the diagnostic criteria and testing methods in order to accurately identify a mitochondrial disorder. In other words, the presence of an elevated lactic acid *without other clinical signs*, such as fatigue, digestive issues, muscle pain or weakness, does not stand alone as a marker for mitochondrial disease.

To some degree, this muddies the waters even further. According to the current *Diagnostic and Statistical Manual of Mental Disorders* (DSM-IV), Autistic Disorder is diagnosed by the presence of multiple characteristics and behaviors under the broader umbrella of Pervasive Developmental Delay (PDD). (More recently, the term PDD has been replaced by the expression "autistic spectrum disorder," or ASD for short.) Mito-

JAMIE

My son Jamie is four years old and has been diagnosed now with epilepsy, autistic traits, asthma, developmental delays, hypotonia, dyspraxia, and GERD. Yet, I've felt, and so has our pediatrician, that we haven't figured out Jamie completely. We are in the early process of working with a Mito specialist and a geneticist who shares our concern that an oxidative phosphorylation defect may be at the root of Jamie's issues.

What an understatement to say that we have had a difficult time getting all the professionals on the same page! Our neurologist will not say autism, the developmental pediatrician will not say Mito, the school system will not say anything, but his pediatrician, whom we have known for ten years, says he is definitely on the autism spectrum, as does his private speech therapist and his occupational therapist. After a year of back and forth with the school system and requesting private evaluations, Jamie receives speech, OT, and has a special education teacher who visits his preschool, but we still don't have a real diagnosis or any idea what the future looks like for him.

chondrial disease is associated with either a spontaneous or genetic mutation in the DNA, but is slippery to diagnose because there are different types of mitochondria present in different areas of the body (i.e., muscle, skin, blood, heart, kidneys, etc.). To assign BOTH of these diagnoses in cooperation with one another adds such complexity that only the most dedicated pediatricians or primary care doctors are able to steer the diagnostic process. To add further confusion to an already confounding diagnostic process, the new *Diagnostic and Statistical Manual of Mental Disorders* (DSM-V) is slated to come out in 2013 and rather profound changes to the ASD diagnostic criteria are expected.

How can a parent know whether or not mitochondrial disease might be part of their child's autism diagnosis? The simplest response is that children with true idiopathic autism (autism with no known cause) do not typically have other health issues in conjunction with the hallmark developmental and behavioral symptoms of ASD.

The Growing Relationship Between Mito and Autism

Some people believe that autism is a neurological disorder that affects brain function, and that the brain of a person with autism is wired differently. Often, MRIs of brains (i.e., brain scans) show differences between children's brains who have autism and brains of typically developing children. There is additional speculation that autism is a genetic disease, as there is a higher tendency to have a child with autism when there is a family history, and a coexisting diagnosis of autism is common with many genetic diseases, such as Down's syndrome, Fragile X syndrome, and Prader-Willi syndrome. Still, others feel that the environment and that environmental toxins or toxic levels of metals, preservatives, or other harmful products found in the air, the earth, or in vaccines are the reasons that the number of children affected by autism is at an alarming high. Similarly, there are many who feel that autism is caused by an allergic reaction, and that allergies to certain foods or types of food (i.e., dairy, wheat, corn syrup) cause an allergic response or abnormal immune reaction in a child, which dramatically affects her development and behavior.

The bottom line is that there is obviously not solid agreement about the cause of autism. In addition, the symptoms that occur, and that often occur at such a young age in a child's life, are very troubling for parents and require significant effort to understand and to manage. Not unlike mitochondrial disease, autism is puzzling and is characterized by behaviors (or symptoms, in the case of Mito) that are atypical or don't make sense. When the hallmark feature of a condition is the confusion it causes for parents and other observers, it makes classification, diagnosis, treatment, and acceptance one thousand times more challenging.

Despite the confusion, there is clear evidence from several perspectives that there definitely exists a group of children with ASD who have mitochondrial disease. In the review article published in 2010 in *Developmental Disabilities Review* (a medical journal), Dr. Richard Haas of University of California, San Diego summarizes the evidence of the co-occurrence of ASD and Mito. Based on epidemiological evidence from published studies, approximately 4 percent of children with ASD are likely to have definite Mito disease, while another 5-8 percent have possible Mito disease (dysfunction that may be more difficult to diagnose). The concept that the two diagnoses co-exist is not new, but is increasingly gaining momentum and research interest as the diagnosis of mitochondrial disease continues to rise in the shadow of the autism boom. In fact, in publications as early as 1998, researchers claimed that marked abnormal mitochondrial function in some autistic children was evidence that the mitochondria could be the cause of inappropriate brain energy metabolism and subsequently be causing the behavioral and developmental symptoms of autism. Additional research in mitochondrial physiology has revealed a relationship between ASD and abnormal mitochondrial function.

What About Vaccines?

Do children with mitochondrial disease have a potential to develop autism or do children with autism have an underlying mitochondrial disorder? There is much speculation regarding the existence of a connection between childhood vaccinations and the onset of autism, but the scientific evidence does not exist at this time to infer a causal relationship between vaccines and autism, even in the known presence of mi-

SAMUEL

My son Samuel is nine and is being tested for Mito. When he was born he needed IV fluids because his blood sugar was very low. No one could figure out why. When he was five months old he contracted RSV and then struggled for months with several bouts of pneumonia. He has suffered from asthma since he was two months old. At age two he had 150 words and at age two and a half he lost them all. Just after his second birthday, he had a virus with a very high fever, which caused febrile seizures. After that initial illness he started to decline, and he continued to have seizures off and on until he was seven years old.

At age three, Nathaniel was diagnosed with autism. At age five he was diagnosed with colitis; he has never had a formed bowl movement in his entire life. At age eight he was diagnosed with type 1 diabetes. Now he suffers from bouts of fatigue; he seems tired just about all the time. His heart rate can range from the thirties all the way up to 188. He spends a good deal of time in the hospital. Most of the time, we (the doctors and his family) are just trying to figure out what is going on with him. Because of his autism, it makes it hard to figure out if he is in pain. We don't know if he doesn't feel the pain or if he just can't tell us. I wish I could help him.

tochondrial disease. The debate again centers around the risks—albeit risks that are often perceived differently by clinicians and parents. To allow a child to not be vaccinated presents the risk of serious infection; the consequences of these infections have been scientifically proven to be very dangerous, even deadly, especially to children with already weakened immune systems. At this time, there is no such evidence to the contrary, and to advise against vaccines would be putting your child, and society at large, at risk. The majority of clinicians are advising parents to vaccinate their children in order to protect them from diseases that would otherwise be life-threatening, *especially* if the child has a metabolic or mitochondrial disease. A childhood illness that could have been prevented by vaccine, such as the mumps, measles, chicken pox, or the flu, would be absolutely devastating for a child with a mitochondrial disorder.

Nonetheless, parents may still be worried about vaccines, or feel guilty or responsible for their child's symptoms, especially if your child began showing signs of autistic regression after her vaccinations. In truth, there are so many "what if's" in the life of a parent advocate! You are trying to be your child's best advocate while trusting the wisdom of doctors and experts involved in your child's care. You are faced with extraordinarily difficult decisions and exhausting situations every day. You are relentlessly your child's voice, your child's champion, your child's interpreter, and your child's healthcare manager. I want to encourage you to be strong in your convictions and follow your instincts. You know your child and the unique nuances of her condition better than anyone else.

However, if you are concerned about the risk of autistic regression and vaccinations for your child, here are some suggested preventive measures:

- Well before the day of the immunizations begin a discussion with your pediatrician about a staggered immunization schedule so that there isn't the opportunity to overload the body or trigger a fever;
- Don't overload your child with immunizations (i.e., more than two or three at one time) in order to "catch-up." It's better to space out the vaccines, waiting at least a month between administration of each batch;
- Reschedule vaccines if your child is sick, or has recently been sick and still isn't "back to normal." This is especially important if your child has had a fever or period of dehydration (from a stomach flu, for example) within the last seven days;
- Be sure your child is well fed and has had plenty of fluids in the twenty-four-hour period before the vaccination appointment;
- Reschedule the vaccines if your child has an unusual rash or diarrhea, even without any other symptoms;
- Consider pre-medicating your child with ibuprofen or acetaminophen prior to the vaccine (to hopefully prevent a possible fever);
- Aggressively avoid fever and dehydration after vaccinations, and don't hesitate to contact your child's doctor at *the first sign* of a temperature over 101 degrees, unusual refusal of food or drink, lethargy, or other unusual behavior.

Several studies have highlighted the risk of fever in children with autism and an OX-PHOS defect (the type of mitochondrial disorder that seems to be most common in children with ASD). In one such study, fever was directly linked as a cause of autistic-related regression (loss of developmental skills, such as speech, eye contact, and social skills) in over 60 percent of the children studied. None showed regression after vaccination unless fever occurred, implying that fever—as opposed to the vaccine itself—is the greater risk factor. This study demonstrates that patients with mitochondrial diseases have an increased risk of loss of skills in the presence of fever or other stressors, such as infection or dehydration. In other words, careful attention to fever management and metabolic support (through good hydration and nutrition) is more important in the child with Mito and ASD than in the child who only has autism. For parents struggling to make sense of the two diagnoses, this is one clear example of how the supportive management of the child who has an underlying mitochondrial disorder (suspected or definitive) needs to be different.

As parents who are navigating the healthcare system with a confusing diagnosis, we are becoming better advocates for our children, and out of necessity we are increasingly proactive about managing their healthcare. For patients with mitochondrial disease and autism, this begins with simple steps such as educating others about germs and good hand washing in order to prevent the spread of illnesses that would be harmful to our children, balancing energy outputs and being creative about structuring our child's day, or learning more about the type of mitochondrial abnormality you are facing. Using passion, we have to help these children. Parents need to join together to send a strong but diplomatic message to the scientific community of what is happening and what we need. The autism community has made great strides in building visibility and awareness over the past several years and the mitochondrial disease community is following in its footsteps.

DAN! Protocol: Overlapping Approaches to Treatment

The Autism Research Institute has developed a treatment approach designed to help reverse developmental and behavioral symptoms of autism called Defeat Autism Now! or DAN! An increasing number of DAN! practitioners are emerging, and the basis of their approach is called "biomedical treatments." The purpose of this chapter is not to educate parents about the DAN! approach, but instead to note the surprising similarities between the biomedical treatment protocol and the most common treatment plan for patients with mitochondrial disease. What parent isn't seeking answers for how to restore their child's health? For whatever reason, many parents are willing to try the DAN! approach, and I have found that the children who respond very well to it are often the same children who are later diagnosed with Mito. The DAN! protocol recommends a diverse collection of treatments that includes changes in diet, use of vitamins, supplements, essential fatty acids, probiotics, and amino acids, as well as chelation therapy and several others. Please note that some of these therapies are controversial and the purpose of this discussion is simply to highlight the overlap between approaches to treatment of both diagnoses.

Of greatest interest to parents concerned or confused about the overlap between an autism and mitochondrial disease diagnosis is the use of supplements in the DAN! protocol, which are administered to treat oxidative stress. Table 8.1 gives a comparison of supplements used for the two conditions.

Table 8.1 Comparison of Supplements Used In Mitochondrial Disease and ASD

Key: ■ frequently prescribed ● not often prescribed ▲ used sometimes		
Supplement	**Used in supporting mitochondrial disease**	**Part of the DAN! protocol for autism**
Co-enzyme Q10	■ used in high doses, typically 5-10 mg/kg	● no evidence of use
B-vitamins	■ especially folic acid and B1 (thiamine) & B2 (riboflavin)	■ especially B6 with Magnesium and B12
Antioxidants	■ vitamin C & E used frequently	■ vitamin C & E used explicitly to "decrease oxidative stress"
Carnitine	■ frequently used, often Mito patients have a carnitine deficiency as well	▲ used sometimes
Creatine	■ thought to improve muscle function	■ thought to be important because of ineffective metathione metabolism
Melatonin	■ used to help with sleep	■ used not only to help with sleep but also thought to be an important part of metathione metabolism
Probiotics	▲ not commonly prescribed, but not contraindicated	■ part of the DAN! protocol to increase immune/gut function
Gluten/Casein free diet	● unusual in children with primary Mito disease but more common in children with Mito and ASD. Some parents report that this makes a big difference in managing their child's neurological symptoms.	■ very common, and often a first-line approach

There is obviously some overlap between the supplements used in the DAN! approach and in a standard "Mito cocktail" (see Chapter 4). Many parents who are seeking answers about mitochondrial disease are familiar with the DAN! protocol but feel that the DAN! doctors are not yet in tune with approaches to treating mitochondrial disease. The striking similarities between the two regimens provide further evidence that there is a cohort of autistic children who respond to therapies that improve their energy metabolism and that decrease oxidative stress and who therefore are potentially more likely to have an OX-PHOS defect. Part of the theory behind use of the biomedical treatment approach to autism is that there is a preexisting weakness in the child's metabolism, and that the child has an inability to detoxify or use antioxidants to remove harmful toxins from the body. The same theory or rationale exists behind the use of the supplements in children (and adults) with mitochondrial disease, and is actually able to be even more targeted when the patient's energy metabolism defect is classified.

ALICE

My name is Alice and I have two young boys who have ASD and a diagnosis of mild OX-PHOS (mitochondrial disease). They have many symptoms of both disorders, including repetitive patterns of behavior (e.g., lining up puzzle pieces), lack of eye contact, eye darting, seeming disinterest in expressing physical affection, chronic diarrhea for two years, severe GI/gut dysfunction/slow GI motility, fatigue, and global delay. The boys have autistic tendencies that "flare up" at different periods in time, especially after a viral illness.

Personally, I would rather not say that a child is "diagnosed with autism." I would say the child is "labeled" autistic. I spend equal amounts of time listening to what people are talking about in both the Mito and autism worlds because I feel uncertain about what the future holds for my two boys. And no doctor can tell me. I am cautiously optimistic though and believe that a parent needs to be informed and know what both fields/ specialists are doing. I follow a DAN! protocol that also includes many supplements and doses recommended as part of the Mito cocktail and it has made a huge difference for both of my boys.

The people I have talked to about the Mito diagnosis are all confused. I try to call it a "disorder of energy production" and emphasize that the boys have historically been fatigued. That helps. Although, our four-year-old went through a period of significant over-activity/ hyperactivity, which really had his teachers confused.

Having the Mito diagnosis feels like a gift, for without it, I think my sons would be lost to me now. They were slipping away from me. The Mito cocktail and the GI/allergy/diet components of DAN! are managing my boys' symptoms at this time. I lose sleep at night thinking about all the children with ASD who are actually kids with undiagnosed OX-PHOS who could be making progress.

Hope for Progress

A great example and parallel to the connection between mitochondrial disease and autism can be found by looking at PKU (phenylketonuria). In the 1960s, Norwegian researchers followed a large group of children with PKU and found that more than 40 percent of PKU infants became autistic in childhood. There was eventually further research, and ultimately there was agreement within the scientific community that some children with PKU develop features of autism or ASD.

Today, there is a treatment for PKU that involves careful elimination of phenylalanine from the child's diet. The incidence of PKU at birth hasn't changed, but the incidence of autism developing in these patients is virtually nonexistent now because the underlying disease (PKU) can be immediately treated following detection by newborn screening. It is my hope that a similar development will occur for our children with autism and a primary mitochondrial disease; that one day it will be treatable.

Key Points from This Chapter

■ While clinicians continue to disagree about the percentage of individuals who have a co-existing diagnosis of ASD and Mito, there is growing evidence that there is a relationship between the two disorders. Based on the medical literature alone, the estimate of children who have ASD and an underlying mitochondrial disorder is anywhere from 4 to 20 percent. However, the most recent epidemiological information published in review articles more specifically suggests that about 4 percent of kids with ASD have a *definitive* mitochondrial disease, while approximately an additional 5 to 8 percent have a *probable or possible* mitochondrial defect.

■ Testing and diagnosis of Mito-autism is difficult, as the tests for each of these diagnoses are tricky and not always definitive. However, there are red flags which, when found in kids with an existing ASD diagnosis, should warrant further testing for a mitochondrial disorder. Some of these red flags include:
  • elevated lactic acid levels, and abnormalities in other metabolic screening tests such as lactate/pyruvate and serum ALT/AST;
  • muscle pain, muscle weakness, muscle fatigue;
  • generalized fatigue, complaints of being tired;
  • difficulty recovering from an illness, fever, or anesthesia; and
  • slow or difficult digestion, persistent nausea or constipation, reflux, and other unusual gastrointestinal disorders.

■ Vaccinations are a cause of concern for many parents, and some parents believe that vaccines caused the onset of skill regression associated with ASD in their child. For children with underlying mitochondrial defects (primarily defects in oxidative phosphorylation, or OX-PHOS), the immune response or fever associated with vaccines was most likely the "trigger" of the regression, and might have occurred in that child after any prolonged stress, such as a high fever, period of illness or dehydration, a surgery requiring anesthesia, and so on.

■ DAN! protocols recommend some of the same supplements that are used in the Mito cocktail to treat Mito patients.

■ The area of autism and Mito-autism has been the focus of much research in recent years and will hopefully help to provide better insight into the relationship between these two diagnoses.

9

Your Mito "Survival Kit"

Never do anything standing that you can do sitting,
or anything sitting that can be done lying down.
— Chinese proverb

All the specific recommendations about living with Mito can be condensed to one piece of advice: "Maximize your energy." Whether this relates to managing symptoms, preventive maintenance through rest or hydration, or working on attitude, it is our goal to be able to *live anyway* with the challenges inherent to this diagnosis. Conserving your energy, for you as an affected adult or for parents advocating for their children, takes place on many, many levels. Energy conservation is physical, emotional, and cerebral. It takes planning, patience, perspective, and persistence. You may be in awe of what you, your children, and your family can manage as years go by. However you handle it, know that you are not alone and it is a constant balancing act shared by every person affected by the disease.

If we could market a "Mito survival kit," what would be inside? A bottle of CoQ10, a network of friends and families to relate to, and practical advice like the following would be a great start!

Pack and Plan Ahead

All of us start out as "Mito rookies" and we all make the same mistake. We leave the house unprepared, wind up doing too much, and then crash. Parents share stories of taking off for the theme park only to watch their child with Mito get hotter, floppier, shakier, and less responsive as the day goes on until they are in a panic and are calling their doctor or going to the ER. Adult patients relate memories of being unable to get up off of the couch or out of bed the "day after" a normal activity like shopping and going out with friends. As we get more experienced, we learn better to pack, pace, and plan ahead.

A good rule of thumb is to always carry fluids (with electrolytes, ideally) and a snack with you. This is especially true of packing for clinic visits, as traffic is often an issue, appointments get delayed, tests get ordered, etc. More patients are left worn out and depleted from clinic appointments than most outings! Plan ahead, expect a delay, and pack extra of everything, including cash, snacks, fluids, medicines, electronics, back-up chargers, and reading material. Some people keep a bag packed and stashed in the car "just in case" with an extra dose of meds, toiletries, clothes, emergency letters, etc. Use a backpack with rolling wheels if you are advocating for yourself and potentially will become fatigued by managing the larger, heavier load. Always bring your child's stroller or wheelchair, even if he can walk short distances (you never know when you'll be sent to the center across the campus or in the opposite end of the hospital for an unexpected test). Likewise, anticipate that outings to special places like the zoo, theme parks, etc. will be more tiring than usual, and plan accordingly. If your affected child has healthy siblings, consider bringing along a friend or sitter who can "tag-team" with the other kids to give the affected child intermittent breaks. Anticipate that the fatigue level will worsen as the day progresses, so plan to do the priority activities first, just in case the others have to be put off.

At the first sign of fatigue (lack of attentiveness, shakes, pain, lethargy)—STOP. Take a break, rehydrate, eat a snack, and rest in a cool place for at least twenty minutes (again, plan ahead the day before where that cool resting spot will be). You can then try the activity again, but if fatigue persists and other symptoms (shaky hands, muscle pain, headache) begin, listen to the cues and stop for prolonged, quiet rest. This implies that adults may need a shorter work day, or need to rest for long periods during the day while children are at school in order to meet their needs in the evenings. Children may not be able to attend a full day of school, and outings/day trips may be shorter than expected. Anticipate travel time getting home as well. If you stay at the park another hour, what will happen on the ride home? For theme park trips, would it be worthwhile to stay at a hotel nearby in order to have a quality rest period during the day, making for an enjoyable and reenergized evening? The goal is to stay ahead of the fatigue, so that you have the opportunity to successfully recharge before the "mitochondrial battery" is totally empty.

Keep Good Records

The sheer volume of paperwork involved in the case history of a typical Mito patient is overwhelming, and could easily fill one or more file boxes. For many families, years of records accumulate, filling up closets and cabinets with test results, clinic notes, interpretations, insurance records, hospitalization notes, etc. Most patients and families prefer not to throw anything away for fear that it will be needed at a later time. However, boxes of medical records and test results, even if organized by year, do very little good for the average patient. I have yet to meet a physician who encourages patients to wheel thirty pounds of medical records into his office at their first appointment. On the other hand, without the patient's medical history, tests might be duplicated, diagnoses and medications might be confused, and important details can get overlooked. Hence, it is important to keep your or your child's medical records, but organization and simplification is key. Even if you don't have a medical background, you can do this.

1. Sort

First, organize everything by year. Then, for each year, organize by type of information: test result, clinic note, medical letter, hospital record, other. Now further sort those categories by month, chronologically. For example, put all test results in order from January to December in one year. Group clinic notes together by doctor, and sort those chronologically by month and year as well. Continue this process with the other categories (medical letter, hospital record, etc.). As you do this, take out any summary pages. Often, the first visit to a new physician will include a detailed note that is organized by a HPI (**h**istory of **p**resent **i**llness) and a SOAP note (**s**ymptoms, **o**bjective info, **a**ssessment, and **p**lan). Make a copy of those pages, and if possible scan those letters and save them in a file on your computer. Keep those copied letters separate, as they can be passed on to new doctors and provide a great snapshot of the issues at that time and simplify the process of documenting years of medical history.

Incidentally, this is a great project for a family member or friend who says, "What can I do to help?" as sorting through this information can be exhausting and overwhelming for many patients, and sometimes is difficult because each record has an emotional memory as well. Once the records are sorted by year, by type, and by month, make two stacks: 1) summary letters and lab test results, and 2) everything else (kept in chronological order). If your records are hundreds of pages long, recognize that you are going to need to keep the summary information only in your medical binder. Some people keep a medical binder for each year, which is fine. However, if you can only sort the records by year as described above, file each year in a box using folders organized either by month or by symptom/doctor's name.

2. Consolidate

Your goal should be to consolidate the paperwork into as little as possible while giving a snapshot of your/your child's history of illness from diagnosis to current date. A hard copy medical binder is helpful, and many patients also keep an electronic copy as well. For less than fifty dollars, you can take the condensed notes, now organized in the medical folder, to an office supply store and have them scan everything and saved to DVD or USB key for you. You can save a copy on your computer, and then keep the USB key or DVD with you. The portability of your medical records in this format can be very helpful when going to appointments or when traveling, and provides a lightweight and organized snapshot of your/your child's medical history and priority symptom areas. Keeping a chronological record like this (again, in a snapshot format) also helps you and your doctors see how symptoms have been progressing, if test findings/lab values have changed, trends in symptoms (especially related to illness, new meds, or hospitalization) and so on without lugging a closet full of records around with you.

3. Prioritize and Summarize

Now you're ready to organize and assemble your binder! An electronic version as well as a hard copy in an actual binder is ideal. Further, put that electronic version online so you can access it from anywhere in an emergency. Google Docs, iDisk, or an email to yourself are all easy options.

Contents of the Medical Binder (Virtual and Hard Copy)

Purchase a three-ring binder along with inserts for separating sections. This is going to be your medical binder and contain only the most important notes, test results, and letters. Your sections may depend on your/your child's symptoms and history, but can typically be classified using the following categories:

Sections One & Two: Basic Information.

The first page of your medical binder should be a contact list that includes contact information for all of your physicians on one page if possible, including email addresses, office phone numbers, pagers, and clinic addresses, if known. On that page, you should also list at least three emergency contacts, with full names and two telephone numbers for each. The second section of your binder should include a copy of your/your child's current insurance card(s), front and back. Be sure you include medical record numbers assigned to you by the hospital or clinic on a separate page as well.

Section Three: Medications.

The third section of your binder should include a list of current medications that is kept up to date at all times (this is very useful in the event of an emergency—you can just hand over the sheet to be copied by the nurse when you check-in and save thirty minutes in the ER). Include the name of each medication (including every ingredient in your Mito cocktail), the prescribing doctor's name, the specific dosage that you or your child takes, as well as the formulation (i.e., 200 mg/5 ml). If your medicines are compounded, you should request from the compounding pharmacist an updated list of all of the different vitamins and supplements included in the compound, along with specific dosage and formulation information for each. Most pharmacies are happy to provide a detailed medication print-out upon request, and usually a quarterly update is sufficient.

Section Four: Diagnosis.

Place the most recent and most comprehensive letter from a physician that summarizes your/your child's history and diagnosis at the front of this section, followed by letters or summary reports from the diagnostic labs/physicians who made the Mito diagnosis. If you are still in the process of being tested for mitochondrial disease, ask for copies of the orders for tests and blood work from your referring physician. This will help ensure that tests are not duplicated in the event of an emergency or during an appointment with a new specialist. [Tip: The first time that you see a new doctor or on the first day of every hospitalization, the admitting doctor is required to dictate an H&P (**hi**story and **p**hysical) which should give a good overview of your medical history and current symptoms. So, if you are overwhelmed with paperwork (or coming up empty-handed) you can always ask for a record of your "intake H&P" from your doctor's office or from the hospital's medical records office.]

Section Five: Emergency Protocols.

Now that you are getting organized, incorporate current protocols or medical letters into your binder in a new section called "emergency protocols." While you or your child are not experiencing an emergency, get these letters completed and signed by your physician (protocol samples, templates, and letters are available at www.MitoAction.org and www.umdf.org). Most patients need at least an emergency room letter and an anesthesia precautions protocol. Some physicians recommend a letter on file for dental emergencies as well (due to the risk of complications related to anesthetics used in dental emergencies). Chapter 5, "Managing and Preventing Symptoms" elaborates further on these emergency documents and situations.

Section Six: Notes from Specialists, Including Summaries of Diagnostic Tests.

Place the most recent copies of clinic notes from your specialists in this section. Remember, we're working toward a snapshot of your most important medical history, so a summary letter or follow-up letter is enough. Consider creating a tab for each specialist if you have several, or label the top of each letter by system (cardiology, immunology, hematology, etc.). Be sure contact information for each specialist is included. It's easier for new physicians to collaborate with your existing doctors when you have done your homework of organizing their recommendations and providing their contact information. Specialists frequently order tests to "rule out" other conditions or to gain better insight into your/your child's symptoms, so it makes sense to attach the results of those tests to each specialist's summary letter, if available.

Section Seven: Hospitalizations.

At the end of every hospital stay, the doctor who sees you or your child on the day you go home will write a "discharge summary" that offers an overview of the reason for the hospitalization and outlines the recommended next steps. Many people with Mito have a revolving door relationship with the hospital and have quite a few medical records that are just related to hospitalizations. For your medical binder, organize the hospital discharge summaries by date, and include one page of summary findings of test results, if available. *Do not* include the lab values that were drawn routinely every day, consult notes, orders for tests, etc. *Do* be sure that the name(s) of the doctors who were instrumental in your/your child's care during that hospitalization are noted accurately in the discharge note, since sometimes the attending on call for the weekend might be someone other than your primary physician or consulting specialist.

Again, if you have the technology to scan all of this info and store it electronically, you can more easily update it and keep it with you. You can even save the information as PDF documents in a file on your smart phone, or save a backup of everything in a free online "cloud" like Google Docs or iCloud, which can be accessed over the Internet anywhere.

Use a Multi-disciplinary Approach to Treatment

There is more to life than the diagnosis of mitochondrial disease! In looking at the big picture, there are a variety of resources and approaches that every family should take advantage of in order to meet the needs of the "whole person" who is affected. For example, consider looking into any or all of the following options in addition to the regimens recommended by your healthcare providers:

- **Adaptive equipment** can be critical in providing support and function to dramatically improve quality of life for adults and children with Mito. Some affected patients are resistant to using wheelchairs or seating devices because they can walk—until they try a custom wheelchair and notice the comfort and support difference! The right adaptive equipment can be extremely helpful in conserving energy and improving you or your child's ability to do things. Physiotherapists and physiatrists are healthcare providers trained in physical medicine and rehabilitation who can help make initial recommendations.
- **Clinical trials** are, for some patients, a way to feel connected to the latest research and to have the opportunity to use some substances that may improve their symptoms while taking part in the trial (ubiquinol, for example). A frequently updated resource with a search function that patients can use to look for clinical trials is www.clinicaltrials.gov. Be sure that you ask questions about reimbursement for travel, access to research data or personal test results, and study requirements when contacting universities and hospitals for more information about clinical trials.
- While children more typically take part in physical therapy, occupational therapy, etc. through early intervention and school-based services, adults can also benefit from **community rehabilitation pro-**

grams. Some rehab programs may be designed to help patients improve their physical skills and endurance related to certain conditions, such as stroke or heart failure. Ask your primary care physician to help you determine eligibility for these programs. For example, can you participate in a cardiac rehab program, even if you did not have a cardiac event? Likewise, some hospitals and rehab centers offer therapeutic swimming programs and yoga for their patients; both have great therapeutic potential for Mito patients (in moderation, of course).

■ **Therapeutic horseback riding** is a unique and multifaceted way for children and adults with Mito to gain strength and confidence while bonding with horses that are specially trained to work as part of a therapeutic program. More information, including where centers are located in North America, can be found at www.pathintl.org (PATH International - Professional Association of Therapeutic Horsemanship International) and www.frdi.net (Federation of Riding for the Disabled International).

■ **Support groups and counseling** are extremely important, especially for parents, adult spouses and patients, and caregivers who feel overwhelmed, are primary caregivers, and have little community support. There are now support groups online and by teleconference offered by MitoAction, as well as in-person meetings in some areas offered by the United Mitochondrial Disease Foundation (UMDF) and some medical centers.

■ **Alternative therapies**, such as biofeedback, acupuncture, acupressure, nutritional approaches, and homeopathic medicine have been used with some success by people with Mito, especially when the symptoms can be directly targeted by the alternative therapy (acupuncture for headaches, for example.)

Maintain the Four Ps

The four Ps are Perspective, Patience, Planning, and Persistence. Every adult patient and caregiver of someone affected by Mito will need to rely on one or more of these four Ps every day. A focus of this book is on finding harmony in your life with Mito, and the four Ps are the instruments that can help you achieve that goal. Remember:

■ **Perspective**: Is this something that you need to act on right now? Is this life or death? Can you get some perspective before you make a decision?

■ **Patience**: When *don't* you need patience while living with Mito? The tube pump broke, the pharmacy lost your prescription, the appointment was delayed for hours, the school "forgot" to give your child his snack, the records were lost, etc. Deep breaths and lots of patience can help you work through the rough moments.

■ **Planning**: Anticipate roadblocks! Just as you would map your trip if you were setting out on a road trip without a GPS, you should map your day to help you anticipate the challenges that may lie ahead. Often, parents of children with Mito, adult patients, and caregivers feel overwhelmed and pressured to make decisions. These decisions can be minor ("Do I take the appointment on Monday or Thursday?") or major ("Do I have a muscle biopsy?"), yet both cause stress. The more that you can do to plan ahead, the better prepared you will be when faced with unexpected roadblocks.

KELLY

*M*y name is Kelly. I am twenty-eight years old and I was diagnosed with Mito four years ago. What am I afraid of? I fear the unknown. There are a lot of scary words used to describe this diagnosis and I have endured and seen others go through scary stuff. I fear that my baseline will decrease. I never know how I will feel each day when I wake up. When I'm having a really "bad" day I often fear that this will become my new "normal."

I cope by staying positive. This disease affects everyone differently and no one can tell me what to expect. I try to keep balance in my life. I allow myself to have bad days—even those whose lives are not affected by Mito have them—but most of the time I remain positive. I have such limited time and energy that I don't want to waste it being negative. I may not be able to do everything I once could, but I have found new hobbies and interests to keep me busy.

Supportive family and friends help. I don't know what I would do without them. It helps me to have a balance of healthy friends and friends who are also affected by mitochondrial disease (these are the only other people who truly get it). It's not like I can ever forget for a moment that I have Mito, but I enjoy hanging out with others who help take my mind off it too. It also helps me to volunteer so that I can help others. I find writing about my thoughts and feelings to be therapeutic as well.

People's lack of understanding about Mito is what hurts the most. With an invisible illness, there are many people who will never "get it." Sometimes people say I look too good to be sick. People can't see all the symptoms I am experiencing or what isn't working correctly inside my body. As a result, some people think you can just "push through" this illness—like that will make it go away. It's upsetting for me to see the support that other people receive when they have a disease that is better known. They get a lot of support and sympathy and people rally around them. If you say you have mitochondrial disease, the common response is, "what's that?" (often even from medical professionals!). People often say things like "there will be a cure soon," but they don't know how little research and how slow going it is for mitochondrial disease, and they don't know how I'm feeling and struggling right now.

■ **Persistence**: You are an advocate by nature if you are dealing with this disease because there are many people who are unaware of the challenges and issues associated with Mito and who will therefore look to you to explain it to them. They may not understand or agree the first time; you'll need persistence to get to where you want to go. As a parent, you can model persistence for your children. As an adult patient, you can practice persistence when it counts, which will help you get the care or services/support that you need.

Now the challenge is to keep the "the four Ps" in practice while you have a smile on your face! (Kind of like patting your head and rubbing your stomach while juggling fire, yes?)

Find the Humor, Even When Things Feel Tragic

An adult Mito patient, Crystal, had the idea to start a group on Facebook called "You know you have Mito when…." This is a great example of living and laughing despite the challenges we face each day as Mito patients and caregivers. Here are a few of the most poignant posts by parents and patients who live with mitochondrial disease.

"You know you have Mito when…"

…you have to buy additional pieces of furniture just to store the growing number of medical supplies in your home.

…you wait weeks to see a specialist but at your appointment you both realize you're too complicated for this doctor and have to hunt down another specialist and wait weeks to see that one.

…when you experience symptoms you can barely describe, let alone find a name for when Googling.

…you make up your own pain scale like: 1 (arterial line placement)…3 (muscle pain)…5 (central jugular line placement)…10 (thankfully, I wasn't conscious…).

…when a simple cold knocks you out for a week.

…when your family spends more money a month on medical "foods" and medicine for one child than on the grocery bill for the whole family of five.

…when, like an expectant mom, you always have a bag packed, just in case you are admitted to the hospital.

…when your child has an MRI or CAT scan and you hear…"Well, that's interesting—I've never seen that before!"

…the same ER resident gets way too excited over seeing you multiple times in the past year for different organ systems.

...your nine-year-old sees a squiggly design on a chair in a public place and exclaims, "Mom look! That looks like mitochondria!"

...when you're filling out paperwork for a new specialist and not only have you checked the "other" box in every single body system, but you've also run out of room on the lines designated for "diagnosis," and "current medication," and "allergies," and "hospitalizations," and "operations."

...when you spend your Friday and Saturday nights researching online.

...you have multiple extra access points to your body.

...when you sleep as much as your cat!

...when your kid gets stopped by airport security to take off his backpack and you have to explain that it is attached to him.

...when you can recall all the blood tests to be drawn and the colored tubes they go in before the resident can ask the attending.

...when a doctor you never met comes into the room and says "Oh! I heard about you in grand rounds during your last inpatient stay."

...when the people in the ER know your names and they don't need to ask for a family history.

...when you think about poops everyday. You have to see them, you have to record them...

...when your child's medical records stacked up are taller than your child.

...when you go into the ER, you give them your protocol letter, and you look out the room door five minutes later to see the ER doctor, several residents, and about three nurses all gathered around a computer with your protocol letter in the middle of them.

...when you instruct the nurse how to draw a blood lactate.

Don't Believe in the Crystal Ball

One of the most difficult aspects of a diagnosis of mitochondrial disease is the uncertainty of the prognosis. Physicians and healthcare providers make predictions about the future or outcome of your or your child's condition in an effort to be fully informative. There is an expectation in today's medical climate that, unlike the days of yore when doctors made house calls and chose to withhold bad news, the patient and immediate family has a right to know all of the relevant information about the patient's condition. However, in the case of mitochondrial disease, this is a slippery slope. So much has changed about our understanding of the breadth of the disease, even in the last few years. Truly, we don't know for sure what the future looks like, even when you are diagnosed with a "well-known" type of mitochondrial disease. Experience and anecdotal stories still play a large part in influencing a physician's expectations about a patient's prognosis. If a physician is relatively inexperienced, his predictions may be grossly inaccurate (either positively or negatively). On the other hand, physicians who work as mitochondrial diagnosticians or specialists might see an above average number of people who are acutely ill, and based on their own experience, can also have a bias in determining your prognosis.

Although the landscape of mitochondrial medicine is changing, many parents, patients, and families have been told that their condition is "so rare that there is little hope," or that "there is no treatment." Information like this trickles down from experience and from interpretation of the medical literature, and while the intent of prognosis is to offer full disclosure, it can be extremely difficult for a stressed and frightened family to hear that their loved one's condition is progressive and incurable. Further, as patients and caregivers, we don't always accurately hear what our physicians are sharing with us, or understand the intent with which it is presented because we are emotionally frazzled. For example, when a physician tells a family that his previous experience with a child with similar symptoms ended in a poor outcome, the family can easily interpret that information as a solid prediction about their own child's future. The physician may intend to communicate, "This is serious and we will be working closely with you to manage your child's disorder because in similar cases, children have become critically ill." The frightened parent hears (interprets), "Your child's case is serious and he is probably going to die because other children like yours have all died." Obviously, the patient or family walks away terrified and distressed by this "bad news," and can easily lose hope and lose perspective by taking the information about prognosis to heart.

Write this on a self-stick note and announce it to yourself and to your family (especially your children or healthy siblings who are also distressed): *"No one–not even the best doctors in the world–can predict OUR future. We will do the best we can with what we have today!"* Many parents and patients who have lived through this terror would agree, it is important and necessary for your sanity and emotional and family well-being to try to let go of the prognosis and focus on your quality of life and on managing your symptoms so that you or your child feels as well as possible day to day, week to week, year to year.

Yes, there are often difficult decisions to make that cause us to face uncomfortable realities; however, the stress of focusing on the prognosis can be literally disabling for an individual or for a family. Finding others who have lived "beyond their prognosis" can be helpful, and fortunately, there are countless children, teens, young adults, and families who can share those stories! To that end, encourage and allow your children to dream. Sometimes, as parents we want to protect our children from disappointment so we try to temper their dreams with reality. Dreams give us hope. Some of the most inspiring young adults who have mitochondrial disease want to be doctors or researchers some day, because they themselves have lived beyond their prognosis and they dream of helping others.

Do What Makes You Happy

Richard Carlson's little book, *Don't Sweat the Small Stuff*, has been a number one bestseller for years. Why does it take so much for us, as a culture, to learn to let go and

GABRIEL

My little boy, Gabriel, was labeled "failure to thrive" at birth. They told us that he had suffered serious brain damage during delivery. On the third day of his stay in the NICU, I was asked to sit down with the doctors who had been caring for him. The metabolic doctor who had been spending a lot of time with him told me that he had a serious genetic defect. She told me that it was a fatal disease and explained that he could not metabolize fats or proteins. She said that no other child born with this disease had lived for longer than six to eight months. She was patient with me when I cried. She said that she wanted to send a muscle fibroblast to a different center that would confirm the disease. She said that Gabriel could be brought home once he could suck on his own and was taken off the tube feeding him through his nose. She told us to give him the best life possible in the next few months. She said it was best "not to resuscitate" should he stop breathing again, because of all of the damage that he had already sustained.

Up to this point, I was in shock and depressed and felt very alone and defeated. But, after spending days with him, watching as he came out of his long sleep, when he finally looked up at me and took formula from a bottle, something changed in my attitude. On the day we were told we could go home, I became an angry, assertive woman–a person I had never been in my whole life. I demanded an apnea monitor to have at home in case he stopped breathing. I insisted that I would breastfeed him and I didn't want the formula. I read all the books I could

do what makes us really happy? His book is filled with bits of advice like, "Let yourself be bored," "Do one thing at a time," and "Live this day as if it might be your last." I have always found it ironic that for people with mitochondrial disease, the diagnosis forces you to practice not sweating the small stuff (in fact, most folks with Mito don't sweat at all!).

When you have a limited amount of energy and potentially a limited amount of time to enjoy your child or enjoy your life, what do you choose to do? One of the greatest gifts that you can allow yourself and your family to receive from this diagnosis is the opportunity to gain perspective and to focus on what is important to you. Maybe you know people who get completely upset when their child doesn't make the soccer team. If you have a child with Mito, you are thankful if he ever even has the opportunity to play soccer at all. You probably know couples who fight about what the weekend plans should be. If you are an adult or spouse caring for someone with Mito, you are thankful if you have opportunity or energy to even have weekend plans.

Let the diagnosis, which has been plunked into your life like an unwelcome houseguest, become an opportunity. Rather than being a burden, let this be a blessing. "Carpe diem" is emblazoned on the programs at college and high school graduations across the country, as we urge our young people to "Seize the day!" Likewise, if you are living with Mito, don't put off the things you want or enjoy. Allow yourself to dream new dreams and to let go of expectations (your own as well as others) that can

find on healing, nutrition, and disease. And I didn't stop there. I sought out a Native American shaman, a Catholic priest who was a faith healer, a chiropractor, and a second opinion from another metabolic doctor.

I found a physician who believed in treating Gabriel, the individual, not the disease. His approach was much more hopeful and that was what I needed to keep going, especially since I was a single parent at this point. He helped me see the little accomplishments that Gabriel was making. We weaned him slowly off of the painkillers that he had been on since birth. We taught him how to eat so that he could grow. We found a school for children with special needs that helped us to help him thrive.

Today, twelve plus years after his birth, Gabriel is of normal height and weight—a handsome devil who is devoted to his family. It has not been an easy road. We have had many bumps and starts. He stopped sleeping (night and day) at about age three. He is incontinent, has many food allergies, and still can only display his discomfort through tantrums or negative behavior. We aggressively modified his diet. We were thankful to get a diagnosis of Asperger's syndrome, which affords me much more knowledge of how to help my son deal with this world that he doesn't really understand, and to help others to understand his world.

I have met wonderful people along the way who are now a part of our lives and Gabriel's world. I feel strongly about the choices I have made for my son, and that they have helped make a difference in his quality of life.

---

be suffocating. When you have a plan, include the people who can help you to make it a reality, such as your doctor, your family, your spouse, friends, etc. Even community advocacy groups can sometimes help you figure out new dreams and how to achieve them, for example, the Special Olympics and organizations that showcase the artwork of people with chronic diseases. There are also a few special foundations that exist for both adults and children that offer the opportunity to have a "wish" granted. The Make-a-Wish Foundation is one such organization—it gives families the opportunity to take a special trip, meet a celebrity, put on a home addition, etc. that will make for special memories and improve quality of life. There are similar organizations for adults that grant wishes, fund special trips, or help with home renovations. In most circumstances, people with mitochondrial disease qualify for support from these foundations with a letter of referral from the patient's metabolic specialist, neurologist, or managing primary physician. Why mention wish trips? Wish trips are an opportunity to make dreams come true, especially for families who don't have the financial means to take a trip. Further, wish-granting organizations often offer supportive mechanisms that make travel for a disabled or chronically ill person easier, such as wheelchair accessible travel and accommodations, portable infusion equipment, etc.

Hobbies are also valuable for adults and kids who live with mitochondrial disease and their caretakers. Again, pursuing a hobby while managing a progressive disease

MARIA

What would have helped before Maria got so sick? Better listening, beginning with her four-month-old appointment all the way through the time she became critically ill eight years later. More attention to detail by everyone, from the feeding team to the specialists. Early diagnosis would have made a difference. She would have received treatment, including a g-tube, much earlier. Had we known of her disease, many of the missteps we made along the way might have been avoided. She probably should not have had such a long commute to preschool, nor ever gone to school all day. We would have understood her inconsistency, so common in mitochondrial disease, which led to her PDD diagnosis. She certainly would not have spent two lonely years in a program for children with autism spectrum disorders. We would have better understood how fatigue, frustration, and pain led to many of her behavioral issues. And throughout Maria's life, we would have strived for greater balance between skill acquisition and fun.

may feel counterintuitive, but in truth, doing something completely unrelated to mitochondrial disease for the pure purpose of relaxation and enjoyment is therapeutic. Adults with Mito may have had meaningful hobbies in the past that can be pursued again, although if rock climbing or waterskiing were your interest, consider less intense alternatives like Hatha yoga, gardening, or geology! Parents of affected children often bitterly argue, reasonably, that there is simply no time for a "hobby." For any parent who has spent sleepless nights in the hospital or at home, this is unfortunately so true. However, without the pursuit of something that gives our mind a break, stress and fatigue can get the best of us.

Think of (and accordingly prioritize the time for) your hobby as "therapy," and consider hobbies that give you health benefits along with distraction (e.g., exercise: jogging, walking, dance, tennis, etc.) or that are "portable" (such as knitting, reading, learning a language, scrapbooking, Sudoku, etc.). Some hobbies allow you to connect with other people who meet simply for the sake of getting together for the same interest, such as an exercise class or book club. For parents and adult patients and caregivers, these are great opportunities to step outside of the daily reminders of the disease and have a shift in focus, even for one hour once a month.

Take Your Time with Difficult Decisions

Moving

Mitochondrial disease is not limited by geography. People all over the world are affected by mitochondrial disorders, but obviously there are not medical centers or support groups in every city or town. A surprising number of families relocate within the first five years of receiving a mitochondrial disease diagnosis in order to be closer to a major medical center where there is greater awareness of and support for the diagnosis. A move is one of the most stressful life events that families can experience, and that stress should be considered when exploring the opportunity for a move. Families who have happily relocated in order to have better access to medical and school services give the following advice:

- Take your time and visit the new place often, during every season.
- Know where your child will go to school and what services are available before committing to the move.
- Ask your doctor directly if he will be available to you and have admitting privileges at the hospital you choose where you relocate.
- Reach out to local Mito groups and try to get advice about available services from other patients or families who live in the area.
- Consider cost of living, state insurance programs, and community services as well as the proximity of major medical centers.

SALLY

It is an unfortunate fact that most of our life with our daughter has been spent in a hospital and sometimes for extended periods of time. It's difficult to move your entire life into one tiny little hospital room, especially if you are like most parents and rarely leave your child's bedside. As our daughter's health continues to decline, with one infection after another, a hospitalization happening once or twice a month, it's difficult to keep a positive outlook on things. There are many times I find myself asking, "Okay God, is this as good as it gets?"

For our family, living in an area where there was a lack of knowledge, direction, or support for mitochondrial disease was so difficult. We found ourselves flying out of state endlessly seeking guidance and leadership. We have been to Boston, Cleveland, Cincinnati, Denver, and Texas. We continue to work on bridging the gap between patient and clinician, but I have to be honest, it is getting better now that we have relocated to an area where there is a mitochondrial specialist and clinic within driving distance! Finally, we can cut the strings from our out-of-state specialists. We have a good metabolic doctor here and are followed very closely. I feel this is key for managing the multitude of symptoms this disease can present.

I want other parents to know how important it is to create balance and quality of life. As a parent of a chronically ill child with an incurable disease, I know there isn't a "one size fits all" approach to finding balance. For us, moving to another state has helped. It gave us the opportunity to be closer to home during hospitalizations and allowed me to meet other people who have become wonderful friends who understand our life and who love and support us.

Managing Many Medical Appointments

This is what happens to a majority of people—adults and children alike—with Mito: After a year or more of pursuing a diagnosis, a diagnosis of mitochondrial disease (some form, to some degree) is confirmed. On the one hand, the diagnosis offers more direction because it is a compass with which to navigate the many symptoms that occur. On the other hand, the label makes you or your child become a "complex" patient, and primary care practitioners and specialists may view every new symptom as a complication of the mitochondrial disorder. Throw in a hospitalization, even for an unrelated illness like the stomach flu, and new symptoms are identified. Lots of tests are ordered and need to be interpreted. Consequently, multiple specialists and their opinions are sought, and the list of doctors involved in your or your child's care grows exponentially each year.

Each subspecialist has his own battery of baseline tests to be completed regularly (MRI, echocardiogram, blood work, exercise function test, vision testing, pulmonary function assessment, etc.). Each test is scheduled on a different day than the initial clinic visit, and there is at least one follow-up appointment to discuss results and to monitor progress of the symptom, adjust medications, etc. Patients and families find themselves booked six to twelve months in advance with multiple doctors, many of whom are in different locations. Each visit brings about more testing, which necessitates future follow-up visits, etc.

There are some families who find themselves involved in at least one clinic visit or outpatient test per week for months on end, even when they are "healthy!" Determining the necessity of these endless appointments and whether the energy expense involved is worth it is a personal decision for every patient and family. Further, your willingness to "invest" in these appointments may adjust over time depending on your own degree of confidence and the appearance of new symptoms. Patients and families often don't realize that they have permission to be involved in the decision-making process for these tests and multiple visits. The following are some questions to ask yourself and your doctors when managing multiple specialists:

- Will this visit with this specialist change the treatment or understanding of my (my child's) condition?
- Will I/my child have better opportunities for services because of this visit?
- Will this test give us information that can be used to modify or improve treatment?
- Will the additional information from this specialist or test do anything other than just provide "more information?"
- Are less frequent follow-up visits a possibility? Why or why not?
- Does every specialist need to be seen regularly, or could they be consulted only when there is a problem related to that symptom area?
- Are baseline tests each year necessary or could they be performed less frequently (especially if they are painful, invasive, costly, or stressful)?

- Would the appointments that we have had gone better or been more productive if the physician had had all of the information first? Could I have better organized my/my child's symptoms and provided better information or documentation?

Further, when thinking about getting the most value out of every specialist appointment, plan ahead by asking these questions at the time of the referral:

- If the specialist orders additional tests, who will communicate the information from these tests to me? To my doctors? Will I get a copy of the results in writing?
- Which doctors will follow me/my child if hospitalized? Who would be available for consult within the same medical system?
- Are consults from multiple medical centers allowed or realistic when hospitalized? If not, who will make decisions about my care when the specialist is unavailable or out of state?

Palliative Care and Hospice

Palliative care is a form of treatment that is focused on managing symptoms so that a patient can experience the best quality of life possible. Palliative care is more commonly part of a patient's treatment plan in situations where invasive tests and even some treatments may compromise the quality of life for a person rather than ease his suffering. Palliative care is not only for patients who are "end-of-life." On the other hand, hospice is a type of care that is focused on supporting patients who are terminally ill. Palliative care and hospice may be scary words for a family to hear because they feel that the words imply that death is near and that the medical team is "giving up." In truth, many patients—children and adults—and their families find their palliative care or hospice teams to be their beacon of light and support when things are the most challenging. It is important to dispel the myth that palliative care is offered only to patients who are terminally ill—meaning expected to die within a year or less. Palliative care is appropriate for many Mito patients who have complex presentations of the disease and whose families strive to make good quality of life decisions for them. A Mito patient may have a palliative care team for years. The family may look to the palliative care team for advice and as a sounding board when an invasive test or procedure is recommended for the patient that may be helpful but may also have side effects. These are very difficult decisions for a child's or adult patient's family to make, and the experience of the palliative care team is invaluable.

The focus for families who choose to involve a palliative or hospice team is on maintaining a good quality of life for the Mito patient and the family as a whole, and does not imply that treatments to help improve symptoms won't be given. In fact, there are some families who share that it was only after becoming involved with palliative care that they actually felt that the whole medical team managed the disease better, was more thoughtful and communicative about decisions, and that the stress of medical appointments and frightening hospitalizations was significantly lowered. Nonetheless, when a physician makes a recommendation that you consider hospice or palliative care, it can be emotionally upsetting. Before you make a decision, request an appointment with someone from the palliative care team to ask your questions, and be honest with him about your wishes and your fears.

Give Back When You Are Able

One way that you can find the silver lining in this disease is to help others who need support. Everyone—parents, patients, family members—who is affected by Mito has periods of time when they really need and benefit from support. Likewise, there are times for most patients, parents, and families when they feel "ok," and can be a source of advice and encouragement for others.

Volunteering

You can volunteer in a variety of ways now, both in person and "virtually." Many people participate in email groups and social media pages that network, give advice, and share resources. You can volunteer virtually by telephone for MitoAction's patient support hotline. You can work with local organizations to organize events, volunteer at the hospital delivering balloons or visiting with patients, share your talents by playing music for people in a rehabilitation center, serve coffee at a walk, etc. As the director of a nonprofit, take my word for it—volunteers are always needed and welcome! Further, being a volunteer is emotionally satisfying and allows you to share something unique and personal that can help other people feel better!

Raising Awareness

Are you a community organizer? You should be part of the efforts to raise awareness about mitochondrial disease! Whether you host an informal reception, plan a big local event, or advocate with your state legislature, your efforts to bring the needs of people who have mitochondrial disease to the forefront have a ripple effect that will help many other families. Don't be afraid to share your personal story. Was getting a diagnosis difficult and costly? Do you battle insurance? How do you feel about the way your life and your family have been affected by mitochondrial disease? Your story is compelling and memorable and brings attention to Mito in a time when many diseases are fighting for the spotlight. Perhaps, when you take the time to call your local newspaper and ask them to do an interview about you or your family's life with Mito, someone else who has not yet been diagnosed will learn about Mito and that will help him get the appropriate diagnosis and care. Perhaps your story will inspire someone thinking of going to medical school to study metabolic and genetic diseases. You never know what can happen, especially when we are all working together to raise awareness for Mito.

JOHN

When my wife died, I didn't know what to do next. I had really enjoyed being a part of the Mito groups while she was alive, but I didn't have that much time to be a volunteer because I was her primary caregiver. When she passed away, we gave green ribbons to everyone who came to her funeral, and asked people to help us to raise awareness about this disease. I found that I felt really compelled to tell her story, and to let people know that Mito affects all of us. She could have gotten a diagnosis sooner if there was better awareness of and recognition of mitochondrial disease.

I know some people shy away from sharing personal information. In fact, I was probably more reserved with the details of our daily lives while my wife was alive. But when I began to tell our story after she died, I was outright shocked at how many people came to my side to support me and my cause. All of the employees in my company got behind me, and we walked as the largest team at the annual Mito Awareness Walk. Now my children are volunteers every year with me and we feel so thankful that we can make a difference. Even more than that, volunteering has made me realize how much I can give even though I thought I had so little to offer. When I see people struggling, I can relate to them, and I feel humbled knowing that I am making a difference.

Being Part of the Mito Community

People who are affected with Mito unanimously agree that there is nothing like being able to connect with someone who knows what it is like to live with mitochondrial disease. Don't be afraid to become part of the mitochondrial disease community, and to look to them for guidance when you need it. You may find a few friends through Internet groups that you will never meet but who are your lifelines when you are in crisis or when you need someone to hear you out and help you make tough decisions. The two things that patients and parents say helped them the most when they were diagnosed are information and support from others with the disease. When you are able to give back, share your energy in ways that satisfy you emotionally and capitalize on your talents and resources. In other words, when you are given something as simple as a smile or a word of encouragement, pass it on!

Key Points from This Chapter

■ **Maximize your energy.** Energy conservation is not just physical. Conserving your energy—this goes for caregivers as well as patients—takes place mentally, emotionally, and physically. Strategically thinking about how to maximize your energy is just as important as financially planning for your future.

■ **Changing your perspective and your priorities is natural as you learn to live well with mitochondrial disease.** What may have been important to you or your family before may not matter anymore. Likewise, the people who were part of your inner circle (family, friends, colleagues) may not be able to be the support system you need when you re-organize your goals and focus on new priorities. See this as an opportunity to welcome new people into your life rather than hanging onto negative (and energy-draining) feelings about friends and family who let you down.

■ **Be a survivor with the four P's: Perspective, Patience, Planning, and Persistence.** It may be a constant balancing act to maintain perspective and to find time to plan as a parent, caregiver, or adult patient; however, these skills are critical to long-term wellness for you and your family. It is likely that as a person affected by mitochondrial disease, you will be discouraged on occasion by the medical system, your child's school, your employer, your family, and your friends. Be patient, and don't give up. Being an advocate is not a part-time position but one that requires daily effort, planning, and persistence!

■ **Take time with difficult decisions, especially when you feel overwhelmed.** Many people today feel pressured and overwhelmed about making decisions, and may become frustrated or make decisions quickly without taking time to really let the options sink in. This stress is even worse when your child is in the hospital or when you are feeling exhausted and overcome with symptoms. Confusion is part of the process of learning what steps to take next when faced with a big decision. Take your time and ask others to respect your need to step back and get some perspective.

■ **Give back.** Your experience, as either a caregiver or as a patient, has molded you in a unique and wonderful way. Take advantage of those experiences and the lessons you have learned by helping others. Volunteer as part of a support program, become active raising awareness or raising money, generate interest in mitochondrial disease by sharing your story with the media, or simply be a good friend to someone else struggling with an illness or disability. The journey of learning to live well with mitochondrial disease has a natural ebb and flow; there will be times when you will be the one in need, and other times when you can give back.

10

Mitochondrial Biochemistry

The scientific community's knowledge about how mitochondria work has grown significantly in the last decade and continues to evolve. While it has been known for some time that mitochondria act as the powerhouse of the cell, the exact mechanism by which ATP is produced is a relatively recent discovery. The biochemistry involved in explaining these details is complex for most people who do not have a biology or science background. A basic explanation of the processes was laid out in Chapter 1, and that is enough for most parents and patients who are new to the world of Mito, and feel understandably overwhelmed. However, many parents, patients, and families want to feel empowered by a deeper understanding of how the mitochondria work, and why a defect in the energy production process at the cellular level can cause such dramatic symptoms. Every tiny step and every molecule needed for the mitochondria's energy-producing reactions is critically important.

This chapter examines the more complex aspects of the biochemistry of mitochondria and is likely to take awhile to absorb, but the glimpse that the next few pages offers into the structure and function of our body's mitochondria is truly fascinating! Readers should refer back to this chapter (along with the glossary at the back of the book) as often as necessary.

The Structure and Function of Mitochondria

When you look at a picture of the mitochondria (Figure 10.1), you see a rod-shaped organelle (a specialized subunit of a cell) composed of an inner and outer membrane.

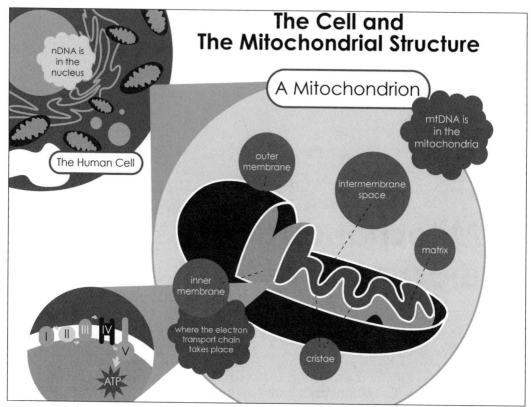

Figure 10.1: The cell and mitochondrial structure.   *Image by Jane Adams*

The membranes are important because they act like conduits, or channels, which allow certain molecules to enter and exit as the energy production process takes place. The inner mitochondrial membrane is where the actual energy production process occurs. The energy molecules produced in the mitochondria are called ATP (adenosine triphosphate). The curved ridge-like structures that you see inside the mitochondria are called cristae; they make it possible for the complex task of energy metabolism to take place by creating more usable surface area for the essential components to operate. The series of reactions within the mitochondria that generate the most energy are called the electron transport chain (ETC). The electron transport chain is essentially an assembly line where molecules move through a series of five complexes, allowing the building blocks (i.e., the molecules broken down from food) to be converted into usable energy currency: ATP. Think of the electron transport chain as a biochemical "conveyor system" that, in a healthy state, produces ATP from the "energy building blocks." The other area of note within the mitochondrial structure is the matrix, which contains the mitochondrial DNA as well as enzyme groups, which are necessary catalysts for the electron transport chain.

How Energy is Made, at a Glance

The primary purpose of the mitochondria is to make energy, which is achieved by a group of metabolic reactions called oxidative phosphorylation (OX-PHOS). These processes take place on the inner mitochondrial membrane via a series of protein complexes called the electron transport chain (ETC). When we eat food for fuel, three steps must occur in the mitochondria for the process of converting food into usable energy to take place. Mitochondrial defects can occur at any point during these steps:

1. **Glycolysis**—Glucose is broken down into two ATP molecules, pyruvate and NADH (this takes place outside of the mitochondria)
2. **Kreb's cycle** (also called Citric Acid Cycle)—Pyruvate is broken down and two more ATP molecules are produced, along with high-energy electrons from NADH and FADH (this takes place within the mitochondria)
3. **OX-PHOS and the Electron Transport Chain** (ETC)—These metabolic reactions use oxygen to transfer high-energy electrons through a series of protein complexes (the ETC) to power and to make an electrochemical gradient, like a battery (ending at Complex V ATPase). The process produces another thirty-four molecules of ATP (this also takes place within the mitochondria)

How Energy is Made, Step by Step

Let's break these steps down even further:

1. Glycolysis
    - Glucose is derived from food and is used to make energy. The other source of energy derived from food is fatty acids. (Sometimes people with mitochondrial disease may have an impaired ability to use fatty acids for energy, a condition called fatty acid oxidation defect.) Typically, however, even in people with Mito, glucose is broken down first to use for energy, and when glucose runs out, fatty acids are utilized next.
    - Glycolysis is the process where one molecule of glucose is broken down further into two molecules of pyruvate. In addition, two molecules of ATP are created in the process. This process occurs outside the mitochondria and does not require oxygen.
    - The breakdown of glucose into pyruvate during glycolysis also results in two by-products, alanine and lactate. In people with mitochondrial disorders, excess alanine and lactate may accumulate in the blood and can be detected by blood tests. (This is significant because abnormal levels of these by-products may serve as a red flag that warrants further testing and consideration of a mitochondrial disease diagnosis.)
    - When each pyruvate molecule binds to a molecule of co-enzyme A, a new molecule is formed: acetyl-CoA. Some people have a deficiency in the enzyme complex that is nec-

essary for this step. The enzyme complex is called pyruvate dehydrogenase (PDH). If part of this enzyme complex is incomplete, the name of the disorder is PDCD (pyruvate dehydrogenase complex deficiency).

2. Kreb's Cycle
   - The next step in the process is the Kreb's cycle. Here, acetyl-CoA is further processed in a series of reactions that create two important high-energy electron carriers: NADH and FADH.

The first two steps, glycolysis and the Kreb's cycle, take glucose and break it down into smaller building blocks that will allow the mitochondria to convert it into energy. These first two steps also produce a little bit of ATP but not enough to amply fuel our bodies' energy needs.

3. OX-PHOS and the Electron Transport Chain (ETC)
   - The third step in the process is where most mitochondrial disorders occur, the electron transport chain.
   - The ETC is a set of five protein complexes, a pathway where the metabolic reactions of oxidative phosphorylation take place. Mitochondrial diseases are also sometimes called OX-PHOS disorders.
   - The name "OX-PHOS" implies what happens in this step: oxygen molecules, proton pumping, electron transfer, and establishment of an electrochemical gradient across the inner mitochondrial membrane allow the ATPase (Complex V) to convert the building blocks of energy (ADP) to ATP. The cell's energy is then stored in the phosphate bond in order to be released and used by the cell as energy.
   - Oxidative phosphorylation is the series of metabolic reactions that occur via aerobic metabolism, a term that suggests that oxygen is present (as compared to anaerobic metabolism; i.e., without oxygen, which happens earlier in glycolysis). Aerobic metabolism is the process of converting food into energy using oxygen, and is considered the most effective way to generate cellular energy. The key word here is aerobic. Oxygen must be present for these reactions to occur!
   - The electron transport chain, where OX-PHOS takes place, is the final and most important step of the energy production process. Indeed, during OX-PHOS, most of the cell's usable energy (thirty-four molecules of ATP) is produced.

The Electron Transport Chain (Complexes I–V)

Let's spend a little more time exploring the electron transport chain (ETC) since it is the pathway that generates the most energy and where defects most commonly occur. The ETC is composed of protein and enzyme groups within the mitochondria (known as Complexes I, II, III, and IV) that have the important job of transferring electrons and altering base molecules, eventually resulting in the formation of ATP. Often, a person's Mito diagnosis is actually a description of the ETC complexes where defects were found, so a patient might say, "I have Complex I and III." Each complex, as mentioned above, is a group of proteins that are linked together like an assembly line. Each step must be completed in its entirety for enough ATP to be produced. The electron transport chain is also called the respiratory chain because it describes "cellular respiration"; in other words, the cell "respires," using oxygen to convert molecules from food into energy.

To understand how transferring electrons through the ETC generates energy, it is important to visualize the concept of a gradient. In this case, a gradient is the difference between the charge inside and outside of a membrane, which generates a force so that energy can be created. The gradient across the mitochondrial membrane drives the flux of particles (protons and electrons) in and out, thereby releasing energy. The ETC is a set of five protein complexes where the metabolic reactions of oxidative phosphorylation take place. The gradient drives electrons and protons (negatively and positively charged molecules) back and forth through the first four complexes. Those particles eventually bind with oxygen, producing water. In the last step of the ETC, Complex V, ATP is generated by the final forceful influx of these particles (protons, specifically) through a "revolving door," or rotor-like mechanism. The force and transfer of the positive and negative particles across the gradient and through this revolving door generates thirty-four molecules of high energy ATP. It takes the force of the charge of the electrons moving through the gradient to "whoosh" through Complex V and generate ATP.

Medical students learn the analogy of a dam when studying the ETC in biochemistry. Trickling water from streams or rivers builds up behind a dam. When the dam opens, the force of the built-up water rushes through the dam and creates energy. The "whoosh" of the water through the dam in this analogy has the force to move turbines, which create energy that can be harnessed as electricity. In the body, the electrons move across the gradient of the complexes while, at the same time, protons are pumped out of the mitochondrial membrane. The build-up of protons outside the membrane and the electrochemical gradient generated by the movement of electrons results in a building up of energy, which ultimately forces an effect like water rushing through the dam into Complex V, where ATP is formed. In this manner, potential electrochemical energy is transformed to *usable* biochemical energy in the form of ATP. Additionally, the positive/negative charge and process is why the analogy of mitochondrial function to a battery is relevant on many levels.

In many ways, mitochondria are like batteries. Not only do they generate energy, but because of the proton/electron transfer in the ETC, they have a positive and negative charge. ATP can be stored as energy, like energy stored in a battery to use later. (Specifically, muscle stores energy in the phosphate bond of phosphocreatine.) However, people with mitochondrial disease have less effective "batteries." A person with Mito has trouble quickly converting stored energy and consequently fatigues quickly. Mito patients also have a lower threshold of stored energy or "reserves" that healthy people can use when needed. This helps us understand why *frequent* "recharging" by eating, drinking, and resting is important for people with Mito!

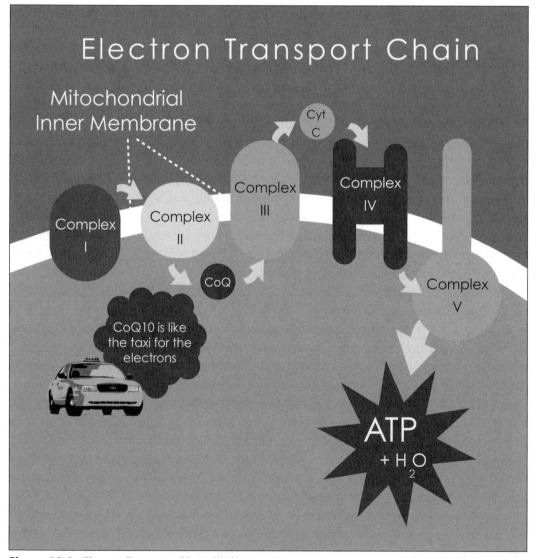

Figure 10.2: Electron Transport Chain (ETC).   *Image by Jane Adams*

Now, let's zoom in and take a closer look at each piece of the ETC (see Figure 10.2). Complex I is a huge enzyme also known as NADH dehydrogenase. High energy electrons (molecules with a negative charge) are transported via a shuttle, Coenzyme Q10 (CoQ10), from Complex I and Complex II to Complex III. At that point, the next "electron taxi," cytochrome c, shuttles the electrons further along to Complex IV. Simultaneously, the energy released from the transfer of these high-energy electrons powers the movement of protons (molecules with a positive charge) to be pumped across the inner membrane of the mitochondria by Complexes I, III, and IV. Finally, the energy gradient that has been created allows the protons to rush back in across the inner membrane of the mitochondria into Complex V.

Complex V is actually a large enzyme group shaped like a mushroom called ATP synthase. It is the final reaction in the metabolic pathway (ETC) and uses the energy generated and stored from the reactions that occurred in the first four complexes to create a usable energy molecule: ATP. At this point, ADP (adenosine diphosphate) is translocated across the membrane to the mitochondrial matrix where ATPase (Complex V) adds phosphate. (Now the term oxidative phosphorylation makes sense.) ADP is an organic compound that is a basic building block of DNA. Most importantly, ADP is converted to ATP for cellular energy during the process of oxidative phosphorylation that takes place within the mitochondria via the electron transport chain. Now ATP is able to be transferred from the mitochondria as usable energy for the body via the cell. Of interest is that Complex V is found in all forms of life and functions the same way in all living things. Because it actually works like a revolving door to create ATP from ADP, we can think of it like a tiny rotary motor.

How Can a Defect in Energy Production Affect Us?

A defect at any point during this process can impact the final quantity of ATP produced. In other words, a deficiency or dysfunction in one or more of the complexes causes an energy shortage within the cells of our bodies. Some defects may be quite significant (i.e., only 5 percent of an enzyme complex is functional), while others may be only mildly deficient. There are actually many causes of mitochondrial dysfunction, including mitochondrial uncoupling, apoptosis, duplication, deletions, and vulnerability due to oxidative damage and toxicity.

In addition, remember that we all have many different types of cells within our bodies (immune cells, blood cells, muscle cells, skin cells, cells that line the inside of our digestive tract, brain cells, etc.). Even in the same individual, certain types of cells (i.e., the mitochondria within those cells) may be more dysfunctional than others. This helps explain why some people with Mito have profound GI distress, while others may have pervasive developmental delay or cognitive difficulty or muscle weakness. Likewise, some adults may have "soft signs" of mitochondrial disease for years before a diagnosis, while others are faced with progressive and devastating symptoms that come on very quickly.

Energy-hungry cells are likely to manifest more obvious problems when there is an energy metabolism defect. For example, skeletal muscle cells require tremendous and sustained amounts of energy, so fatigue, muscle pain, weakness, and cramping would more readily appear when a person with Mito exceeds her available energy supply. Moreover, over time this energy deficit can result in cell malfunction and damage. Although all of our bodies' systems are dependent on the energy created by the process of oxidative phosphorylation, the threshold for impact by an OX-PHOS defect may be more crucial for some organ systems than for others. This explanation helps us understand why more energy-dependent body systems, such as the central nervous system and gastrointestinal system, would be most affected by a mitochondrial defect.

Nonetheless, mitochondrial researchers and clinicians believe that OX-PHOS function is not the exclusive component that predicts a person's clinical presentation, symptoms, ability, or lifespan. Many factors, including defects in the genes that code other mitochondrial processes, also play a large role in how effectively (or ineffectively) ATP can be produced, and how our cells adapt. (More about this in Chapter 2 on diagnosis.)

Free Radicals—A Common Link between Diseases of Aging & Mitochondrial Diseases

Mitochondrial function (i.e., effectiveness and efficiency of producing energy) is impaired in two groups of people: the elderly and people with mitochondrial disease. Further, some symptoms of mitochondrial disease (even in children) mimic the natural aging process in several ways. How is this possible? How can symptoms in children, teens, and previously healthy adults have similarities to the diseases of aging? We know that the mitochondria are responsible for many activities within the body, but their primary purpose is to make energy. Remember that the usable energy currency is called ATP. The mitochondria are able to convert the food that we eat into energy that the body can use. When the mitochondria don't work effectively or efficiently, less energy is produced. Inefficient mitochondria don't work as effectively as they should, like an assembly line that is missing a part and cannot keep up. This inefficiency in the mitochondria creates an accumulation of harmful by-products, like unwanted waste, called free radicals. When free radicals accumulate in cells, they cause damage.

For healthy mitochondria, with the perfect balance of energy input to energy output, harmful free radicals are able to be overcome by the normal activities of our cells. However, for children and adults who have a dysfunction in their mitochondria, production and accumulation of these harmful by-products is thought to occur at an increased rate. In circumstances when the mitochondria do not function properly, the mitochondria are not able to keep up. Free radicals, as well as other metabolic by-products, can accumulate. Meanwhile, the energy production process cannot speed up to accommodate the dysfunction. Dr. Bruce Cohen is a leader in clinical mitochon-

Recap: Important Energy Production Terms

Glucose: Glucose is derived from food and ultimately, along with fats and proteins, is converted into energy. During glycolysis, glucose is broken down into pyruvate, which is then converted into energy in the next step of energy synthesis in the mitochondria.

ATP (adenosine triphosphate): The star of the show, ATP is the energy molecule that we all want more of! Thirty-six ATP molecules per unit of glucose are the result of normal energy metabolism.

ADP (adenosine diphosphate): ADP is the "understudy" to ATP. ADP grabs an additional phosphate and becomes ATP during the reaction that takes place in Complex V of the electron transport chain. Adenosine diphosphate (ADP) becomes adenosine triphosphate (ATP) when phosphorylation takes place (in other words, another phosphate is added for a grand total of three).

Coenzyme Q10 (CoQ10): Also known as ubiquinone, CoQ10 is a "taxi driver" for the high-energy electrons that need to move along through the electron transport chain between Complexes I and II, and onto Complex III. High doses of CoQ10 are often taken as a supplement by children and adults with mitochondrial disease in order to improve mitochondrial function.

Cytochrome c: Also a "taxi driver" for high-energy electrons, cytochrome c shuttles electrons from Complex III to IV.

NADH & FADH2: These proteins hold high-energy electrons, which move through the electron transport chain to ultimately create ATP. NADH is found in Complex I; FADH2 is associated with Complex II.

Oxygen (O2): The presence of oxygen is necessary for the reactions within the electron transport chain to occur. Oxygen "accepts" electrons during these reactions and produces water. Without oxygen, the electron transport chain cannot occur. The presence of oxygen is what makes this energy production pathway so effective (because energy can be produced other ways, but is much less efficient).

Electrons: Molecules with a negative charge. Electrons are transferred along the electron transport chain and are eventually bound to oxygen. As this occurs, an electrochemical gradient is created across the mitochondrial membrane.

Protons: Molecules with a positive charge. Protons are pumped across the mitochondrial inner membrane, building up a force like water in a dam that rushes back into Complex V, creating ATP.

drial medicine and uses the analogy that, like a car engine, mitochondria can only burn fuel at a certain rate, and reach a set limit where the energy-producing reactions cannot go any faster. In fact, even if one were able to provide additional oxygen or fuel for the mitochondria, the electron transport chain has a maximum speed and capacity to use these molecules. Accordingly, during the process of using oxygen to convert the molecules from food into molecules that can be used for energy (oxidative phosphorylation), defective mitochondria generate more harmful free radicals. This in turn can lead to more rapid cellular and organ dysfunction over time.

The idea that dysfunctional mitochondria are not able to burn fuel effectively actually helps to explain two important premises of mitochondrial disease diagnosis and management. First, defective mitochondria not only generate more free radicals, but also cause more metabolic by-products of all types to be dumped into the cell. Think of a fire that doesn't burn efficiently and subsequently produces a lot of smoke and little heat. The overabundance of these by-products—not only free radicals but also naturally occurring metabolic by-products such as lactic acid, pyruvic acid, and amino acids such as alanine—can build-up in the blood. In the presence of mitochondrial dysfunction, abnormally high blood (serum) levels of these by-products can be measured and are considered red flags for mitochondrial disease. This is especially true when the mitochondria are required to work harder, such as during periods of illness, fever, or physiological stress. It makes sense then that a number of children and adults with Mito have elevated lactate (serum lactic acid, a metabolic by-product) levels during an illness or hospitalization, even if their levels are near normal at other times. In other words, when the mitochondria are ineffectively converting food into usable energy, an excess of these by-products is pumped out into the blood and results in abnormally high lactate levels. The accumulation of these by-products can contribute to a person's Mito symptoms, such as muscle pain or fatigue, but are otherwise not detectable except through specific blood and urine laboratory tests.

Second, the accumulation of harmful free radicals is thought to be neutralized by another type of molecule called antioxidants. Antioxidants are scavenger molecules that "eat up" the excess free radicals that contribute to disease and neurologic diseases of aging. Some antioxidant enzymes exist naturally in our bodies, such as glutathione. However, use of the enzymes in most forms is not helpful because the enzymes are broken down in the stomach and are unable to be used by the cells. Instead, many of the supplements used by physicians to treat children and adults with mitochondrial disease are antioxidant compounds, including Vitamin C, alpha-lipoic acid, selenium, and, most commonly, coenzyme Q10.

Left unmanaged, researchers suggest that high levels of harmful free radicals can contribute to cell damage and contribute to disease. (In fact, many "anti-aging" supplements and products contain ingredients that are antioxidants.) People with mitochondrial disease often take supplemental antioxidants intended to help "clean up" an abundance of harmful free radicals that could cause further harm to an already fragile system. Usually these supplements are compounded together as part of the "Mito cocktail," which is explained fully in Chapter 4 on treatment.

Key Points from This Chapter

■ Oxidative phosphorylation is a series of metabolic reactions that takes place via five protein complexes (the electron transport chain) inside the mitochondria. The energy made in the mitochondria is used by the cell to fuel all systems of the body and is called ATP.

■ Energy in the form of ADP is released when the positive and negative particles proceed through the first four complexes in the ETC. The energy thus created is stored in the mitochondrial membrane, and is tapped after enough energy has built up to create a gradient, or force, to move to the final complex (Complex V ATPase) where ADP is converted to the final energy molecule, ATP.

■ Mitochondria play a key role in the process of aging and are susceptible to damage by harmful by-products called free radicals. Antioxidant compounds combat the cellular damage caused by free radicals.

■ There are many potential opportunities for mitochondrial dysfunction to occur during the process of breaking down food into energy, and both the place where the defect occurs and the degree of defect makes a difference in how symptoms manifest. This helps to explain why there is such a spectrum of clinical presentation among patients with Mito.

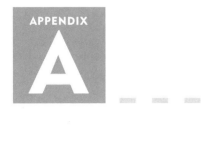

Glossary

Acetyl CoA: A necessary molecule in metabolism that conveys the carbon atoms to the Kreb's (citric acid) cycle to be oxidized for energy.

Acupressure: Alternative medicine technique that uses the fingers, elbows, or feet to apply pressure to key points to the surface of the skin to stimulate the body's self curative abilities.

Acupuncture: Alternative medicine technique that employs the use of needles that are inserted and manipulated at key points in the body.

Acute: Sharp, sudden, severe.

Adaptive equipment: Devices or tools specially made to assist disabled persons with daily living activities to support independence, such as walking, reading, hearing, eating, bathing, dressing, grooming, driving.

Adenosine diphosphate (ADP): An adenosine compound containing two phosphoric acid groups. ADP is the precursor to ATP in the energy production process within the cell.

Adenosine triphosphate (ATP): A compound containing three phosphoric acid groups. An enzyme found in all cells, but particularly in muscle cells. When this substance is split by enzyme action, energy is produced. The energy of the muscle is stored in this compound.

ADP: *See* Adenosine diphosphate.

Aerobic metabolism: Provides most of the energy for long duration exercise by using oxygen to convert nutrients to energy. Relies on the circulatory system to transport oxygen to the working muscles for endurance exercise.

ALA: *See* Alpha lipoic acid.

Alalia: *See* Speech delay.

Alanine: Nonessential amino acid used by the body to build protein.

Alopecia: Absence or loss of hair, especially of the head.

Alpers' disease: Progressive degenerative disease of the central nervous system mostly seen in infants and children. Caused by genetic mutations in the POLG gene.

Alpha lipoic acid (ALA): Fatty acid antioxidant made by the body and found in every cell. Needed by the body to produce energy for the body's normal functions by converting glucose (blood sugar) into energy.

Amino acid proteins: Building blocks of proteins and the intermediates of metabolism. Building blocks of biological molecules.

Aminoglycoside antibiotics: Antibiotic effective against certain bacteria.

Amnesia: Loss of memory.

Anaerobic metabolism: Provides energy by the partial breakdown of carbohydrates without the need for oxygen. Produces energy for short, high intensity bursts of activity before the lactic acid builds up resulting in muscle pain, burning, and fatigue making it difficult to maintain such intensity. *See also* Glycolysis.

Anesthesia protocol: Medication and procedure alerts for patients receiving anesthesia (drug that reduces or prevents pain).

Anorexia: Eating disorder characterized by below average, unhealthy body weight and obsessive fear of gaining weight.

Anoxia: Complete deprivation of oxygen supply.

Antioxidants: Molecules found in food or in the body that prevent or slow oxidative cell damage. Some supplements, like CoQ10, have antioxidant properties. Some foods are high in antioxidants, especially grains, legumes, and brightly colored fruits and vegetables.

Antiretrovirals: Medications used to treat viral and retro viral infections caused by viruses such as HIV.

Anxiety: A normal reaction to stress that creates a physiological and psychological state which may result in feelings of fear, worry, uneasiness, or dread.

Apnea: Temporary cessation of breathing.

ASD: *See* Autism spectrum disorders.

Ataxia: Defective muscular coordination, especially manifested when voluntary muscular movements are attempted. Tremors.

Atonic seizure: Sudden loss of muscle tone and strength causing the person to suddenly fall down. Also called drop attack or drop seizure. *See also* Epilepsy; Seizure.

ATP: *See* Adenosine triphosphate.

Autism: A disorder of brain development characterized by impaired social and communication skills with a limited range of interests and restricted and repetitive behaviors. *See also* Autism spectrum disorders (ASD); Pervasive developmental disorder (PDD).

Autism spectrum disorders (ASD): A range of psychological conditions characterized by widespread abnormalities of social interactions and communication, as well as restricted interests and repetitive behavior. *See also* Autism; Pervasive developmental disorder (PDD).

Autistic regression: Term used to describe the state of a child when he appears to develop typically but then starts to lose speech and social skills between 15 and 30 months and is subsequently diagnosed with autism.

Autonomic dysfunction: *See* Dysautonomia.

Autonomic nervous system: The part of the nervous system that is concerned with control of involuntary bodily functions such as increased heart rate or pupil dilation.

Autosomal dominant (Dominant inheritance): Disease caused when one parent passes on the mutated gene.

Autosomal recessive (Recessive inheritance): Disease caused when both parents pass on a specific genetic mutation.

Baseline: A known or initial value with which subsequent values of what is being measured can be compared.

Beckman oral motor techniques: Oral motor therapy that strengthens and activates the muscles of the face and mouth needed for chewing and swallowing.

Beta blockers: Drugs that treat heart rhythm disorders, high blood pressure, migraines, panic attacks, or glaucoma.

Biochemical testing: Measuring the amount or activity of a particular enzyme or protein in a sample of blood, urine, or tissue.

Biofeedback: Alternative therapy practice that trains individuals to improve their health by controlling certain bodily functions that happen involuntarily, such as heart rate or blood pressure. Often used for chronic pain or migraine headaches.

Biomedical treatments: From biological and medical, pertains to the application of natural sciences to the study of medicine, frequently used for autism.

Bipolar disorder: Manic-depressive disorder: brain disorder that causes unusual mood shifts, energy, and activity levels. Usually characterized by intense emotional moods that may fluctuate from overly joyous and overexcited to extreme sadness and hopelessness.

Blood lactate: Lactic acid that appears in the blood as a result of intense exercise indicating insufficient oxygen is available to fuel that exercise and results in muscle fatigue.

Buccal swab test: Cheek swab, method of rubbing the inside of the cheek with a soft swab to collect cheek cells for DNA testing.

Cardiac ultrasound: *See* Echocardiogram (ECHO).

Cardiomyopathies: Abnormalities or disease of the heart muscle.

Carnitine: An amino acid produced by the liver and kidneys that helps the body turn fat into energy.

Carnitine transport: Transfer of long chain fatty acids into the mitochondria for beta oxidation (to extract energy from fat: metabolism).

Casein: Principal protein in milk that supplies the amino acids necessary for growth and development.

CBT: *See* Cognitive behavioral therapy.

Cellular respiration: Metabolic reactions that take place in the cells of organisms to convert biochemical energy from nutrients into ATP, energy.

Central nervous system (CNS): The majority of the nervous system that consists of the brain and spinal cord. It integrates information received from and coordinates activity for all parts of the body.

Cerebral palsy: Loss of sensation or loss of ability to move or to control movement resulting from developmental defects in brain or trauma at birth.

Chelation therapy: The recognized treatment for removing heavy metals (such as lead) from the body.

Chromosomal DNA: *See* Nuclear DNA.

Chromosome: Organized structure of DNA and protein found in cells.

Chronic: Recurring frequently, continuing a long time, persistent, does not easily go away.

Chronic progressive external opthalmoplegia (CPEO): Slowly progressing disease characterized first by drooping eyelids and eventual inability/difficulty moving the eye.

Citric acid cycle: *See* Kreb's cycle.

Classic symptoms or syndrome: "Red flags" or typical complaints associated with a particular disease.

Clinical presentation: The interpretation of physical signs or symptoms to determine a diagnosis.

CNS: *See* Central nervous system.

Coenzyme Q10 (CoQ10): Oil soluble, vitamin-like substance found in most mitochondria cells, assists in the body's generation of energy.

Cognition: The process of thought, processing information, concept development, knowledge.

Cognitive behavioral therapy (CBT): Mental health counseling that assists the patient in becoming aware of inaccurate or negative thinking so they may view and respond to challenging situations more clearly and effectively.

Cognitive degeneration: Slow, progressive deterioration and dysfunction of brain systems.

Cognitive delay: A significant lag in reasoning, thinking, problem solving, and judgment.

Colitis: Inflammation of the colon.

Complex I: NADH dehydrogenase: The first enzyme in the mitochondrial respiratory chain. Used to power the synthesis of ATP, energy production in the cell.

Complex II: succinate dehydrogenase: Second enzyme in the mitochondrial respiratory chain and a component of the Krebs cycle. Injects electrons into the respiratory chain for energy conservation at a lower level than NADH.

Complex III: cytochrome bc1: Third enzyme in the mitochondrial respiratory chain. Able to increase production of ROS (reactive oxygen species) during hypoxia (state in which the whole or a region of the body is deprived of adequate oxygen supply).

Complex IV (Cytochrome c oxidase): Fourth enzyme in the mitochondrial respiratory chain. *See also* COX.

CoQ10: *See* Coenzyme Q10.

COX (Cytochrome c oxidase, Complex IV): A large enzyme complex, COX is the fourth complex in the electron transport chain and is a crucial step in the synthesis of ATP. Mutations within the COX assembly (Complex IV) are often more severe than other mitochondrial defects and are associated with several genetic mutations and syndromes including SURF1, Leigh's Syndrome, and leukodystrophy.

CPEO: *See* Chronic progressive external opthalmoplegia.

Creatine: An organic acid produced by the body that helps to supply energy to all cells in the body, especially muscle.

Cristae: Folds within the inner membrane of the mitochondria.

CVS: *See* Cyclic vomiting syndrome.

Cyclic vomiting syndrome (CVS): Disorder that causes recurrent episodes of intense nausea, vomiting, and tiredness.

Cytochrome c: Acts as a carrier of electrons between complexes III and IV in the electron transport chain.

Cytopathy: Disorder of a cell.

D5: Fluid solution of a balance of salt and sugar in distilled water used for intravenous fluid replenishment during emergencies and surgery.

DAN: Abbreviation for Defeat Autism Now from the Autism Research Institute committed to finding effective treatments for autism.

Dehydration: Excessive loss of body fluid.

Dementia: Irreversible deterioration of a person's mental state with absence or reduction of intellectual abilities.

Deoxyribonucleic acid (DNA): Chemical basis of heredity and the carrier of genetic information for organisms.

Depakote: *See* Valproic acid.

Depression: Mood disorder characterized by feelings of sadness, loss, anger, or frustration that interfere with daily life for long periods of time.

Developmental delay: A term used to describe the condition of a child aged three to nine who is not achieving new skills in the typical time frame and/or is exhibiting behaviors that are not appropriate for his age. Can affect psychomotor, physical, cognitive, social, emotional, communication, or adaptive growth and development. *See also* Individuals with Disabilities Education Act.

Diprivan: *See* Propofol.

DNA: *See* Deoxyribonucleic acid.

Dominant inheritance. *See* Autosomal dominant.

Down syndrome: A common genetic disorder in which a person is born with forty-seven rather than forty-six chromosomes in all or some of his cells, resulting in developmental delays, low muscle tone, characteristic physical features, and other effects.

Dysautonomia (Autonomic dysfunction): Any disease or malfunction of the autonomic nervous system.

Dysmotility: Muscles of the gastrointestinal tract do not work normally.

Dysphasia: Trouble swallowing.

Dyspnea: Shortness of breath either at rest or during exercise.

Dyspraxia: Specific disorder in the area of motor skill development.

Early intervention: Infant/toddler/child evaluations and therapies or any action that may modify medical or developmental diagnoses.

Echocardiogram (ECHO, cardiac ultrasound): Imaging technique that uses standard ultrasound techniques that can show two dimensional images of the heart/cardiovascular system.

Electrolytes: Salts in the body that conduct electricity and are found in body fluids, tissues, and blood.

Electron: A molecule with a negative charge. Electrons are transferred along the electron transport chain and are eventually bound to oxygen. As this occurs, an electrochemical gradient is created across the mitochondrial membrane. *See also* Proton.

Electron transport chain (ETC): Series of reactions within the mitochondria that generate energy. *See also* Respiratory chain.

Encephalopathy: Any disorder, disease, or dysfunction of the brain.

Energetics: Science of study of energy, especially in relation to human use of energy in form of food and expenditure of energy.

ENS: *See* Enteric nervous system.

Enteral nutrition: Alternative means of obtaining nutrition through a feeding tube directly into the digestive tract if the oral means of feeding cannot be sustained but the person has a functioning gastrointestinal tract.

Enteric nervous system (ENS): Part of the nervous system that controls the gastrointestinal system.

Enzymes: Special proteins that facilitate all the biochemical reactions in the body.

Enzymology: Branch of science that studies the biochemical nature of enzymes and their actions.

Epidemiology: Science that defines and explains the interrelationships of factors that determine disease frequency and distribution.

Epilepsy: Brain disorder that causes spontaneous, repeated seizures caused by abnormally excited electrical signals in the brain. *See also* Seizure.

Erythromycin: Antibiotic used to treat certain bacterial infections such as pneumonia, bronchitis, diphtheria, whooping cough, lung, skin, ear, intestine, and urinary tract infections.

ETC: *See* Electron transport chain.

Exercise function test: Assessment that provides specific information of the individual systems involved during exercise, such as cardiac, pulmonary, hematologic, musculoskeletal.

Exercise intolerance: Lack of ability to endure physical exertion/exercise at the expected level or duration. Characterized by fatigue, exhaustion, muscle pain, cramps, weakness, or breathlessness.

Factitious disorder: *See* Fictitious symptom disorder.

FADH: *See* Flavine adenine dinucleotide.

Failure to thrive (FTT): A descriptive term used to identify children whose current weight or rate of weight gain is significantly below that of other children of the same age and sex.

Fatty acid: A type of molecule found in lipids (fats). May be saturated, unsaturated, and/or an essential fatty acid. Metabolism of fatty acids may be impaired in some mitochondrial disorders.

Fatty acid oxidation defect: A defect in one of the enzymes involved in fatty acid metabolism.

Fatty oxidation disorder (FOD): genetic metabolic deficiencies in which the body is unable to break down fatty acids to make energy because an enzyme is missing or not working.

Febrile: significant rise in body temperature, fever.

Fibroblasts: Type of cell found in connective tissue that produces collagen.

Fictitious symptom disorder (Factitious disorder): Mental illness characterized by a person feigning or creating physical or mental symptoms for the purpose of assuming the sick role.

Fine motor: Skills pertaining to small muscles, especially in the hand and related to manual dexterity and coordination.

Flavine adenine dinucleotide (FADH): An electron acceptor in the metabolic process.

FOD: *See* Fatty oxidation disorder.

Fragile X syndrome: A genetic condition involving changes in part of the X chromosome. A genetic condition resulting in a range of physical and intellectual limitations with emotional and behavioral features that can be mild to severe.

Free radical: A type of molecule formed as a natural by-product of oxygen reactions within the body which, when over-produced or accumulated within tissues, can be harmful. *See also* antioxidants.

FTT: *See* Failure to thrive.

Gabapentin: *See* Neurontin.

Gastric dismotility: Abnormal contractions of the muscles in the gut wall result in slow and uncoordinated movement of food through the digestive tract.

Gastrointestinal (GI): Refers to the stomach and small and large intestines.

Gastronomy tube: *See* G tube.

Gastroparesis: A disorder that affects the ability of the stomach to empty its contents normally but there is no blockage.

Gene: The basic unit of heredity. Each gene occupies a certain place on a chromosome; heredity traits are controlled by pairs of genes in the same position on a pair of chromosomes. A human has thousands of genes. *See also* Genetic, Genetic disease, and Genomic sequencing.

Genetic: Pertaining to heredity and reproduction.

Genetic counseling: Process by which patients or relatives at risk of genetically inherited disorders are advised of the consequences or nature of the disorder, the probability of developing or transmitting it, and the options open to them for management or family planning.

Genetic disease: Inherited disease caused by mutation in a person's genes.

Genome: In molecular biology and genetics, genome is the entirety of an organism's hereditary information.

Genomic sequencing: Laboratory process that determines the complete DNA sequence of an organism's hereditary information. Genetic diseases can sometimes be identified by genomic sequencing.

GERD: Gastroesophageal reflux disease characterized when the liquid content of the stomach backs up or refluxes into the esophagus. *See also* Reflux.

GI: *See* Gastrointestinal.

Global delay: Term that describes a condition that occurs during the developmental period of a child's life—birth to 18 years. Characterized by lower intellectual functioning and accompanied by limited communication, self care, home living, vocational, academic, and leisure skills.

Glucophage: *See* Metformin.

Glucose: Sugar, the most important carbohydrate in the body's metabolism formed during digestion.

Glutathione metabolism: Production and use of glutathione in the body. Glutathione is a naturally occuring anti-oxidant produced by the body in the cell that helps scavenge free radicals, protecting the cells from damage.

Gluten: Protein found in wheat, rye, and barley.

Glycolysis: Metabolic process that converts glucose into molecules that can be used by the mitochondria to produce energy. *See also* Anaerobic metabolism.

Gross motor: Skills pertaining to the large muscles as in balancing, running, throwing.

G tube (Gastronomy tube): Alternative means of nutritional support through a feeding tube surgically inserted through a small incision in the abdomen into the stomach to provide long term nutrition.

Heat intolerance: Inability to feel comfortable in high external temperatures and humidity.

Hemophilia: Inherited, rare bleeding disorder characterized by unusually long time for blood to clot.

Heteroplasmy: Situation in which, within a single cell, there is a mixture of mitochondria, some containing normal DNA, some containing mutant DNA.

Histological testing (Histochemical testing): Microscopic tissue examination. Tissue is most commonly obtained via a surgical procedure where a small biopsy sample is taken from the muscle or other organs.

Homeopathic medicine (Homeopathy): Alternative form of medicine that seeks to stimulate the body's ability to heal itself by giving small doses of highly diluted substances that produce similar symptoms in healthy people.

Homeostasis: The body's ability to physiologically regulate its inner environment to ensure stability in response to the outer environment, i.e., changes in temperature, exposure, toxins, etc.

Hospice: Type of care that focuses on the comfort and quality of life to support the patient and families when dealing with a life limiting illness.

Hydration: Amount of water or other fluids consumed per day.

Hypochondria: Condition characterized by a person having excessive preoccupation, worry, and undue alarm about having a serious illness with no medical basis.

Hypoglycemia: Term used to describe the condition that occurs when blood sugar (glucose) is too low.

Hypotonia: Loss of tone in the muscles, pertains to defective muscular tone or tension.

Hypoxia: Condition in which whole body or a region of the body is deprived of adequate oxygen supply.

ID: *See* Intellectual disability.

IDEA: *See* Individuals with Disabilities Education Act.

Idiopathic: Disease without recognizable cause, pertaining to conditions without clear origins.

IEP: *See* Individualized Education Program.

IFSP: *See* Individual Family Service Plan.

Immunodeficiency: Body's immune system has decreased ability or total inability to fight infectious diseases.

Impairment: A medical condition that leads to disability. Any loss or abnormality of physiological, psychological or anatomical structure or function.

Individual Family Service Plan (IFSP): Mandated by the Individuals with Disabilities Education Act (IDEA). Plan that documents and guides early intervention process for children with disabilities and their families. Contains information about the services necessary to facilitate a child's development and enhance the family's capacity to facilitate the child's development. *See also* Individuals with Disabilities Education Act.

Individualized Education Program (IEP): Mandated by the Individuals with Disabilities Education Act (IDEA). Plan to meet the unique educational needs of one child with disabilities, coordinated to include parents, therapists, teachers, and any related professionals so child may reach educational goals easier than they otherwise would. *See also* Individuals with Disabilities Education Act.

Individuals with Disabilities Education Act (IDEA): US Federal Law that governs how states and public agencies provide special education, special related services, and early intervention to children with disabilities ages birth to 18 or 21.

Insensible fluid loss: Term to describe water that leaves the body through breathing and the skin.

Intellectual disability (ID): (formerly mental retardation) A condition that results in cognitive skills that fall below the average range as well as significant difficulties in acquiring the skills needed to function independently in the environment. Causes may or may not be genetic.

Ischemia: Condition in which blood flow and thus oxygen is restricted to a part of the body, organ, or tissue.

Ischuria: *See* Urinary retention.

Jejunostomy tube: *See* J tube.

Jejunum: Upper section of the small intestine which is just below the stomach.

J tube (Jejunostomy tube): Alternative means of nutritional support through a feeding tube surgically implanted into the upper section of the small intestine to bypass the stomach and be fed directly into the intestinal tract.

Kearns Sayre Syndrome: Also known as oculocraniosomatic disease. A mitochondrial myopathy characterized by isolated involvement of the muscles controlling eyelid and eye movement.

Ketogenic diet: High fat, adequate protein, low carbohydrate diet used to treat hard to control seizures in children.

Kidney dysfunction: Slow loss of kidney function that removes waste and excess water from the body.

Kreb's cycle (Citric acid cycle): A series of enzyme catalyzed chemical reactions important in all living cells that use oxygen as part of cellular respiration. Occurs in the matrix of the mitochondria.

Lactate: *See* Lactic acid.

Lactated ringer's (LR): Liquid solution of electrolytes in distilled water used for intravenous fluid replenishment during emergencies or surgery.

Lactic acid (Lactate, Milk acid): A colorless syrupy liquid formed in milk by the fermentation of the sugars by micro-organisms. Formed during muscular activity by the breakdown of glycogen.

Lactic acidosis: Condition when the level of lactic acid builds up in the body faster than it can be removed. Produced when oxygen levels in the body drop and characterized by nausea and weakness.

Leiber hereditary optic neuropathy (LHON): Condition mitochondrially inherited from the mother characterized by degeneration and loss of central vision.

Leigh's disease/syndrome: Mitochondrial disease usually starting in the first year of life with floppiness, wobbliness, vomiting, involuntary writhing movements, hyperventilation, loss of motor and verbal milestones, spasticity, hearing loss, vision loss, carbohydrate intolerance, high lactic acid.

Lethargy: A condition of sluggishness or stupor.

Leukodsytrophy: Group of disorders characterized by degeneration or hardening of the white matter of the brain.

LHON: *See* Leiber hereditary optic neuropathy.

LR: *See* Lactated ringer's.

Magnetic resonance imaging (MRI): A medical imaging technique used in radiology to visualize detailed internal structures.

Magnetic resonance spectroscopy (MRS): A medical imaging technique used in radiology.

Malabsorption: Abnormality or difficulty absorbing nutrients from food in the gastrointestinal tract.

Malaise: General feeling of illness or discomfort.

Malignant hyperthermia (MH): Inherited, life threatening condition that causes rapid rise in body temperature and severe muscle contractions when the person is exposed to general anesthesia drugs.

Malnutrition: Condition that occurs when the body is not receiving enough nutrients.

Maternal mitochondrial DNA mutation inheritance (mtDNA): DNA of mitochondrial origin inherited from the mother.

Matrix: Part of the mitochondria enclosed by the innermost membrane, which contains the mitochondrial DNA as well as high concentration of enzymes.

Meditation: Alternative therapy practice that trains the mind to self-induce a level of consciousness to achieve benefit, such as reduction of stress or pain.

MELAS: *See* Mitochondrial encephalopathy lactic acidosis and stroke.

Melatonin: Hormone produced by the pineal gland in the brain that regulates sleep and wake cycles.

Mendelian inheritance: Copy of each gene comes from the mother and father.

Meningitis: Inflammation of the membranes of the spinal cord or brain.

Mental retardation: *See* Intellectual disability.

MERRF: *See* Myoclonic epilepsy and ragged red fiber disease.

Metabolic: Physical and chemical changes that take place within an organism, all energy and material transformations within living cells.

Metabolic crisis: Rapid failure of physical and mental functions possibly resulting in death.

Metabolism: *See* Aerobic metabolism; Glutathione metabolism; Metabolic.

Metformin (Glucophage): Oral, anti-diabetic drug used to treat type 2 diabetes.

MH: *See* Malignant hyperthermia.

Migraines: Very painful headache characterized by pulsing or throbbing in one area of the head and often accompanied by nausea and vomiting and sensitivity to light and sound.

Milk acid: *See* Lactic acid.

MIRAS: *See* Mitochondrial recessive ataxia syndrome.

Mito cocktail: Term for variety of vitamins and supplements commonly used by patients diagnosed with mitochondrial disorders.

Mitochondria (Mitochondrion, s.): Microscopic organelles that create energy for the cells in living things. Mitochondria are known as the powerhouse of the cell, and are not only important in energy production but also play a role in protein regulation and fat metabolism as well. Mitochondria use oxygen to release energy through a process called cellular respiration. *See also* Cellular respiration.

Mitochondrial disorder: Dysfunction of the mitochondria which are slender, microscopic filaments in cells that are the source of energy in the cell and are involved in protein synthesis and fats metabolism.

Mitochondrial encephalopathy lactic acidosis and stroke (MELAS): Disease caused by defect in the mitochondrial genes inherited from the female parent. Affects many of the body's systems, particularly the brain, nervous system, and muscles.

Mitochondrial neurogastrointestinal encephalopathy (MNGIE): Disease that affects several parts of the body, particularly the digestive system, and nervous system.

Mitochondrial oxidative stress: State where free radical molecules are produced in large numbers and cause damage to nearby cells.

Mitochondrial recessive ataxia syndrome (MIRAS): Mitochondrial disease resulting from POLG mutation and recessive inheritance. Symptoms include epilepsy, encephalopathy, balance difficulties, psychiatric symptoms, cognitive impairment, eye disorders.

MNGIE: *See* Mitochondrial neurogastrointestinal encephalopathy.

Molecular diagnosis: All tests and methods used to identify a disease or a predisposition to a disease by analyzing the DNA.

Molecular DNA sequencing: Molecular genetics is the study of the agents (molecules) that pass information from generation to generation. These molecules are our genes and are long polymers (large molecules composed of repeating structural units) of deoxyribonucleic acid or DNA. DNA consists of four chemical building blocks placed in a unique order to code for all the genes in living organisms. DNA sequencing is the scientific study by geneticists to compare DNA sequence from a healthy person to the same DNA sequence from an afflicted person.

Molecular testing: Used in DNA testing, examination of specific genes to detect abnormality.

Motility: Ability to move spontaneously.

Motor delay: Lag in a child's ability to develop muscular coordination. May be characterized by floppiness, clumsiness, weakness, poor muscle tone, irregular gait, or delayed speech. May be a sign of neurological dysfunction.

Motor movement disorders: Term used to describe variety of types of dysfunctions that result in movement irregularities. May be hypokinetic (impaired movement in one or more areas of the body) or hyperkinetic (excessive movements that are unplanned.)

MRI: *See* Magnetic resonance imaging.

MRS: *See* Magnetic resonance spectroscopy.

mtDNA: *See* Maternal mitochondrial DNA mutation inheritance.

Muscle biopsy: Minor surgical procedure using a needle or small incision to remove a small sample of muscle tissue which is examined microscopically to determine a diagnosis.

Mutation (genetic): Changes in a genomic sequence. May be sudden and spontaneous changes in the cell caused by radiation, viruses, mutagenic chemicals, or transposons as well as errors that occur during DNA replication.

Myasthenia gravis: Disease characterized by muscular weakness and progressive fatigue.

Myoclonic epilepsy and ragged red fiber disease (MERRF): Disorder that affects many parts of the body, especially muscles and nervous system. Characterized by muscle twitches, weakness and stiffness, seizures, coordination difficulties, loss of sensation in the extremities, and deterioration of mental function.

Myoclonic seizure: Brief, jerking, rapid contraction and relaxation of muscles, usually on both sides of the body. *See also* Epilepsy.

Myoclonus: Brief, involuntary twitching or spasms of a muscle or group of muscles.

Myopathy: Disease or abnormal condition of muscles.

NADH Dehydrogenase: Located in the inner mitochondrial membrane, it is first enzyme (Complex I) of the mitochondrial electron transport chain.

NARP: *See* Neuropathy, ataxia, and retinitis pigmentosa.

nDNA: *See* Nuclear DNA.

Neuromuscular: Pertaining to or affecting both nerves and muscles.

Neurontin (Gabapentin): Pharmaceutical drug used to treat seizures and nerve pain.

Neuropathic pain: State of chronic pain accompanied by tissue injury and damaged nerve fibers.

Neuropathy: *See* Peripheral neuropathy.

Neuropathy, ataxia, and retinitis pigmentosa (NARP): Mitochondrial disease featuring weakness of the muscles near the trunk, wobbliness, retinal disease, seizures, and developmental delay.

Neuropsychological evaluation (NPE): Assessment of cognitive functioning and behavior. Areas assessed typically include motor, orientation, new learning, memory, intelligence, language, visual perception and decision, reasoning, judgment skills. May also contribute to the diagnosis of a cognitive deficit and the localization of abnormalities in the central nervous system.

Neuropsychological issues: The study of brain functioning and its relationship to behavior and learning.

Neuropsychological testing: Use of scientifically objective tests to evaluate brain function. May cover the range from simple motor performance to complex reasoning and problem solving.

Neuropsychology: Branch of medicine that studies the structure and function of the brain as it relates to reasoning, thinking, emotions, and behaviors.

Neutropenia: Disorder characterized by an abnormally low number of white blood cells.

NPE: *See* Neuropsychological evaluation.

NPO: Nothing by mouth/fasting.

Nuclear DNA (nDNA, Chromosomal DNA): DNA that make up 22 out of 23 chromosomes usually associated with genetic diseases.

Obsessive compulsive disorder (OCD): An anxiety disorder characterized by intrusive thoughts that produce uneasiness, fear, worry, apprehension, or repetitive behaviors.

Occupational therapy: Use of work-related skills to treat or train the physically or emotionally ill in self-care, work, play, and leisure time task performance skills.

OCD: *See* Obsessive compulsive disorder.

Oculocraniosomatic disease: *See* Kearns Sayre Syndrome.

OHI: *See* Other health impairment.

Optic nerve atrophy: Damage to the optic nerve—the nerve that carries images of what we see from the eye to the brain.

Organelle: A specialized structure within a cell that performs a specific function.

Organic acidemias: Term used to classify a group of metabolic disorders that disrupt normal amino acid metabolism.

Osmotic laxatives: Short term remedy for constipation that works by pulling large amounts of water into the large intestine thus making stools soft and loose.

Other health impairment (OHI): Physical or mental impairments that can affect a child's performance in school.

Oxidative phosphorylation (OX-PHOS): Metabolic pathway that uses energy released by the oxidation of nutrients to supply energy for metabolism.

Oxidative stress: Term to describe the level of damage in a cell, tissue, or organ caused by the by-products (free radicals) produced as a result of normal, essential metabolic reactions such as the body's ability to combine digested food with the air we breathe to produce energy.

OX-PHOS: *See* Oxidative phosphorylation.

Palliative: Medical care or treatment that focuses on reducing the severity of symptoms rather than treating the disease itself or providing a cure.

Pancreatic enzyme deficiency (Pancreatic insufficiency): Result when the pancreas does not secrete enough chemicals and digestive enzymes for normal digestion to occur.

Pancreatic insufficiency: *See* Pancreatic enzyme deficiency.

Paresthesia: Sensation of pricking, tingling, or numbness of the skin.

Paroxysmal neuropathies: Short, sharp, electric-like pains.

PDCD: *See* Pyruvate dehydrogenase complex deficiency.

PDD: *See* Pervasive developmental disorder.

PDH: *See* Pyruvate dehydrogenase complex.

Peripheral nervous system (PNS): Communications network made up of nerves and ganglia within the body that transmits information from the brain and spinal cord (central nervous system) to every other part of the body.

Peripheral neuropathy: Disorders caused by damage to the nerves of the peripheral nervous system which distorts and may interrupt messages between the brain and the rest of the body. Often characterized by pain and numbness in the hands and feet.

Pervasive developmental disorder (PDD): Group of disorders usually characterized by delays in the development of communication and socialization skills. *See also* Autism; Autism spectrum disorders (ASD).

Petit mal seizure: Brief disturbance of brain function due to abnormal electrical activity in the brain which results in a brief state of unawareness or staring. May be called an absence seizure. *See also* Epilepsy; Seizure.

Phenotype: The observable physical or biochemical characteristics of an organism. Can be determined by both genetic makeup and environmental influences.

Phenylalanine: An essential amino acid formed from protein.

Phenylketonuria (PKU): A recessive hereditary disease caused by the body's failure to oxidize an amino acid because of a defective enzyme.

Physiatrist (Rehabilitation physician): Physician who is an expert in nerve, muscle, and bone injuries or illnesses that affect how a person moves. Specializes in diagnosing and treating pain and restoring maximum function lost through illness, injury, or disability.

Physical therapy: Rehabilitation to promote restoration of function and prevention of disability concerned with circulation, strength, muscles, and motion.

Physiotherapist: Healthcare professional who works to improve movement and function of patients with physical difficulties as a result of illness, injury, disability, or aging.

PKU: *See* Phenylketonuria.

Plasma alanine: Major gluconeogenic amino acid used to make glucose in the liver.

POLG: *See* Polymerase subunit gamma.

Polymerase subunit gamma (POLG): Gene involved in mitochondrial DNA replication and repair. Mutations are associated with several mitochondrial diseases.

PNS: *See* Peripheral nervous system.

Prader-Willi syndrome: Uncommon genetic disorder characterized by poor muscle tone, floppiness, low levels of sex hormones, constant feeling of hunger.

Primary diagnosis (Principal diagnosis): Main condition established after study of signs and symptoms by the physician to be the primary cause of a health condition.

Primary generalized seizure: Seizures with no apparent cause that impair consciousness and distort the electrical activity of the whole or a large portion of the brain. *See also* Epilepsy; Seizure.

Principal diagnosis: *See* Primary diagnosis.

Probiotics: Small organisms that help maintain the natural balance of microflora in the intestines.

Prognosis: Medical terminology used to describe the course of the illness or disease and predict the outcome.

Propofol (Diprivan): Short acting drug that reduces anxiety, promotes sleep or loss of consciousness, and is used for general anesthesia or sedation.

Proton: A molecule with a positive charge. Protons are pumped across the mitochondrial inner membrane, building up a force like water in a dam that rushes back into Complex V, creating ATP. *See also* Electron.

Pseudo obstruction: Symptoms of intestinal blockage without any apparent obstruction resulting in small or large intestines losing their ability to contract and push food, stool, and air through the gastrointestinal tract.

Psychotropic medication: Any medication or chemical substance that acts upon the central nervous system and affects the mind, emotions, and behavior.

Ptosis: Dropping or drooping of the upper or lower eyelid.

Pulmonary function assessment: Test used to measure the lungs' capacity to move air in and out, hold air, and exchange oxygen and carbon dioxide.

Pyruvate: *See* Pyruvic acid.

Pyruvate dehydrogenase complex (PDH): Defect in enzyme involved in fatty acid metabolism.

Pyruvate dehydrogenase complex deficiency (PDCD): Neurodegenerative disorder associated with abnormal mitochondrial metabolism that derives energy from carbohydrates. Disruption of this cycle deprives the body of energy.

Pyruvic acid (Pyruvate): An organic acid produced in the metabolism of carbohydrates, fats, and amino acids. A product of sugar metabolism.

Quadriparesis: Weakness of all four limbs.

Ragged red fibers (RRF): Abnormal muscle cells.

Reactive oxygen species (ROS): Chemically reactive molecules containing oxygen. Strong oxidants that can damage other molecules and cell structures of which they are part. Mitochondrial membranes of the cell are highly susceptible.

Recessive inheritance: *See* Autosomal recessive.

Reflux: Condition when the contents of the stomach leak backwards from the stomach into the esophagus (tube from the mouth to the stomach). *See also* GERD.

Refractory to treatment: Resistant, unresponsive to treatment or cure.

Regression: Turning back or a return to a former state.

Rehabilitation physician: *See* Physiatrist.

Renal tubular acidosis: A condition that occurs when the kidneys fail to properly remove acid in the urine, leaving the blood too acidic.

Respiratory chain: Another term for the electron transport chain, the group of protein and enzyme complexes in the mitochondrial matrix where ATP is produced. Sometimes mitochondrial diseases are called respiratory chain disorders. *See also* Electron transport chain (ETC).

Respiratory syncytial virus (RSV): Very common, highly contagious virus that causes respiratory tract infections. RSV, along with other highly contagious viruses, is very dangerous for infants and young children with mitochondrial disease.

Restorative rest: Periods of inactivity, rest, or even daydreaming that enable the body to rejuvenate.

ROS: *See* Reactive oxygen species.

RRF: *See* Ragged red fibers.

RSV: *See* Respiratory syncytial virus.

Schizophrenia: Mental disorder characterized by difficulty to tell the difference between real and unreal experiences, think logically, have normal reactions, and behave normally in social situations.

Secondary diagnosis: Other medically related problems the patient may have that may or may not be related to or contribute to the primary diagnosis.

Seizure: Physical change in behavior caused by abnormal electrical activity in the brain. Some seizures are characterized by loss of awareness or consciousness or twitching or shaking of the body. *See also* Atonic seizure; Epilepsy.

Selective serotonin reuptake inhibitor (SSRI): Psychotropic drugs used as antidepressants to treat depression or anxiety disorders.

Sensorineural deafness: Hearing loss that occurs from damage to the inner ear, the nerve that runs from the ear to the brain.

Sensory integration disorder: *See* Sensory processing disorder.

Sensory neuropathy: Damage to the sensory nerve which may produce loss of sensation, tingling, numbness, and pain.

Sensory processing disorder (SPD, Sensory integration disorder): Neurological disorder resulting from the brain's inability to process certain information received from the body's five sensory systems—sight, sound, taste, smell, touch including temperature, position, and pain.

Serum ALT/AST: Test that measures the amount of this enzyme in the blood to determine if the liver is damaged or diseased.

Short bowel syndrome: A condition in which nutrients are not properly absorbed due to intestinal disease or surgical removal of a large portion of the small intestine.

Skeletal muscles: Muscle tissue that is attached to bone and is responsible for movement and supporting the skeleton.

Smooth muscle dysfunction: Irregular performance of involuntary muscles found in digestive tract, respiratory passages, urinary and genital ducts, urinary bladder, gallbladder, or walls of blood vessels.

Soft signs: Minor symptoms that suggest, but do not confirm, a diagnosis.

Speech delay (Alalia): A delay in the development of the actual process and use of making sounds using organs and mechanisms that produce speech.

Speech/language/oral-motor therapy: Study, diagnosis, and treatment of defects and disorders of the voice and spoken communication skills involving the larynx, mouth, lips, chest, and abdominal muscles.

SSRI: *See* Selective serotonin reuptake inhibitor.

Stamina: Endurance, capability to sustain prolonged effort.

Statins: Class of drug used to lower cholesterol levels.

Stroke: Interruption of blood supply to any part of the brain which results in brain cells dying.

Swallow dysfunction: Irregularity of ability to cause or enable the passage of something from the mouth through the throat and esophagus into the stomach by muscular action.

Swallow study: Evaluation of the cause of difficulty or inability to swallow.

Synapse: Point of junction between two neurons (brain cells).

Tachycardia: Abnormally rapid heart beat.

TENS therapy: *See* Transcutaneous electrical nerve stimulation (TENS) therapy.

Total parenteral nutrition (TPN): Using intravenous nutrition formula to bypass the normal eating and digestion process.

Toxicity: The degree to which an organism can be damaged by a poisonous substance.

Toxins: A poisonous substance produced by living cells or organisms that is capable of causing disease when introduced into body tissues.

TPN: *See* Total parenteral nutrition.

Transcutaneous electrical nerve stimulation (TENS) therapy: An alternative treatment therapy available for managing pain. A TENS unit is a portable battery operated device that sends electrical impulses to certain parts of the body to block pain signals.

Urinary retention (Ischuria): Lack of ability to urinate or to completely empty the bladder.

Vagal nerve stimulation (VNS): Type of treatment to treat seizures in which short bursts of electrical energy are directed to the brain via the vagus nerve, a large nerve in the neck. A small device is implanted under the skin with leads to the neck. *See also* Epilepsy.

Valproic acid (Depakote): Drug used to treat seizures or anxiety and mood disorders.

VNS: *See* Vagal nerve stimulation.

X-linked genetic inheritance: Gene causing the trait or disorder is located on the X chromosome.

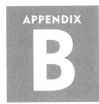
Physicians and Centers Offering Care and Testing for Patients with Mitochondrial Disease

denotes that the physician is part of a dedicated mitochondrial center or program

Labs Offering Mitochondrial Disease Testing

- **Clinical Biochemical Genetics**
  John M. Shoffner, MD
  Medical Neuro Genetics
  1 Dunwoody Parks, Suite 250
  Atlanta, GA 30338
  Phone: (678) 225-0222
  www.medicalneurogenetics.com/bios.asp

- **Gene Dx**
  207 Perry Parkway
  Gaithersburg, MD 20887
  Phone: (301) 519-2100
  Fax: (301) 519-2892
  Email: genedx@genedx.com
  www.genedx.com

- **Medical Genetics Laboratories**
  Baylor College of Medicine
  One Baylor Plaza, NAB 2015
  Houston, TX 77030
  Client Services: (800) 411-GENE (4363)
  Fax: (713) 798-2787
  Email: genetictest@bcm.edu
  www.bcm.edu/geneticlabs

- **MEDomics**
  Steve Sommer, MD
  Founder and President
  426 N. San Gabriel Ave.
  Azusa, CA 91702
  Phone: (626) 804-3645
  Fax: (626) 529-0907
  Email: info@medomics.com
  www.medomics.com

- **MitoMed Diagnostic Laboratory**
  University of California, Irvine
  2014 Hewitt Hall
  Irvine, CA 92697
  Phone: (949) 824-1886
  Fax: (949) 824-3007
  Email: mdl.lab@uci.edu
  www.mammag.uci.edu/foswiki/bin/view/
  MITOMED/MITOMEDClinicalLaboratory

- **Transgenomic**
  Craig Tuttle
  Chief Executive Officer, President
  12325 Emmet St.
  Omaha, NE 68164
  Phone: (888) 813-7253; (402) 452-5400
  Fax: (402) 452-5401
  Email: info@transgenomic.com
  www.transgenomic.com

Physicians and Centers by Region

NORTHEAST

- **Darius J. Adams, MD***
Children's Hospital/Albany Medical Center
47 New Scotland Ave., Suite MC88
A240
Albany, NY 12208
Phone: (518) 262-5120
Fax: (518) 262-5924
www.amc.edu

- **Julian Ambrus, MD**
Buffalo General Hospital
100 High St.
Buffalo, NY 14203
Phone: (716) 859-2985
Fax: (716) 859-1249
www.buffalo.edu/

- **Irina Anselm, MD***
Assistant professor in Neurology
New England Medical Center
300 Longwood Ave.
Fegan 11
Boston, MA 02115
Phone: (617) 355-2758
Fax: (617-730-0285)
www.childrenshospital.org

- **Gerard Berry, MD, PhD***
Director, Metabolism Program
Professor of Pediatrics, Harvard Medical School
Children's Hospital Boston
Genetics/Metabolism
300 Longwood Ave.
CLS 14
Boston, MA 02115
Phone: (617) 355-4316
Fax: (617) 730-0466
www.childrenshospital.org

■ **Basil Darras, MD***
Associate Neurologist in Chief for Clinical Services
Director, Neuromuscular Program
Children's Hospital Boston
Fegan 11
300 Longwood Ave.
Boston, MA 02115
Phone: (617) 355-8235
Fax: (617) 730-0279
www.childrenshospital.org

■ **Darryl Devivo, MD**
Pediatric Neurology-Board Certified
New York Presbyterian Hospital
710 West 168th St.
NI 101
New York, NY 10032
Phone: (212) 305-5244
http://nyp.org

■ **Salvatore DiMauro, MD***
Lucy G. Moses Professor of Neurology
Director Emeritus, H. Houston Merritt Clinical Research Center for
    Muscular Dystrophy and Related Diseases
Columbia University
630 W 168th St., #4-424B
New York, NY 10032
www.cumc.columbia.edu/dept/neurology

■ **Marni Falk, MD***
Pediatrics Department, Human Genetics and Molecular Biology
The Children's Hospital of Philadelphia
ARC 1002c
3615 Civic Center Blvd.
Philadelphia, PA 19104
Phone: (215) 590-4564
http://stokes.chop.edu

■ **Amy Goldstein, MD***
Pediatric Neurologist
University of Pittsburgh School of Medicine
Division of Child Neurology
4401 Penn Ave., Floor 2

Pittsburgh, PA 15224
Phone: (412) 692-5520
Fax: (412) 692-6787
www.chp.edu/CHP/Home

■ **Michio Hirano, MD***
Professor of Neurology and Pathology & Cell Biology Neuromuscular Disease
Columbia University Medical Center
710 West 168th St.
New York, NY 10032
Phone: (212) 305-1048
www.cumc.columbia.edu/dept/neurology

■ **David Holtzman, MD, PhD**
Mass General Hospital for Children
Pediatric Neurology
55 Fruit St.
YAW 6
Boston, MA 02114 -2696
Phone: (617) 726-3402
Fax: (617) 724-9610
www.massgeneral.org

■ **Staci Kallish, DO***
Pediatrics, Genetics and Metabolism
Clinical and Biochemical Geneticist
Tufts Medical Center/Floating Hospital for Children
800 Washington St.
Mailbox #340
Boston, MA 02111
Phone: (617) 636-8100
Fax: (617) 636-0745
www.tuftsmedicalcenter.org

■ **Mark S. Korson, MD***
Chief of Metabolism Service, Director of Metabolic Disorders Clinic
Tufts Medical Center/Floating Hospital for Children
800 Washington St.
Mailbox #434
Boston, MA 02111
Phone: (617) 636-8100
Fax: (617) 636-0745
www.tuftsmedicalcenter.org

■ **Katherine Sims, MD***
Director, Neurogenetics and Mitochondrial Disorders Clinic
Massachusetts General Hospital
55 Fruit St.
Boston, MA 02114
Phone: (617) 726-5718
Fax: (617) 724-9620
www.massgeneral.org

SOUTHEAST

■ **Carol Greene, MD**
Director, Pediatric Genetics Clinic
Co-Director, Adult Genetics Clinic
Certification in Medical Genetics and Pediatrics
University of Maryland
22 South Greene St.
Baltimore, MD 21201
Phone: (800) 492-5538
www.umm.edu

■ **Andrea Gropman, MD**
Faculty, Neurology; Principal Investigator, Children's Research Institute
Children's National Medical Center
Center for Neuroscience Research (CNR)
111 Michigan Ave., NW
Washington, DC 20010-2970
Phone: 202-476-3511
Email: agropman@childrensnational.org
www.childrensnational.org

■ **Richard Kelley, MD, PhD**
Director, Division of Metabolism at Kennedy Krieger Institute
Pediatrics and Clinical Genetics
Kennedy Krieger Institute
707 N. Broadway
Baltimore, MD 21205
Phone: (443) 923-7600
Fax: (443) 923-7696

■ **Fran Kendall, MD***
Genetics Specialist Physician
Virtual Medical Practice, LLC
5579 Chamblee Dunwoody Rd.

Suite 110
Atlanta, GA 30338
Phone: (404) 720-0820
www.virtualmdpractice.com

NORTH CENTRAL

▪ **Bruce H. Cohen, MD***
Akron Children's Hospital
NeuroDevelopmental Science Center
Considine Professional Building
215 W. Bowery St., Suite 4400
Akron, OH 44308
Phone: (330) 543-8050
Fax: (330) 543-8054
www.akronchildrens.org

▪ **Shawn McCandless, MD, PhD**
Department of Genetics
School of Medicine
Case Western Reserve University
Biomedical Research Building 622
2109 Adelbert Rd.
Cleveland, OH 44106-4955
Tel: (216) 844-1612
Fax: (216) 368-3432
Email: shawn.mccandless@case.edu
www.case.edu

▪ **Marvin Natowicz, MD, PhD***
Clinical Pathology
Cleveland Clinic Main Campus
Mail Code NE5
9500 Euclid Ave.
Cleveland, OH 44195
Phone: (216) 636-1768
http://my.clevelandclinic.org

▪ **Sumit Parikh, MD***
Center for Pediatric Neurology
Cleveland Clinic Main Campus
Mail Code S71
9500 Euclid Ave.
Cleveland, OH 44195

Phone: (216) 444-5559
http://my.clevelandclinic.org

- **Arthur Zinn, MD**
  Director, Metabolic Service, UHCMC
  University Hospitals of Cleveland
  Center for Human Genetics
  11100 Euclid Ave., #1500
  Cleveland, OH 44106
  Phone: (216) 844-3936
  www.uhhospitals.org

SOUTH CENTRAL

- **Pauline Filipek, MD**
  Pediatric Neurology
  University of Texas-Houston Medical School
  Autism Center at the Children's Learning Institute
  7000 Fannin St., Suite 2453
  Houston, TX 77030
  Phone: (713) 500-3600
  Fax: (713) 383-1482
  www.childrenslearninginstitute.org

- **Ronald Haller, MD, PhD**
  Internal Medicine and Neurology
  Southwestern Medical Center
  7232 Greenville Ave.
  Suite 435
  Dallas, TX 75231
  Phone: (241) 345-4611
  www.utsouthwestern.edu

- **Mary Kay Koenig, MD***
  Assistant Professor, Departments of Pediatrics and Neurology
  Division of Child & Adolescent Neurology
  Mitochondrial Clinic Director
  Tuberous Sclerosis Center Co-Director
  University of Texas-Houston Medical School
  6431 Fannin St., MSB 3.153
  Houston, Texas 77030
  Phone: (713) 500-7113
  Fax: (713) 500-7101
  http://ped1.med.uth.tmc.edu

■ **Dmitriy Niyazov, MD**
Ochsner Children's Health Center
1315 Jefferson Hwy.
New Orleans, LA 70121
Phone: (504) 842-3900
www.ochsner.org

■ **Fernando Scaglia, MD**
Associate Professor, Department of Molecular and Human Genetics
Baylor College of Medicine
Department of Molecular and Human Genetics
Baylor College of Medicine
One Baylor Plaza, MS BCM225
Houston, TX 77030
Phone: 832-822-4280
Fax: 832-825-4294
http://www.bcm.edu

NORTHWEST

■ **Suman Jayadev, MD**
Acting Assistant Professor of Neurology
Research Affiliate, Center on Human Development and Disability
University of Washington Medical Center
1959 NE Pacific St.
Box # 356465
Seattle, WA 98195
Phone: (206) 221-2930
Fax: (206) 685-8100
http://depts.washington.edu/neurolog/welcome.html

■ **Eric E. Kraus, MD**
Associate Professor of Neurology
University of Washington Medical Center
1959 NE Pacific St.
Box # 356465
Seattle, WA 98195
Phone: (206) 598-0216
Fax: (206) 598-7698
http://depts.washington.edu/neurolog/welcome.html

■ **Russell P. Saneto, DO, PhD***
Associate Professor, Neurology
Center for Clinical and Translational Research
Seattle Children's Hospital
B-5552-Neurology
4800 Sand Point Way NE
Seattle, WA 98105
Phone: (206) 987-2078
www.seattlechildrens.org

■ **Michael Weiss, MD**
Associate Professor of Neurology
University Washington Medical Center
1959 NE Pacific St.
Box # 356115
Seattle, WA 98195
Phone: (206) 598-7688
Fax: (206) 598-7698
http://depts.washington.edu/neurolog/welcome.html

MIDWEST

■ **Bryan Hainline, MD, PhD**
J. W. Riley Children's Hospital, Indiana University
702 Barnhill Dr., Rm 0907
Indianapolis, IN 46202
Phone: (317) 274-3966
Fax: (317) 278-0936

■ **Wendy Peltier, MD**
Associate Professor of Neurology
Medical College of Wisconsin
9200 West Wisconsin Ave.
Milwaukee, WI 53226
Phone: (414) 805-8710
Fax: (414) 955-0115
www.mcw.edu

■ **Laurence Walsh, MD**
Medical Geneticist, Neurodevelopmental disabilities
IU Medical Genetics Services Inc.
702 Barnhill Dr., #1340
Indianapolis, IN 46202
Phone: (317) 274-8800

WEST

- **Jose Abdenur, MD**
  Medical Director of Metabolic Services and the PSF Chief of the Metabolic
    Disorders Division
  Children's Hospital of Orange County
  455 South Main St.
  Orange, CA 92868
  Phone: (714) 532-8852
  Fax: (714) 532-8362
  www.chocpsf.com

- **Bruce Barshop, MD, PhD**
  Clinical Biochemical Genetics
  UCSD Bio-Chemical Genetics Lab
  9500 Gilman Dr.
  La Jolla, CA 92093
  Phone: (619) 543-5237
  http://biochemgen.ucsd.edu

- **Richard Boles, MD***
  Associate Professor of Pediatrics/Director of the Metabolic and
    Mitochondrial Disorders Clinic
  Children's Hospital Los Angeles Medical General
  4650 West Sunset Boulevard
  Los Angeles, CA 90027
  Phone: (323) 361-2178
  Fax: (323) 361-1172
  www.childrenshospitallamedicalgroup.org ; www.curemito.org

- **Greg Enns, MD***
  Associate Professor
  Director, Biochemical Genetics Program
  Lucille Packard Children's Hospital at Stanford
  Medical Genetics Division
  300 Pasteur Dr.
  H315 MC 5208
  Stanford, CA 94305
  Phone: (650) 723-6858
  Fax: (650) 498-4555
  www.lpch.org

■ **J. Jay Gargus, MD, PhD**
Genetics, Metabolic Disorders
Children's Hospital of Orange County
455 S. Main St.
Orange, CA 92868
Phone: (714) 532-7982
Fax: (949) 824-1762
www.choc.com

■ **Richard H. Haas, MD***
Pediatric Neurologist/Professor
University of California San Diego School of Medicine
9500 Gilman Dr., # 0935
La Jolla, CA 92093-0935
Phone: (858) 822-6705
Fax : (858) 822-6707
http://som.ucsd.edu

■ **Taosheng Huang, MD***
Director, MitoMed Diagnostic Lab School of Medicine
University of California, Irvine
314 Sprague Hall
Mail Code: 3950
Irvine, CA 92697
Phone: (949) 824-9346
Fax: (949) 824-9776
Email: huangts@uci.edu
www.faculty.uci.edu

■ **Robert K. Naviaux, MD, PhD***
Children's Specialists of San Diego Associate Professor In Residence
UC San Diego School of Medicine
The Mitochondrial and Metabolic Disease Center
200 W. Arbor Dr., #8467
San Diego, CA 92103

CANADA

- **Gabriela Horvath, MD**
  BC Children's Hospital
  Rm K3-200
  4480 Oak St.
  Vancouver BC V6H 3V4
  Canada
  Phone: (604) 875-2880
  www.bcchildrens.ca

- **Anna Lehman, MA, MD**
  Assistant Professor, Department of Medical Genetics
  Clinical Geneticist, Provincial Medical Genetics Programme
  Child & Family Research Institute (CFRI)
  Dept of Medical Genetics, C234
  4500 Oak St.
  Vancouver BC V6H3N1
  Canada
  Phone: 604-875-2345 x6785
  Fax: 604-875-2376
  Email: alehman@cw.bc.ca
  www.cfri.ca

- **Sandra Sirrs, MD**
  Medical Director
  Adult Metabolic Diseases Clinic
  Vancouver General Hospital
  Diamond Health Care Centre
  2775 Laurel St., 4th floor
  Vancouver BC V5Z 1M9
  Canada
  Phone: (604) 875-5965
  Email: sandra.sirrs@vch.ca

- **Mark Tarnopolsky, MD**
  Professor, Division of Neurology, Department Pediatrics and Medicine
  Head, Neuromuscular and Neurometabolic Disease
  McMaster University
  Health Sciences Centre
  Room 2H26
  1200 Main St. W. Hamilton
  Ontario L8N 3Z5
  Canada

Phone: (905) 521-2100 x 75226
Fax: (905) 577-8380
Email: tarnopol@mcmaster.ca
www.fhs.mcmaster.ca/medicine

This list is updated periodically online at http://www.mitoaction.org/forums/list-mito-specialists

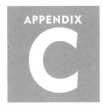
Useful Websites for Support and Information

There are endless resources available on the Internet; the following is a list of patient and personal favorites.

Organizations and Foundations for Mitochondrial Diseases and Genetic Disorders:

www.MitoAction.org
Support, education, and outreach for people living with mitochondrial disease. Email support@MitoAction.org to request a copy of MitoAction's free DVD series and a Mito awareness kit, or call their toll-free number 888-648-6228.

www.UMDF.org
The United Mitochondrial Disease Foundation

www.CLIMB.org
Children living with inherited metabolic diseases; located in the UK

www.MitoCanada.org
Support, research, and awareness in Canada for mitochondrial disorders

www.amdf.org/au
Australian Mitochondrial Disease Foundation

www.rarediseases.org
The National Organization for Rare Diseases

www.geneticalliance.org
Offers advocacy, education, and empowerment for people suffering from genetic disorders.

www.curemito.org
The Mitochondrial Dysautonomia and Functional Disorders Alliance

www.globalgenesproject.org
Supports world rare disease awareness campaigns

www.fodsupport.org
Support for those with fatty oxidation disorders

Clinical Organizations, Explanations of Medical Terms, Treatment, and Testing

http://sigs.nih.gov/mito
The National Institute of Health Mitochondrial Research Interest Group

www.virtualmdpractice.com
Dr. Fran Kendall's medical practice dedicated to clinical mitochondrial disease management

www.MEDomics.com
Supplier of diagnostic testing for mitochondrial disorders

www.transgenomic.com
Transgenomic Labs, supplier of diagnostic testing for mitochondrial disorders

www.bcm.edu/geneticlabs
Medical Genetics Laboratories at Baylor College of Medicine, supplier of diagnostic testing for mitochondrial disorders

www.genedx.com/site/neurology
Gene Dx offers comprehensive genetic testing for neurological disorders

biochemgen.ucsd.edu
Mitochondrial and Metabolic Disease Center at University of California San Diego

www.mitosoc.org
The Mitochondrial Medicine Society

www.pubmed.gov
US National Library of Medicine citation database

www.clinicaltrials.gov
US National Institute of Health Clinical Trial database

www.OMIM.org
Online catalog of human genetic disorders

www.edisonpharma.com
Edison Pharma, dedicated to developing treatments for rare diseases

www.nsgc.org
National Society of Genetic Counselors

www.ncbi.nlm.nih.gov
National Center for Biotechnology Information

Patient, Parent, and Family Support

www.complexchild.com
Complex Child e-magazine for parents of special needs children

www.patientadvocate.org
The Patient Advocate Foundation

www.parentcenternetwork.org
Website helping parents of special needs children connect to other parents

www.oley.org
Support for those living on home TPN (total parenteral nutrition)

www.madisonfoundation.org
Connecting parents of children with metabolic diseases around the world

www.health.groups.yahoo.com
Search for "mitochondrial disease" or for specific diagnoses to find a list of email list-servs that you can join. Some are public, some are private, most are moderated by a parent or adult patient.

www.mitoaction.org/red-tape
A collection of "cut the red tape" articles offering specific advice on issues such as reimbursement, family grants, wish trips, service dogs, disability, social security, etc.

www.parentcenternetwork.org/parentcenterlisting.html
Parent Technical Assistance Center Network's map of parent centers in the United States

www.narha.org
The North American Riding for Handicapped Association

www.fdri.net
The Federation for Disabled Riding International

www.epilepsyfoundation.org
"Living with Epilepsy" offers resources for parents and for caregivers about managing seizure disorders.

www.youtube.com/mitoaction
A collection of "real" patient, child, and family videos to help illustrate living with mitochondrial disease and assist in explaining the science. Requests for copies on DVD can be directed to info@mitoaction.org.

Special Education

www.mitoaction.org/education
Comprehensive listing of special education requirements by age, templates for letters, sample IEPs, sample health care plans, and sample symptom checklists and daily progress reports.

www.homeschool.com
Everything parents need to know about homeschooling their child(ren)

www.ifspweb.com
Nebraska University's comprehensive explanation of the US Individualized Family Service Plan

www.wrightslaw.com
Detailed explanations of the IDEA law and special education terms and services

www.specialeducationadvisor.com
Special Education Advisor offering explanations of terms and children's special education rights

http://www.parentcenternetwork.org/parentcenterlisting.html
Parent-to-parent network provides information to parents about the available services, processes, and providers that your child is eligible to use through his IFSP in your state.

Autism

http://www.autism-society.org
The Autism Society exists to improve the lives of all affected by autism by increasing public awareness about the day-to-day issues faced by people on the spectrum, advocating for appropriate services for individuals across the lifespan, and providing the latest information regarding treatment, education, research, and advocacy.

http://www.autismdigest.com
An online digest of magazines that provides practical, actionable information to help parents and professionals improve the quality of life and quality of care for individuals on the autism spectrum.

Emergency Protocols

http://www.mitoaction.org/guide/table-contents
"Protocols for Emergency Management" provide several customizable protocols that provide specific recommendations about use of anesthesia, fluids, and fasting in emergency situations for people with Mito.

http://www.emdn-mitonet.co.uk/PDF/mitoane.pdf
European Mitochondrial Disease Network's downloadable PDF of the UMDF's 1998 article about anesthesia precautions, written by Bruce Cohen MD, John Shoffner MD, and Glenn DeBauer MD.

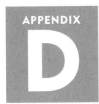

Sample Individualized Education Program (IEP)

The following is a real IEP for a real seven-year-old child with mitochondrial disease. Parents and teachers should take note that it is provided here as an example only; the very idea of a standardized IEP is counterintuitive to the purpose of an IEP (hence the word "Individualized" in the name). Every child's goals and needs are different; this is true even amongst siblings or children who have very similar diagnoses and abilities.

Note in the sample IEP provided that the emphasis is on both big picture goals as well as very specific goals for the child. Note also the opportunity for parents to contribute their vision for their child as well as the information provided by teachers about the child's progress. Parents can help their child's IEP team by keeping focused on their vision of health and safety, and by helping the team understand what an important role they play in helping their child stay safe and healthy.

More information, including examples of additional goals and accommodations, health care plans, symptom checklists, progress reports, and so on, can be found online at www.mitoaction.org/education.

School District Name: ~~Tilyaem Public schools~~

School District Address: ~~WP community home hartford, 6a 04003~~

School District Contact Person/Phone #: ~~Dilew Marker / 86.wh.wr. ollr~~

Student Information

Last Name:	~~Eagle~~	Form Date:	10/6/2008
First Name:	Eva	Date of Birth:	~~06.wha~~
Middle Name:	Christina	Age:	7
Local ID:	1319991266	Grade:	Kindergarten
State ID:	1034399115	Place of Birth:	
Primary Lang:	English	Language of Instruction:	English
Home Address:	~~Philandsbury Street~~	Gender:	Female
Town/City: ~~Paughim~~ State: ~~MA~~ Zip: ~~01ljpr~~		School Year:	2008-2009
Home Phone:	~~7h.-3hml.ds1~~	Year of Graduation:	2026

If 18 or older:
- ☐ Acting on Own Behalf
- ☐ Shared Decision-Making
- ☐ Court Appointed Guardian:
- ☐ Delegated Decision-Making

Parent/Guardian #1 Information

Name:	~~BeCaghnwya2~~	Home Phone:	~~fwll9h44992~~
Home Address 1:	~~BeCaghnwya2~~	Other Phone:	
Home Address 2:		Cell Phone:	
Town/City: ~~Vaughim~~ State: ~~Ma~~ Zip: ~~01jmr~~		Relationship To Student:	Mother
Parent email:		Primary Language:	English

Parent/Guardian #2 Information

Name:	~~BeCaghnwya2~~	Home Phone:	~~7tljhbhhr4tktC~~
Home Address 1:	~~3Paghnlw4 3A~~	Other Phone:	
Home Address 2:		Cell Phone:	
Town/City: ~~Vaughim~~ State: ~~Ma~~ Zip: ~~01jh42~~		Relationship To Student:	Father
Parent email:		Primary Language:	

Meeting Information

Date of Meeting:	6/3/2010	Type of Meeting:	Reevaluation
Next Scheduled annual review:	6/2/2011	Next Scheduled 3-year eval:	5/31/2013

Assigned School Information
(Complete after a placement decision has been made.)

School:	~~mawar. Latyhwwhwl.~~	School Program:	
Address:	~~3vhwawwhTuLl. 4rwww.h. 210~~	Telephone:	~~jl. 2whr.~~
Contact Person: ~~Caghwnwm~~ Role: Program Director Phone: ~~4l.wpl. w9h~~			

Cost share placement: ○ Yes ● No ○ N/A If yes, please specify agency:

Use with Special Education Eligibility Determination and Individualized Education Plan Form

School District Name:
School District Address:
School District Contact Person/Phone #:

Individualized Education Program

IEP From: 6/3/2010   **To:** 6/2/2011

Student Name: Eva   DOB: ID#: 1034399115

Parent and/or Student Concerns

What concern(s) does the parent and/or student want to see addressed in this IEP to enhance the student's education?

Our greatest concern for Eva in the big picture is maintaining her health and fostering an environment that is safe and allows her to continue to make progress physically, emotionally, socially, and cognitively. Eva's mitochondrial disease diagnosis puts her at greater risk for fatigue from over-exertion and regression or loss of skills from even a minor illness. Eva has remained healthy and strong over this past school year. Our family commends the teachers and the ██████ for their hard work in helping Eva to stay healthy and safe, and for continuing to know how and when to push her to grow.

Student Strengths and Key Evaluation Results Summary

What are the student's educational strengths, interest areas, significant personal attributes and personal accomplishments?
What is the student's type of disability(ies), general education performance including MCAS/district test results, achievement towards goals and lack of expected progress, if any?

Eva is social, happy, engaging 6.3 year- old who is willing to work toward a goal. She presents with a diagnosis of Mitochondrial disease and Leigh's disease. She thrives on positive interaction with others, and seems proud of herself as she learns new things or can accomplish tasks independently. Eva has developmentally made a lot of progress, and takes part regularly in imaginative play alone or with friends. Eva is found eligible for special education services under the category p of multiple disabilities.

Eva has made wonderful gains in the bathroom. She is wearing underwear throughout the school day with minimal accidents, less than once per week. She uses an adapted potty chair to go to the bathroom but is working on using the regular adapted toilet. She helps to wipe and knows where to put the wipe, although requires some assistance to be sure of total cleanliness. She is able to help pull up and down her pants and underwear with minimal to moderate assistance, depending on the pants and their location. Eva knows the sequence of steps to wash her hands but requires physical assistance to turn on and off the water and get the soap due to their location. She is able to scrub them and rinse them as well as dry them off with 100% accuracy. She inconsistently asks for the bathroom when she feels the urge to go but is taken on a regular basis.

Test Results: Education: Eva was assessed using sections of the Brigance Diagnostic Inventory of Early Development, classroom observations, classroom notes and teacher report. Eva demonstrates overall higher scores in areas of emerging academic skills such as shapes, colors and letters. This is evident through her ability to identify colors; red, blue, green, yellow, orange, purple, brown, black, pink, gray, and white, shapes; circle, square, triangle, rectangle, diamond, oval, star and heart, uppercase letters, name body parts; mouth, eyes, nose, feet, hair, tongue, head, ears, hands, legs, arms, stomach, teeth, back, toes, chin, knees, neck, chest and shoulders, as well as her ability to count up to number 18 and recite the alphabet. She is able to point to more body parts than she can name including heels, ankles, wrist, waist, and thumbs. She also demonstrates higher scores in social and emotional development skills. This is evident through her concern for peers, ability to play cooperatively, imaginative play, awareness of "good" and "bad" behavior, and her turn taking skills. All of the previous sections scored as an average of five to six years old. It is noted that certain sections of the Brigance assessment reflect what things mean to her. When asked questions regarding, "what do you do in different situations", "Use of objects", "Function of community helpers", and "Knows where to go for services". She answered questions honestly and in the manner that she observes them or how they have meaning to her. This is noted to be a very appropriate skill and shows how she views her own personal environment. She also demonstrates splinter skills in many areas of the assessment.

Physical Therapy: Eva has made significant gains in her strength and endurance over the past two years which has allowed her to continue to develop and refine gross motor skills. This is noted in her improved ability to move in and out of various positions on the floor, sit and play on the floor without support for extended periods of time, transfer up and down from the floor with support of a person or object, and walk with increasing independence for increased distances throughout her day using her gait trainer.

Testing- Speech: Eva's overall language development is at a 2 year 6 month level with scattered skills up to 4 years. Her speech is intelligible to familiar listeners within known context. She is able to produce several early emerging sounds in initial, medial, and final positions, but her misarticulations are marked by substitutions, omissions, velar fronting, stopping, and consonant cluster reductions for sounds that are more difficult to produce (e.g., k, g, s, v, th, z, j, sh, ch). Eva's utterances are made up of 1-4 words (mean length of utterance-MLU 2.2). She uses speech for labeling, greetings/partings, gaining attention, commenting, requesting, negating, answering questions, indicating help, and expressing basic needs (hunger/thirst/ bathroom). She currently uses pronouns, plurals, prepositions, and verbs including –ing. She does not currently use possessive 's' or the past tense form of verbs. Eva is now starting to comment about what is occurring in pictures of a book and what she is currently doing.

School District Name: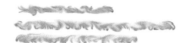

School District Address:

School District Contact Person/Phone #:

Fine motor/ADL: Eva demonstrates many strong fine motor skills despite her decreased hand strength and ataxic quality to her movements. She is able to participate more in ADL activities throughout her day, this includes self feeding, assisting with toileting routine and hygiene tasks.

Eva's parents commented that she has developmentally made a lot of gains in the last year. She is much more aware of herself, her environment and the people around her. She is very motivated to make choices and to do things independently. This is the first year that we have seen these gains in Eva, and we (her parents) feel that we should build on this in our goals for her in the next year. She is social, engaging, playful and happy most of the time. She thrives from small groups and one-on-one attention and loves learning. She is motivated and will practice new things, such as new words or fine motor tasks (including feeding herself). Her mobility is still a challenge for Eva at home, as she can crawl everywhere she would like to go but is not safe in a walker independently in the house, and fatigues so easily that the walker is not functional for anything except short distances in other situations.

In the coming year, we feel that Eva would benefit from continuing to build on the OT, PT, and speech goals from this year. The intensity, frequency and consistency of these therapies are, from our perspective, an ongoing source of Eva's success and growth. She has shown interest in friends and classmates this year and would benefit from being in a classroom where she can have meaningful interactions with her teachers and meaningful play and relationships with her classmates. We would also like to see Eva learn more independent play skills. Specifically, Eva plays well alone on the floor with toys, but is interested in more complex activities such as the computer. If she were able to play independently using the computer, we believe that this would be a skill that would help her be more satisfied when playing without help at home and would serve her well in the future. We are thrilled with Eva's progress toilet-training at school, and feel that any and all focus on independence with functional ADLs is also very important.

It is expected that she will meet her goals within the IEP year. It is anticipated that she will participate in the MCAS Alt assessment in the spring of 2014.

Vision Statement: What is the vision for this student?

Consider the next 1 to 5 year period when developing this statement. Beginning no later than age 14, the statement should be based on the student's preferences and interests, and should include desired outcomes in adult living, post-secondary and working environments.

Our vision for Eva is that she continue to be healthy and to make slow but significant progress each year. Quality of life is our greatest goal for Eva due to the uncertainty of her prognosis. Meaningful relationships and activities are becoming more important for Eva; therefore it is our vision that in the coming years Eva will develop relationships with friends who she can socialize with in and out of school. She will be able to communicate with her peers, her teachers, and with other children and adults who do not know her as well. She will have the ability to move appropriately and independently to get to the place that she wants to go without significant fatigue or restriction. She will be consistently toilet trained at home and at school, and be able to feed herself with minimal help. She will be able to communicate her needs, including fatigue, pain and hunger or thirst. She will understand safety and have learned to compensate or recognize some of her limitations (for example, understanding that she could fall if she leans forward in a chair, or to be able to compensate for significant ataxia in her feeding or play).

We are very grateful to _____ and the _____ for the opportunity to see Eva thrive and make such wonderful progress. Thank you!

Individualized Education Program

IEP Dates: from 06/03/2010 **to** 06/02/2011

Student Name: Eva ~~~~~   **DOB:** ~~~~   **State ID Number:** 1034399115

Present Level of Educational Performance
A: General Curriculum

Check all that apply:

☑ English Language Arts

☑ History and Social Studies

☑ Science and Technology

☑ Mathematics

☑ Other Curriculum Areas

General curriculum area(s) affected by this student's disability(ies):
Consider the language, composition, literature (including reading) and media strands.

Consider the history, geography, economic and civics and government strands.

Consider the inquiry, domains of science, technology and science, technology and human affairs strand.

Consider the number sense, patterns, relations and functions, geometry and measurement and statistics and probability strands.

Specify: preschool/kindergarten curriculum

How does the disability(ies) affect progress in the curriculum area(s)?
Due to developmental delays and health issues, Eva is unable to access the general curriculum. She requires an intensive, therapeutic program that includes substantial accommodations and modifications to access learning as well as her environment.

What type(s) of accommodation, *if any*, is necessary for the student to make effective progress?
A multi-sensory, thematic unit based curriculum.
Individual or small group instruction.
Opportunities for rest and frequent snacks/drinks, as needed.
Minimal distractions.
A.F.O's, walker, stroller/wheelchair and adaptive seating, stander
Photographs and picture symbols
Flip and talk communication book
Adapted utensils as needed, open cup with straw

What type(s) of specially designed instruction, *if any*, is necessary for the student to make effective progress?
Check the necessary instructional modification(s) and describe how such modification(s) will be made.

☑ Content

Multisensory thematic based functional curriculum adapted for her level (based on the Massachusetts Curriculum Frameworks).

☑ Methodology/Delivery of Instruction

Small group or individual, slow pace, predictable routines, latency time for responses, multiple trials of tasks.

☑ Performance Criteria

Progress reports, data collection, teacher notes, teacher observation, participation in activities, task completion, level of prompts and assistance required.

Individualized Education Program

IEP Dates: from 06/03/2010 **to** 06/02/2011

Student Name: Eva 🔲   **DOB:** 🔲   **State ID Number:** 1034399115

Present Levels of Educational Performance
B: General Considerations

Check all that apply.

☑ Adapted Physical Education   ☐ Assistive tech devices/services   ☐ Behavior

☐ Braille needs (blind/visually impaired)   ☑ Communication (all students)   ☐ Communication (deaf/hard of hearing students)

☐ Extra curriculum activities   ☐ Language needs (LEP students)   ☑ Nonacademic activities

☐ Social/emotional needs   ☐ Travel training   ☐ Skill development related to vocational preparation or experience

☑ Other: O.T. , P.T.

Age-Specific Considerations

☐ For children ages 3 to 5 - participation in appropriate activities

☐ For children ages 14+ (or younger if appropriate) - student's course of study

☐ For children ages 16 (or younger if appropriate) to 22 - transition to post-school activities including community experiences, employment objectives, other post school adult living objectives and, if appropriate, daily living skills

Other Considerations

How does the disability(ies) affect progress in the indicated area(s) of other educational needs?:

Due to developmental delays and health issues, Eva is unable to access the general curriculum. She requires an intensive, therapeutic program that includes substantial accommodations and modifications to access learning as well as her environment.

What type(s) of accommodation, *if any*, is necessary for the student to make effective progress?:

A multi-sensory, thematic unit based curriculum.
Individual or small group instruction.
Opportunities for rest and frequent snacks/drinks, as needed.
Minimal distractions.
A.F.O's, walker, stroller/wheelchair, adaptive seating, stander
Photographs and picture symbols
Flip and talk communication book
Adapted utensils as needed, open cup with straw

What type(s) of specially designed instruction, *if any*, is necessary for the student to make effective progress?
Check the necessary instructional modification(s) and describe how such modification(s) will be made.

☑ Content

Multisensory thematic based functional curriculum adapted for her level (based on the Massachusetts Curriculum Frameworks).

☑ Methodology/Delivery of Instruction

Small group or individual, slow pace, predictable routines, latency time for responses, multiple trials of tasks.

☑ Performance Criteria

Progress reports, data collection, teacher notes, teacher observation, participation in activities, task completion, level of prompts and assistance required.

Individualized Education Program

IEP Dates: from 06/03/2010 **to** 06/02/2011

Student Name: Eva ~~~ **DOB:** ~~~ **State ID Number:** 1034399115

Student Goal

Goal Number:
Specific Goal Focus:
Current Performance Level: What can the student currently do?

Measurable Annual Goal: What challenging, yet attainable, goal can we expect the student to meet by the end of this IEP Period? How will we know that the student has reached this goal?

Benchmarks/Objectives: What will the student need to do to complete this goal?

Individualized Education Program

IEP Dates: from 06/03/2010 **to** 06/02/2011

Student Name: Eva ~~■■■■■~~   **DOB:** ~~■■■■■~~   **State ID Number:** 1034399115

Student Goal

Goal Number: 1
Specific Goal Focus: Communication
Current Performance Level: What can the student currently do?

A speech and language assessment was completed as part of a 3 year re-evaluation to determine Eva's current skills and develop appropriate goals. Eva's overall language development is at a 2 year 6 month level with scattered skills up to 4 years. Her speech is intelligible to familiar listeners within known context. She is able to produce several early emerging sounds in initial, medial, and final positions, but her misarticulations are marked by substitutions, omissions, velar fronting, stopping, and consonant cluster reductions for sounds that are more difficult to produce (e.g., k, g, s, v, th, z, j, sh, ch). Eva's utterances are made up of 1-5 words (mean length of utterance-MLU 2.2). She uses speech for labeling, greetings/partings, gaining attention, commenting, requesting, negating, answering questions, indicating help, and expressing basic needs (hunger/thirst/ bathroom). She currently uses pronouns, plurals, prepositions, and verbs including –ing. She does not currently use possessive 's' or the past tense form of verbs. Eva is now starting to comment about what is occurring in pictures of a book and what she is currently doing. Eva follows one step directions, two step related directions, but demonstrates difficulty with two step unrelated directions. Often times she performs the final step. Eva is able to identify pictures of familiar objects and verbs. She knows several body parts, colors, letters, numbers, and shapes.

Measurable Annual Goal: What challenging, yet attainable, goal can we expect the student to meet by the end of this IEP Period? How will we know that the student has reached this goal?

Eva will increase her sentence length to maximize expressive language skills during daily activities.

Benchmarks/Objectives: What will the student need to do to complete this goal?

1. Eva will produce 2 four word sentences to describe what is occurring in a picture of a familiar storybook in 4 out of 5 opportunities 80% of the time across a 4 week period.
2. Eva will produce a 4 word sentence to describe what she is doing in 4 out of 5 opportunities 80% of the time across a 4 week period .
3. Eva will use past tense verbs to express what she did in a recent activity in 3 out of 5 opportunities 50% of the time across a 4 week period.

Individualized Education Program

IEP Dates: from 06/03/2010 **to** 06/02/2011

Student Name: Eva ~~~~~~   **DOB:** ~~~~~~   **State ID Number:** 1034399115

Student Goal

Goal Number: 2
Specific Goal Focus: Cognitive Development
Current Performance Level: What can the student currently do?

Eva is able to identify all uppercase letters out of a choice of three letters. She is able to identify her shapes and colors accurately 100% of the time. Eva can count up to number 18 on a regular basis and continues to work on accurate identification of numbers 1-10 as well as 1:1 correspondence of numbers one through five. She is more accurate with 1:1 correspondence for numbers two through five; she tends to want to count orally once number one is present. She understands the quantitative concepts of many/one, little/big, empty/full and light/heavy. She also shows understanding of the directional and positional concepts of close/open, front/back, in/out, behind/in front of, bottom/top, over/under, up/down, forward/backward, away from/toward, low/high and right/left. It is important to note that Eva shows more understanding of these concepts when they relate to her, such as when she is walking and having her perform the task i.e. forward/back. Eva is able to point to many body parts when asked and is able to identify a variety of them as well. She is also able to classify a number of things such as; animals, toys, clothes, foods, pets, numbers, things to read, shapes, and fruits by naming appropriate things under each category. Eva is able to recite the spelling of her name. She continues to work on spelling her name out accurately by matching all of the letters in her name or spelling out her name if a model of her name is present. Eva has just started to complete a simple pattern as seen at circle (a,b,a,b) with great accuracy. Eva has started to show interest in money when she plays with the cash register and is able to match change to each other or to its specific money bag with moderate assistance.

Measurable Annual Goal: What challenging, yet attainable, goal can we expect the student to meet by the end of this IEP Period? How will we know that the student has reached this goal?

Eva will continue to improve her overall cognitive development and emerging academic skills.

Benchmarks/Objectives: What will the student need to do to complete this goal?

1. Eva will identify lowercase letters a-z, out of a choice of 3 letters in 3 out of 5 opportunities for four consecutive weeks.
2. Eva will spell out her first and last name (in all capitals) without a model or matching in 3 out of 5 opportunities for four consecutive weeks.
3. Eva will count out 1-5 objects using 1:1 correspondence with similar manipulatives (all the same shape and color) 100% of the time for four consecutive weeks.
4. Eva will name money: penny, nickel, dime, quarter and dollar in 3 out of 5 opportunities for four consecutive weeks.

Individualized Education Program

IEP Dates: from 06/03/2010 **to** 06/02/2011

Student Name: Eva ![]   **DOB:** ![]   **State ID Number:** 1034399115

Student Goal

Goal Number: 3
Specific Goal Focus: Gross Motor

Current Performance Level: What can the student currently do?

Eva has continued to make significant skills with her walking skills. In the school setting she walks either with support given by her teacher/staff or using her gait trainer (KidWalk). The KidWalk is a weight bearing assisted gait trainer that is set up to provide needed support through Eva's trunk. In it her arms are free for functional use while walking. Eva uses the gait trainer for functional mobility throughout her day at school to walk to and from the bathroom, therapies and for walks throughout the school setting with her classmates and teachers.

Without the gait trainer, Eva is able to walk short distances with assistance/ support through her trunk and/or her hands. During therapy sessions, Eva is also using a full weight bearing pediatric rolling walker to walk for short distances with assistance. She is able to stand and orientate herself within the walker with verbal cues and assistance to steady the walker. At this time Eva requires assistance to help her complete turns and also at times to control and maintain her balance within the walker.

Measurable Annual Goal: What challenging, yet attainable, goal can we expect the student to meet by the end of this IEP Period? How will we know that the student has reached this goal?

Eva will walk for short functional distances with a full weight bearing walker with supervision at least 2X/day with 80% consistency over a four week period.

Benchmarks/Objectives: What will the student need to do to complete this goal?

1. Eva will stand from a chair and orientate herself within a walker 2X/day with 80% consistency over a four week period.
2. Once standing, Eva will turn herself and the walker and proceed to walk 2X/day with 80% consistency over a four week period.
3. Eva will walk a distance of 30 feet with a full weight bearing walker 2X/day with 80% consistency over a four week period.
4. Eva will turn while walking with a walker to navigate around corners and obstacles 2X/day with 80% consistency over a four week period.

Individualized Education Program

IEP Dates: from 06/03/2010 **to** 06/02/2011

Student Name: Eva 🖉

DOB: 🖉   **State ID Number:** 1034399115

Student Goal

Goal Number: 4
Specific Goal Focus: Fine Motor
Current Performance Level: What can the student currently do?

Eva has continued to work hard and make nice progress in the areas of fine motor as it affects her classroom work, self help skills, and play skills. Eva has appeared to enjoy the many sensory based activities including movement or vestibular with the swings and tactile activities. Eva demonstrates overall decreased muscle strength In her upper extremities however has shown gains in this area. This is observed when using the swings; Eva will assist with maintaining her balance using her arms as well as propel the swing by pushing and pulling with her arms.

Eva very much enjoys assisting in choosing activities performed during her therapy time and is motivated to complete many tasks independently.   In regards to fine motor activities, Eva typically will choose to play with her dolls or use manipulatives such as play dough, beads or puzzles. She also enjoys activities with crayons or markers to work on her pre writing skills. Eva appears to be right sided dominant. She will typically begin each activity with her right hand however is observed to often switch hands to use her left periodically. Eva uses a variety of grasp patters with her hands. She does demonstrate decreased hand and grasp strength with hyper mobility at the joints of her fingers and thumb. Eva often will pickup items using a raking palmer grasp with her whole hand. This provides her with more stability. She is also observed to use a lateral pinch with her thumb adducted to the side of her index finger when picking up smaller items. Eva uses bulb crayons for coloring or drawing activities. She is able to imitate vertical and horizontal lines and will color in circular motions. At this time she is unable to draw just one circle. She is demonstrating good pre writing skills and will continue to work on beginning to form letters with these basic lines.

Eva has also continued to improve with her ability to participate in self help tasks including brushing her hair, dressing, and clothes management while toileting. When toileting, Eva will assist with pulling up/down her pants given minimal to moderate assistance. She stands at the grab bar in the bathroom and will hold on with one hand to maintain her balance while using the other hand to manage her clothing.

Measurable Annual Goal: What challenging, yet attainable, goal can we expect the student to meet by the end of this IEP Period? How will we know that the student has reached this goal?

Eva will complete various daily classroom activities (including eating, toileting routine, pre-writing activities, and play activities) demonstrating improved fine motor skills as seen by successfully completing the following objectives:

Benchmarks/Objectives: What will the student need to do to complete this goal?

1. Eva will demonstrate the ability to accurately form letters in her name given a visual demonstration and visual guidelines 3 out of 4 opportunities for 4 consecutive weeks.
2. Eva will draw a circle with fair approximation to choose objects on a worksheet 3 out of 4 opportunities for 4 consecutive weeks.
3. When toileting, Eva will manage her clothing by pulling up/down her pants given prompts only 3 out of 4 opportunities for 4 consecutive weeks.

Individualized Education Program

IEP Dates: from 06/03/2010 **to** 06/02/2011

Student Name: Eva ███████   **DOB:** ███████   **State ID Number:** 1034399115

Service Delivery

What are the total service delivery needs of this student?

Include services, related services, program modifications and supports (including positive behavioral supports, school personnel and/or parent training/supports). Services should assist the student in reaching IEP goals, to be involved, and progress in the general curriculum, to participate in extracurricular/nonacademic activities and to allow the student to participate with nondisabled students while working towards IEP goals.

School District Cycle: ◉ N/A   ○ 5 day   ○ 6 day   ○ 10 day   ○ Other

A. Consultation (Indirect Services to School Personnel and Parents)

Focus on Goal #	Type of Service	Type of Personnel	Start Date	End Date	Frequency and Duration
1	Communication (individual)	Speech and Language Pathologist			1 x 15 min/week
3	Physical Therapy Consultation	Physical Therapist			1 x 15 min/week
4	Occupational Therapy	OTR/COTA			1 x 15 min/week

B. Special Education and Related Services in General Education Classroom (Direct Service)

Focus on Goal #	Type of Service	Type of Personnel	Start Date	End Date	Frequency and Duration

C. Special Education and Related Services in Other Settings (Direct Service)

Focus on Goal #	Type of Service	Type of Personnel	Start Date	End Date	Frequency and Duration
1-4	Extended School Year	Special Education Teacher, Paraprofessional			23 hrs/week
2	Academics	Special Education Teacher, Paraprofessional			28 hrs/week

Individualized Education Program

IEP Dates: from 06/03/2010 **to** 06/02/2011

Student Name: Eva ~~███~~   **DOB:** ~~███~~   **State ID Number:** 1034399115

Nonparticipation Justification

Is the student removed from the general education classroom at any time? (Refer to IEP 5 - Service Delivery, Section C)

☐ No   ☑ Yes

If yes, why is removal considered critical to the student's program?

Eva requires an intensive therapy program to meet her needs. She requires a longer school day and year in order to maintain acquired skills. Her curriculum is highly individualized and requires a dense staff to student ratio throughout the day.

> IDEA 2004 Regulation 20 U.S.C. §612 (a) (5).550: "... removal of children with disabilities from the regular educational environment occurs **only when** the nature or severity of the disability of a child is such that education in regular classes with the use of supplementary aids and services cannot be achieved satisfactorily." (Emphasis added.)

Schedule Modification

Shorter: Does this student require a shorter school day or school year?

☑ No   ☐ Yes - shorter day   ☐ Yes - shorter year   If yes, answer the questions below.

Longer: Does this student require a longer school day or school year to prevent substantial loss of previously learned skills and / or substantial difficulty in relearning skills?

☐ No   ☐ Yes - longer day   ☑ Yes - longer year   If yes, answer the questions below.

How will the student's schedule be modified? Why is this schedule modification being recommended?
If a longer day or year is recommended, how will school district coordinate services across program components?

Summer Program to maintain his current skill level and prevent regression.
The Collaborative Day runs during the school year from 9am-3:30pm, Mon-Fri.
Summer program is provided at the SSEC Community Program, SSEC Community Program during the summer will run from 7/6/09-8/19/09 Mon-Thurs from 9am-2:45pm. Therapies delivered on a maintenance level.

Transportation Services

Does the student require transportation as a result of the disability(ies)?

○ No   Regular transportation will be provided in the same manner as it would be provided for students without disabilities.
         If the child is placed away from the local school, transportation will be provided.

◉ Yes   Special transportation will be provided in the following manner:

☐ on a regular transportation vehicle with the following modifications and/or specialized equipment and precautions:

☑ on a special transportation vehicle with the following modifications and/or specialized equipment and precautions:
wheelchair van provided by ~~███~~ Public Schools

> After the team makes a transportation decision and after a placement decision has been made, a parent may choose to provide transportation and may be eligible for reimbursement under certain circumstances. Any parent who plans to transport their child to school should notify the school district contact person.

Individualized Education Program

IEP Dates: from 06/03/2010 **to** 06/02/2011

Student Name: Eva ~~████~~   **DOB:** ~~████~~   **State ID Number:** 1034399115

State or District-Wide Assessments

Identify state or district wide assessments planned for this IEP period.

1.   4.
2.   5.
3.   6.

Fill out the table below. Consider any state or district-wide assessment to be administered during the time span covered by this IEP. For each content area, identify the student's assessment participation status by putting an 'X' in the corresponding box for columns 1, 2, or 3.

Content Area	1. Assessment participation: Student participates in on-demand testing under routine conditions in this content area.	2. Assessment participation: Student participates in on-demand testing with accommodations in this content area. (see (1) below)	3. Assessment participation: Student participates in alternate assessment in this content area. (see (2) below)
	Column 1	**Column 2**	**Column 3**
English Language Arts	☐	☐	☐
History and Social Sciences	☐	☐	☐
Mathematics	☐	☐	☐
Science and Technology	☐	☐	☐
Reading	☐	☐	☐

(1) For each content area identified by an X in column 2 above: note in space below, the content area and describe the accommodations necessary for participation in the on-demand testing. Any accommodations used for assessment part of his/her instructional program.

(2) For each content area identified by an X in column 3 above: note in the space below, the content area, why the on-demand assessment is not appropriate and how that content area will be alternately assessed. Make sure to include the learning standards that will be addressed in each content area, the recommended assessment method(s) and the recommended evaluation and reporting method(s) for the student's performance on the alternate assessment.

Individualized Education Program

IEP Dates: from 06/03/2010 **to** 06/02/2011

Student Name: Eva ~~████~~   **DOB:** ~~████~~   **State ID Number:** 1034399115

Additional Information

☐ Include the following transition information: the anticipated graduation date; a statement of interagency responsibilities or needed linkages; the discussion of transfer of rights at least one year before age of majority; and a recommendation for a Chapter 688 Referral.

☐ Document efforts to obtain participation if a parent and if student did not attend meeting or provide input.

☐ Record other relevant IEP information not previously stated.

Response Section
School Assurance

I certify that the goals in this IEP are those recommended by the Team and that the indicated services will be provided.

_____   _____

Signature and Role of LEA Representative   Date

Parent Options / Responses

It is important that the district knows your decision as soon as possible. Please indicate your response by checking at least one (1) box and returning a signed copy to the district. Thank you.

☐ I accept the IEP as developed   ☐ I reject the IEP as developed.

☐ I reject the following portions of the IEP with the understanding that any portion(s) that I do not reject will be considered accepted and implemented immediately. Rejected portions are as follows:

☐ I request a meeting to discuss the rejected IEP or rejected portion(s).

_____   _____

Signature of Parent, Guardian, Educational Surrogate Parent, Student 18 and Over*   Date

Required signature once a student reaches 18 unless there is a court appointed guardian.

Parent Comment: I would like to make the following comment(s) but realize any comment(s) made that suggest changes to the proposed IEP will not be implemented unless the IEP is amended.

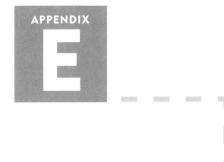

Recommended Sources for Coenzyme Q10 and Mito Cocktail Ingredients

Acton Pharmacy is located in Massachusetts and is a compounding pharmacy with a long history of helping families with mitochondrial disease. Ubiquinone is offered to patients as part of a compound, and can be purchased as a liquid or in capsule form. Saad Dinno is the owner and compounding pharmacist. www.actonpharmacy.com

America's Compounding Center (ACC) is located in Massachusetts but is licensed in many states and offers shipping options to families outside of MA. Both ubiquinone and ubiquinol are available through ACC. Arthur Margolis is the owner and compounding pharmacist. www.accrx.com

Epic4Health sells the Tischon formulation of ubiquinol, researched and formulated for people with mitochondrial disorders. Call and mention that you are a patient or parent of an affected child for a discount. www.epic4health.com

The International Academy of Compounding Pharmacists represents more than 2,000 specialty compounding pharmacists and technicians. Patients can search for a compounding pharmacist by geographic area. Be sure to ask each pharmacy for their experience with mitochondrial disease, and if they have none, consider asking them to call one of the experienced compounding pharmacists listed above. www.iacprx.org

Pine Pharmacy is located in western New York and is a family-owned compounding pharmacy with an interest in patients with mitochondrial disease. Owner Al Muto and his son offer an effervescent formula that can be mixed with water, as well as an over-the-counter "Mito Mix" for adult patients who do not have insurance coverage. www.pinepharmacy.com

Sigma-Tau Pharmaceuticals is the maker of the brand name product Carnitor®, which is levocarnitine. Carnitor comes in IV, tablets, and oral solution and is indicated for use in primary and secondary (as is most common for mitochondrial disorders) l-carnitine deficiency. http://www.sigmatau.com

Solace Nutrition has a long history of producing medical foods, including special formulas and supplements used by patients who have metabolic diseases. They offer Cyto-Q, which is ubiquinol (the more potent form of CoQ10), as well as several other special formulations helpful to people with Mito. www.solacenutrition.com

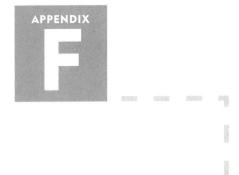

Selected Bibliography

Autism

Has Your Child with Autistic Symptoms Been Properly Screened for a Subset of Mitochondrial Disease Known as OXPHOS?...Probably Not. Davi A. (2010). The Autism File- Global, issue 36.

The Journey from ASD to a mitochondrial disease diagnosis: Symptoms, testing, treatments and responses to a mitochondrial cocktail- Families Stories- Part II. Davi A. (2011). The Autism File-Global, issue 38.

Mitochondrial dysfunction in autism. Giulivi C, Zhang YF, Omanska-Klusek A, Ross-Inta C, Wong S, Hertz-Picciotto I, Tassone F, Pessah IN.

Abstract

CONTEXT: Impaired mitochondrial function may influence processes highly dependent on energy, such as neurodevelopment, and contribute to autism. No studies have evaluated mitochondrial dysfunction and mitochondrial DNA (mtDNA) abnormalities in a well-defined population of children with autism.

OBJECTIVE: To evaluate mitochondrial defects in children with autism.

DESIGN, SETTING, AND PATIENTS: Observational study using data collected from patients aged 2 to 5 years who were a subset of children participating in the Childhood Autism Risk From Genes and Environment study in California, which is a population-based, case-control investigation with confirmed autism cases and age-matched, genetically unrelated, typically developing controls, that was launched in 2003 and is still ongoing. Mitochondrial dysfunction and mtDNA abnormalities were evaluated in lymphocytes from 10 children with autism and 10 controls.

MAIN OUTCOME MEASURES: Oxidative phosphorylation capacity, mtDNA copy number and deletions, mitochondrial rate of hydrogen peroxide production, and plasma lactate and pyruvate.

RESULTS: The reduced nicotinamide adenine dinucleotide (NADH) oxidase activity (normalized to citrate synthase activity) in lymphocytic mitochondria from children with autism was significantly lower compared with controls (mean, 4.4 [95% confidence interval {CI}, 2.8-6.0] vs 12 [95% CI, 8-16], respectively; P = .001). The majority of children with autism (6 of 10) had complex I activity below control range values. Higher plasma pyruvate levels were found in children with autism compared with controls (0.23 mM [95% CI, 0.15-0.31 mM] vs 0.08 mM [95% CI, 0.04-0.12 mM], respectively; P = .02). Eight of 10 cases had higher pyruvate levels but only 2 cases had higher lactate levels compared with controls. These results were consistent with the lower pyruvate dehydrogenase activity observed in children with autism compared with controls (1.0 [95% CI, 0.6-1.4] nmol × [min × mg protein](-1) vs 2.3 [95% CI, 1.7-2.9] nmol × [min × mg protein](-1), respectively; P = .01). Children with autism had higher mitochondrial rates of hydrogen peroxide production compared with controls (0.34 [95% CI, 0.26-0.42] nmol × [min × mg of protein](-1) vs 0.16 [95% CI, 0.12-0.20] nmol × [min × mg protein](-1) by complex III; P = .02). Mitochondrial DNA overreplication was found in 5 cases (mean ratio of mtDNA to nuclear DNA: 239 [95% CI, 217-239] vs 179 [95% CI, 165-193] in controls; P = 10(-4)). Deletions at the segment of cytochrome b were observed in 2 cases (ratio of cytochrome b to ND1: 0.80 [95% CI, 0.68-0.92] vs 0.99 [95% CI, 0.93-1.05] for controls; P = .01).

CONCLUSION: In this exploratory study, children with autism were more likely to have mitochondrial dysfunction, mtDNA overreplication, and mtDNA deletions than typically developing children.

Autism and mitochondrial disease. Haas RH. Research in Developmental Disabilities Rev. 2010 Jun;16(2):144-53.
  Abstract
    Autism spectrum disorder (ASD) as defined by the revised Diagnostic and Statistical Manual of Mental Disorders: DSM IVTR criteria (American Psychiatric

Association [2000] Washington, DC: American Psychiatric Publishing) as impairment before the age of 3 in language development and socialization with the development of repetitive behaviors appears to be increased in incidence and prevalence. Similarly, mitochondrial disorders are increasingly recognized. Although overlap between these disorders is to be expected, accumulating clinical, genetic, and biochemical evidence suggests that mitochondrial dysfunction in ASD is more commonly seen than expected. Some patients with ASD phenotypes clearly have genetic-based primary mitochondrial disease. This review will examine the data linking autism and mitochondria.

Bridging the Gap between Mitochondrial Disease and Autism. Kendall F. Autism Science Digest. 2011 April. www.virtualmdpractice.com

Fever plus mitochondrial disease could be risk factors for autistic regression. Shoffner J, Hyams L, Langley GN, Cossette S, Mylacraine L, Dale J, Ollis L, Kuoch S, Bennett K, Aliberti A, Hyland K. Journal of Child Neurology. 2010 Apr;25(4):429-34. Epub 2009 Sep 22.

Abstract

Autistic spectrum disorders encompass etiologically heterogeneous persons, with many genetic causes. A subgroup of these individuals has mitochondrial disease. Because a variety of metabolic disorders, including mitochondrial disease, show regression with fever, a retrospective chart review was performed and identified 28 patients who met diagnostic criteria for autistic spectrum disorders and mitochondrial disease. Autistic regression occurred in 60.7% (17 of 28), a statistically significant increase over the general autistic spectrum disorder population (P < .0001). Of the 17 individuals with autistic regression, 70.6% (12 of 17) regressed with fever and 29.4% (5 of 17) regressed without identifiable linkage to fever or vaccinations. None showed regression with vaccination unless a febrile response was present. Although the study is small, a subgroup of patients with mitochondrial disease may be at risk of autistic regression with fever. Although recommended vaccinations schedules are appropriate in mitochondrial disease, fever management appears important for decreasing regression risk.

Diagnosis of Mitochondrial Disease

Diagnostic criteria for respiratory chain disorders in adults and children. Bernier FP, Boneh A, Dennett X, Chow CW, Cleary MA, Thorburn DR. Neurology. 2002 Nov 12;59(9):1406-11.

Abstract

BACKGROUND: Respiratory chain (RC) disorders are clinically, biochemically, and molecularly heterogeneous. The lack of standardized diagnostic criteria poses difficulties in evaluating diagnostic methodologies.

OBJECTIVE: To assess proposed adult RC diagnostic criteria that classify patients into "definite," "probable," or "possible" categories.

METHODS: The authors applied the adult RC diagnostic criteria retrospectively to 146 consecutive children referred for investigation of a suspected RC disorder. Data were collected from hospital, genetics, and laboratory records, and the diagnoses predicted by the adult criteria were compared with the previously assigned assessments.

RESULTS: The authors identified three major difficulties in applying the adult criteria: lack of pediatric-specific criteria; difficulty in segregating continuous data into circumscribed major and minor criteria; and lack of additivity of clinical features or enzyme tests. They therefore modified the adult criteria to allow for pediatric clinical and histologic features and for more sensitive coding of RC enzyme and functional studies. Reanalysis of the patients' data resulted in congruence between the diagnostic certainty previously assigned by the authors' center and that defined by the new general RC diagnostic criteria in 99% of patients.

CONCLUSIONS: These general diagnostic criteria appear to improve the sensitivity of the adult criteria. They need further assessment in prospective clinical and epidemiologic studies.

The in-depth evaluation of suspected mitochondrial disease. Mitochondrial Medicine Society's Committee on Diagnosis, Haas RH, Parikh S, Falk MJ, Saneto RP, Wolf NI, Darin N, Wong LJ, Cohen BH, Naviaux RK. Molecular Genetics and Metabolism. 2008 May;94(1):16-37. Epub 2008 Feb 1.

Abstract

Mitochondrial disease confirmation and establishment of a specific molecular diagnosis requires extensive clinical and laboratory evaluation. Dual genome origins of mitochondrial disease, multi-organ system manifestations, and an ever increasing spectrum of recognized phenotypes represent the main diagnostic challenges. To overcome these obstacles, compiling information from a variety of diagnostic laboratory modalities can often provide sufficient evidence to establish an etiology. These include blood and tissue histochemical and analyte measurements, neuroimaging, provocative testing, enzymatic assays of tissue samples and cultured cells, as well as DNA analysis. As interpretation of results from these multifaceted investigations can become quite complex, the Diagnostic Committee of the Mitochondrial Medicine Society developed this review to provide an overview of currently available and emerging methodologies for the diagnosis of primary mitochondrial disease, with a focus on disorders characterized by impairment of oxidative phosphorylation. The aim of this work is to facilitate the diagnosis of mitochondrial disease by geneticists, neurologists, and other metabolic specialists who face the challenge of evaluating patients of all ages with suspected mitochondrial disease.

Mitochondrial disease criteria: Diagnostic applications in children. Morava E, van den Heuvel L, Hol F, de Vries MC, Hogeveen M, Rodenburg RJ, Smeitink JA. Neurology. 2006 Nov 28;67(10):1823-6.

Abstract

BACKGROUND: Based on a previous prospective clinical and biochemical study, a consensus mitochondrial disease scoring system was established to facilitate the diagnosis in patients with a suspected mitochondrial disorder.

OBJECTIVE: To evaluate the specificity of the diagnostic system, we applied the mitochondrial disease score in 61 children with a multisystem disease and a suspected oxidative phosphorylation disorder who underwent a muscle biopsy and were consecutively diagnosed with a genetic mutation.

METHODS: We evaluated data of 44 children diagnosed with a disorder in oxidative phosphorylation, carrying a mutation in the mitochondrial or nuclear DNA. We compared them with 17 children who, based on the clinical and metabolic features, also had a muscle biopsy but were finally diagnosed with a nonmitochondrial multisystem disorder by further genetic analysis.

RESULTS: All children with a genetically established diagnosis of a primary oxidative phosphorylation disorder had a mitochondrial disease score above 6 (probable mitochondrial disorder), and 73% of the children had a score above 8 (definite mitochondrial disorder) at evaluation of the muscle biopsy. In the nonmitochondrial multisystem disorder group, the score was significantly lower, and no patients reached a score comparable with a definite respiratory chain disorder.

CONCLUSIONS: The mitochondrial disease criteria system has a high specificity to distinguish between mitochondrial and other multisystem disorders. The method could also be applied in children with a suspected mitochondrial disorder, prior to performing a muscle biopsy.

Mitochondrial Medicine

Pharmacologic effects on mitochondrial function. Cohen BH. Developmental Disabilities Research Reviews. 2010 Jun;16(2):189-99.

Abstract

The vast majority of energy necessary for cellular function is produced in mitochondria. Free-radical production and apoptosis are other critical mitochondrial functions. The complex structure, electrochemical properties of the inner mitochondrial membrane (IMM), and genetic control from both mitochondrial DNA (mtDNA) and nuclear DNA (nDNA) are some of the unique features that explain why the mitochondria are vulnerable to environmental injury. Because of similarity to bacterial translational machinery, mtDNA translation is likewise vulnerable to inhibition by some antibiotics. The mechanism of mtDNA replication, which is required for normal mitochondrial maintenance and duplication, is inhibited by a relatively new class of drugs used to treat AIDS. The electrochemical gradient maintained by the IMM is vulnerable to many drugs that are weak organic acids at physiological pH, resulting in excessive free-radical generation and uncoupling of oxidative phosphorylation. Many of these drugs can cause clinical injury in otherwise healthy people, but there are also examples where particular gene mutations may predispose to increased drug toxicity. The spectrum of drug-induced mitochondrial dysfunction extends across many drug classes. It is hoped that preclinical pharmacogenetic and functional studies of mitochondrial toxicity, along with personalized genomic medicine, will improve both our understanding of mitochondrial drug toxicity and patient safety.

Multisystem manifestations of mitochondrial disorders. Di Donato S. Journal of Neurology. 2009 May;256(5):693-710. Epub 2009 Mar 1.

Abstract

Mitochondria are cytoplasmic organelles in eukaryotic cells that accomplish several distinct vital functions, including oxidative phosphorylation, metabolic anaplerotic and degradative pathways, and integration of signaling for apoptosis. Impaired oxidative phosphorylation, the common final pathway of mitochondrial metabolism, results in a variety of clinical manifestations, and the term mitochondrial disorders is currently ascribed to (mostly) genetic diseases of the respiratory chain associated with mitochondrial DNA mutation or nuclear DNA mutations. Genetic disorders with impaired oxidative phosphorylation are extremely heterogeneous, as their clinical presentation ranges from lesions of single tissues or specialized structures, such as the optic nerve in the mitochondrial DNA-associated Leber's hereditary optic neuropathy and in the nuclear DNA-associated dominant optic atrophy, to more widespread pathologies, including myopathies, peripheral neuropathies, encephalomyopathies, cardiopathies, or complex multisystem disorders. The age at onset ranges from neonatal to adult life. This review focuses on mitochondrial diseases that find significant expression outside the central nervous system and the peripheral neuromuscular system, and manifest with substantial clinical signs and symptoms in tissues and organs such as the heart, endocrine system, liver, kidney, blood, and gastrointestinal tract. The available information on putative genotype-phenotype correlations and the related pathogenic mechanisms are summarized when appropriate.

A history of mitochondrial diseases. DiMauro S. Journal of Inherited Metabolic Diseases. 2010 May 21. [Epub ahead of print]

Abstract

This article reviews the development of mitochondrial medicine from the premolecular era (1962-1988), when mitochondrial diseases were defined on the basis of clinical examination, muscle biopsy, and biochemical criteria, through the molecular era, when the full complexity of these disorders became evident. In a chronological order, I have followed the introduction of new pathogenic concepts that have shaped a rational genetic classification of these clinically heterogeneous disorders. Thus, mitochondrial DNA (mtDNA)-related diseases can be divided into two main groups: those that impair mitochondrial protein synthesis in toto, and those that affect specific respiratory chain proteins. Mutations in nuclear DNA can affect components of respiratory chain complexes (direct hits) or assembly proteins (indirect hits), but they can also impair mtDNA integrity (multiple mtDNA mutations), replication (mtDNA depletion), or mtDNA translation. Besides these disorders that affect the respiratory chain directly, defects in other mitochondrial functions may also affect oxidative phosphorylation, including problems in mitochondrial protein import, alterations of the inner mitochondrial membrane lipid composition, and defects of mitochondrial dynamics. The enormous and still ongoing progress in our understanding of mitochondrial medicine was made possible by the intense collaboration of an international cadre of "mitochondriacs." Having published my first paper on a patient with mitochondrial myopathy 37 years ago (DiMauro et al., 1973), I feel qualified to write a history of the mitochondrial diseases, a fascinating, still evolving, and continuously puzzling area of medicine. In each section, I follow a chronological order of the salient discoveries and I show only the portraits of distinguished deceased mitochondriacs and those whose names became eponyms of mitochondrial diseases.

Historical perspective on mitochondrial medicine. DiMauro S, Garone C. Developmental Disabilities Research Review. 2010 Jun;16(2):106-13.

Abstract

In this review, we trace the origins and follow the development of mitochondrial medicine from the premolecular era (1962-1988) based on clinical clues, muscle morphology, and biochemistry into the molecular era that started in 1988 and is still advancing at a brisk pace. We have tried to stress conceptual advances, such as endosymbiosis, uniparental inheritance, intergenomic signaling and its defects, and mitochondrial dynamics. We hope that this historical review also provides an update on mitochondrial medicine, although we fully realize that the speed of progress in this area makes any such endeavor akin to writing on water.

Mitochondrial disorders in the nervous system. DiMauro S, Schon EA. Annual Review Neurosciences. 2008;31:91-123.

Abstract

Mitochondrial diseases (encephalomyopathies) have traditionally been ascribed to defects of the respiratory chain, which has helped researchers explain their genetic and clinical complexity. However, other mitochondrial functions are greatly important for the nervous system, including protein importation, organellar dynamics, and programmed cell death. Defects in genes controlling these functions are attracting increasing attention as causes not only of neurological (and psychiatric) diseases but also of age-related neurodegenerative disorders. After discussing some pathogenic conundrums regarding the neurological manifestations of the respiratory chain defects, we review altered mitochondrial dynamics in the etiology of specific neurological diseases and in the physiopathology of more common neurodegenerative disorders.

Mitochondrial disorders and general anaesthesia: a case series and review. Footitt EJ, Sinha MD, Raiman JA, Dhawan A, Moganasundram S, Champion MP. British Journal Anaesthesia. 2008 Apr;100(4):436-41.

Abstract

Patients with mitochondrial disease are at risk of metabolic decompensation and often require general anaesthesia (GA) as part of their diagnostic work up and subsequent management. However, the evidence base for the use of GA is limited and inconclusive. We have documented the practice and outcome in the use of GA in paediatric patients with mitochondrial disease using a retrospective case review study of 38 mitochondrial patients who had undergone 58 anaesthetics within the regional metabolic service for the period 1989-2005. A variety of anaesthetic agents were used and the pattern of use reflects that seen in standard paediatric practice. There were no episodes of malignant hyperthermia and no documented intraoperative events attributable to the GA. Three post-operative adverse events were noted; one episode of hypovolaemia, one episode of acute on chronic renal failure, and one episode of metabolic decompensation 12 h post-muscle biopsy. Despite theoretical concern about this group of patients, adverse events after GA are rare and in most cases unrelated to the anaesthesia. Further prospective studies of GA in mitochondrial disease are required to create evidence-based clinical guidelines for safe practice.

Mitochondrial disease: a practical approach for primary care physicians. Haas RH, Parikh S, Falk MJ, Saneto RP, Wolf NI, Darin N, Cohen BH. Pediatrics. 2007 Dec;120(6):1326-33.

Abstract

Notorious variability in the presentation of mitochondrial disease in the infant and young child complicates its clinical diagnosis. Mitochondrial disease is not a single entity but, rather, a heterogeneous group of disorders characterized by impaired energy production due to genetically based oxidative phosphorylation dysfunction. Together, these disorders constitute the most common neurometabolic disease of childhood with an estimated minimal risk of developing mitochondrial disease of 1 in 5000. Diagnostic difficulty results from not only the variable and often nonspecific presentation of these disorders but also from the absence of a reliable biomarker specific for the screening or diagnosis of mitochondrial disease. A simplified and standardized approach to facilitate the clinical recognition of mitochondrial disease by primary physicians is needed. With this article we aimed to improve the clinical recognition of mitochondrial disease by primary care providers and empower the generalist to initiate appropriate baseline diagnostic testing before determining the need for specialist referral. This is particularly important in light of the international shortage of metabolism specialists to comprehensively evaluate this large and complex disease population. It is hoped that greater familiarity among primary care physicians with the protean manifestations of mitochondrial disease will facilitate the proper diagnosis and management of this growing cohort of pediatric patients who present across all specialties.

Presentation and diagnosis of mitochondrial disorders in children. Koenig MK. Pediatric Neurology. 2008 May;38(5):305-13.

Abstract

The first disorder of mitochondrial function was described by Luft in 1959. Over the ensuing decades, multiple cases of mitochondrial dysfunction were reported, and the term "mitochondrial disorder" arose to describe any defect in the mitochondrial electron transport chain. The sequence of the mitochondrial genome was elucidated in 1981 by Anderson et al., and during the next 20 years, >200 pathogenic point mutations, deletions, insertions, and rearrangements were described. Most of the original cases were adults, and the diagnosis of a mitochondrial disorder in an adult patient became relatively straightforward. Adults present with well-defined "mitochondrial syndromes" and generally carry mitochondrial DNA mutations that are easily identified. Children with mitochondrial disorders are much harder to define. Children are more likely to have a nuclear DNA mutation, whereas the "classic" syndromic findings tend to be absent. This review describes both the varying presentations of mitochondrial disorders and the common laboratory, imaging, and pathologic findings related to children.

Prevalence of mitochondrial DNA disease in adults. Schaefer AM, et al, Annals of Neurology. 2008; 63:35-39.

Abstract

OBJECTIVE: Diverse and variable clinical features, a loose genotype-phenotype relationship, and presentation to different medical specialties have all hindered attempts to gauge the epidemiological impact of mitochondrial DNA (mtDNA) disease. Nevertheless, a clear understanding of its prevalence remains an important goal, particularly about planning appropriate clinical services. Consequently, the aim of this study was to accurately define the prevalence of mtDNA disease (primary mutation occurs in mtDNA) in the working-age population of the North East of England.

METHODS: Adults with suspected mitochondrial disease in the North East of England were referred to a single neurology center for investigation from 1990 to 2004. Those with pathogenic mtDNA mutations were identified and pedigree analysis performed. For the midyear period of 2001, we calculated the minimum point prevalence of mtDNA disease for adults of working age (>16 and <60/65 years for female/male patients, respectively).

RESULTS: In this population, we found that 9.2 in 100,000 people have clinically manifest mtDNA disease, making this one of the commonest inherited neuromuscular disorders. In addition, a further 16.5 in 100,000 children and adults younger than retirement age are at risk for development of mtDNA disease.

INTERPRETATION: Through detailed pedigree analysis and active family tracing, we have been able to provide revised minimum prevalence figures for mtDNA disease. These estimates confirm that mtDNA disease is a common cause of chronic morbidity and is more prevalent than has been previously appreciated.

Symptoms of Mitochondrial Disease

Mitochondrial cytopathy in adults: what we know so far. Cohen BH, Gold DR. Erratum in: Cleveland Clinic Journal of Medicine 2001 Sep;68(9):746.

Abstract

Mitochondrial cytopathies are a diverse group of inherited and acquired disorders that result in inadequate energy production. They can be caused by inheritable genetic mutations, acquired somatic mutations, exposure to toxins (including some prescription medications), and the aging process itself. In addition, a number of well-described diseases can decrease mitochondrial energy production; these include hyperthyroidism, hypothyroidism, and hyperlipidemia.

Autonomic dysfunction presenting as orthostatic intolerance in patients suffering from mitochondrial cytopathy. Kanjwal K, Karabin B, Kanjwal Y, Saeed B, Grubb BP. Clinical Cardiology. 2010 Oct;33(10):626-9.

Abstract

BACKGROUND: Disturbances in autonomic nervous system function have been reported to occur in patients suffering from mitochondrial cytopathies. However, there is paucity of literature on the occurrence of orthostatic intolerance (OI) in these patients. We report on a series of patients diagnosed with mitochondrial cytopathy who developed features of autonomic dysfunction in the form of OI.

METHODS: This was a single-center report on a series of 6 patients who were followed in our clinic for orthostatic intolerance. All of these patients had a diagnosis of mitochondrial cytopathy on the basis of muscle biopsy and were being followed at a center specializing in the treatment of mitochondrial disorders. This study was approved by our local institutional review board. Each of the patients had suffered from symptoms of fatigue, palpitations, near syncope, and syncope. The diagnosis of OI was confirmed by head-up tilt test. Collected data included demographic information, presenting symptoms, laboratory data, tilt-table response, and treatment outcomes.

RESULTS: Six patients (3 females) were identified for inclusion in this report. The mean age of the group was 48 ± 8 years (range, 40-60 years). All of these patients underwent head-up tilt-table testing and all had a positive response that reproduced their clinical symptoms. Among those having an abnormal tilt-table pattern, 1 had a neurocardiogenic response, 1 had a dysautonomic response, and 4 had a postural orthostatic tachycardia response. All but 1 patient reported marked symptom relief with pharmacotherapy. The patient who failed pharmacotherapy received a dual-chamber closed-loop pacemaker and subsequently reported marked improvement in her symptoms with elimination of her syncope.

CONCLUSIONS: Orthostatic intolerance might be a significant feature of autonomic nervous system dysfunction in patients suffering from mito-chondrial cytopathy.

Clinical implications of mitochondrial disease. Muravchick S. Advanced Drug De-livery Review. 2008 Oct-Nov;60(13-14):1553-60. Epub 2008 Jul 4.
Abstract
The terms mitochondrial myopathy, mitochondrial cytopathy, and inher-ited mitochondrial encephalomyopathy encompass a large grouping of syndromes produced either by genetically transmitted or acquired dis-ruption of mitochondrial energy production or biosensor function. Many of these disorders are clinically apparent during infancy, but for some the metabolic signs of oxidative stress may not appear until the young or middle adult years. Initially thought to be a rare disorder, it now appears that mitochondrial dysfunction is relatively common but often unrecog-nized because symptoms are extremely variable and usually insidious in onset. It has also become apparent that mitochondrial dysfunction is a component of many common cardiovascular and neurological disease states and of physiologic aging. Recent advances in our understanding of the mechanisms of mitochondrial dysfunction may explain and link a wide variety of clinical phenomena. This review summarizes the current knowledge regarding the clinical implications of inherited and acquired mitochondrial disease, the effects of anesthetics on mitochondrial func-tion, and the extent to which mitochondrial bioenergetic state deter-mines anesthetic requirement and potential anesthetic toxicity.

The spectrum of mitochondrial disease, in Mitochondrial and Metabolic Disor-ders: a primary care physician's guide. Naviaux RK. Psy-Ed Corp., Oradell, NJ, pp. 3-10, 1997. Cleveland Clinic Journal of Medicine. 2001 Jul;68(7):625-6, 629-42.

The neurologic manifestations of mitochondrial disease. Parikh S. Developmen-tal Disabilities Research Reviews. 2010 Jun;16(2):120-8.
Abstract
The nervous system contains some of the body's most metabolically de-manding cells that are highly dependent on ATP produced via mitochon-drial oxidative phosphorylation. Thus, the neurological system is consis-tently involved in patients with mitochondrial disease. Symptoms differ depending on the part of the nervous system affected. Although almost any neurological symptom can be due to mitochondrial disease, there are select symptoms that are more suggestive of a mitochondrial problem.

Certain symptoms that have become sine qua non with underlying mitochondrial cytopathies can serve as diagnostic "red flags." Here, the typical and atypical presentations of mitochondrial disease in the nervous system are reviewed, focusing on "red flag" neurological symptoms as well as associated symptoms that can occur in, but are not specific to, mitochondrial disease. The multitudes of mitochondrial syndromes are not reviewed in-depth, though a select few are discussed in some detail.

The role of mitochondrial dysfunction in psychiatric disease. Scaglia F. Developmental Disabilities Research Reviews. 2010 Jun;16(2):136-43.

Abstract

Mitochondrial respiratory chain disorders are a group of genetically and clinically heterogeneous disorders caused by the biochemical complexity of mitochondrial respiration and the fact that two genomes, one mitochondrial and one nuclear, encode the components of the respiratory chain. These disorders can manifest at birth or present later in life. They result, at least in part, in defective production of ATP. Typically, mitochondrial disorders affect tissues with high energetic demands such as skeletal muscle, cardiac muscle, and the central nervous system. Neurological dysfunction is the most frequent clinical presentation of these disorders. The central nervous system is highly dependent on oxidative metabolism, and particular mitochondrial disorders are accompanied by focal brain necrosis (Leigh disease), dementia, or static encephalopathy. Furthermore, many children with mitochondrial encephalomyopathies present with more subtle and indolent signs including focal cognitive deficits of memory, perception, and language. Some subjects with mitochondrial disorders may also exhibit nonverbal cognitive impairment, compromised visuospatial abilities, and short-term memory deficits associated with working memory that likely reflect defects in synaptic plasticity. Psychiatric features are found within the clinical spectrum of mitochondrial syndromes. It is increasingly recognized that mitochondrial dysfunction may be associated with neuropsychiatric abnormalities such as dementia, major depression, and bipolar disorder. Furthermore, several lines of evidence suggest that there is involvement of mitochondrial dysfunction in schizophrenia, including documented alterations in brain energy metabolism, electron transport chain activity, and expression of genes involved in mitochondrial function. The purpose of this review article is to summarize the psychiatric features observed in mitochondrial cytopathies and discuss possible mechanisms of dysfunctional cellular energy metabolism that underlie the pathophysiology of major subsets of psychiatric disorders.

Mitochondrial dysfunction in neurodegenerative diseases. Schapira AH. Neuro-chemical Research. 2008 Dec;33(12):2502-9. Epub 2008 Nov 8.

Abstract

Mitochondria play a pivotal role in mammalian cell metabolism, hosting a number of important biochemical pathways including oxidative phosphorylation. As might be expected from this fundamental contribution to cell function, abnormalities of mitochondrial metabolism are a common cause of human disease. Primary mutations of mitochondrial DNA result in a diverse group of disorders often collectively referred to as the mitochondrial encephalomyopathies. Perhaps more importantly in numerical terms are those neurodegenerative diseases caused by mutations of nuclear genes encoding mitochondrial proteins. Finally there are mitochondrial abnormalities induced by secondary events, e.g., oxidative stress that may contribute to senescence, and environmental toxins that may cause disease either alone or in combination with a genetic predisposition.

Treatment of Mitochondrial Disorders

A modern approach to the treatment of mitochondrial disease. Parikh S, Saneto R, Falk MJ, Anselm I, Cohen BH, Haas R., Medicine Society TM. Curr Treat Options Neurol. 2009 Nov;11(6):414-30.

Abstract

The treatment of mitochondrial disease varies considerably. Most experts use a combination of vitamins, optimize patients' nutrition and general health, and prevent worsening of symptoms during times of illness and physiologic stress. We agree with this approach, and we agree that therapies using vitamins and cofactors have value, though there is debate about the choice of these agents and the doses prescribed. Despite the paucity of high-quality scientific evidence, these therapies are relatively harmless, may alleviate select clinical symptoms, and theoretically may offer a means of staving off disease progression. Like many other mitochondrial medicine physicians, we have observed significant (and at times life-altering) clinical responses to such pharmacologic interventions. However, it is not yet proven that these therapies truly alter the course of the disease, and some experts may choose not to use these medications at all. At present, the evidence of their effectiveness does not rise to the level required for universal use. Based on our clinical experience and judgment, however, we agree that a therapeutic trial of coenzyme Q10, along with other antioxidants, should be attempted. Although individual specialists differ as to the exact drug cocktail, a common approach involves combinations of antioxidants that may have a synergistic effect. Because almost all relevant therapies are classified as medical foods or over-the-counter supplements, most physicians also attempt to balance the apparent clinical benefit of mitochondrial cocktails with the cost burden that these supplements pose for the family.

Coenzyme Q and mitochondrial disease. Quinzii CM, Hirano M. Developmental Disabilities Research Reviews. 2010 Jun;16(2):183-8.

Abstract

Coenzyme Q(10) (CoQ(10)) is an essential electron carrier in the mitochondrial respiratory chain and an important antioxidant. Deficiency of CoQ(10) is a clinically and molecularly heterogeneous syndrome, which, to date, has been found to be autosomal recessive in inheritance and generally responsive to CoQ(10) supplementation. CoQ(10) deficiency has been associated with five major clinical phenotypes: (1) encephalomyopathy, (2) severe infantile multisystemic disease, (3) cerebellar ataxia, (4) isolated myopathy, and (5) nephrotic syndrome. In a few patients, pathogenic mutations have been identified in genes involved in the biosynthesis of CoQ(10) (primary CoQ(10) deficiencies) or in genes not directly related to CoQ(10) biosynthesis (secondary CoQ(10) deficiencies). Respiratory chain defects, ROS production, and apoptosis contribute to the pathogenesis of primary CoQ(10) deficiencies. In vitro and in vivo studies are necessary to further understand the pathogenesis of the disease and to develop more effective therapies.

The mitochondrial cocktail: Rationale for combined nutraceutical therapy in mitochondrial cytopathies. Tarnopolsky MA. Advanced Drug Delivery. Rev. 2008 Oct-Nov;60(13-14):1561-7. Epub 2008 Jul 4.

Abstract

Mitochondrial cytopathies ultimately lead to a reduction in aerobic energy transduction, depletion of alternative energy stores, increased oxidative stress, apoptosis, and necrosis. Specific combinations of nutraceutical compounds can target many of the aforementioned biochemical pathways. Antioxidants combined with cofactors that can bypass specific electron transport chain defects and the provision of alternative energy sources represents a specific targeted strategy. To date, there has been only one randomized double-blind clinical trial using a combination nutraceutial therapy and it showed that the combination of creatine monohydrate, coenzyme Q10, and alpha-lipoic acid reduced lactate and markers of oxidative stress in patients with mitochondrial cytopathies. Future studies need to use larger numbers of patients with well-defined clinical and surrogate marker outcomes to clarify the potential role for combination nutraceuticals ("mitochondrial cocktail") as a therapy for mitochondrial cytopathies.

Mitochondrial myopathies: Diagnosis, exercise intolerance, and treatment options. Tarnopolsky MA, Raha S. Medical Science Sports Exercise 2005 Dec;37(12):2086-93.

Abstract

Mitochondrial myopathies are caused by genetic mutations that directly influence the functioning of the electron transport chain (ETC). It is estimated that 1 of 8,000 people have pathology inducing mutations affecting mitochondrial function. Diagnosis often requires a multifaceted approach with measurements of serum lactate and pyruvate, urine organic acids, magnetic resonance spectroscopy (MRS), muscle histology and ultrastructure, enzymology, genetic analysis, and exercise testing. The ubiquitous distribution of the mitochondria in the human body explains the multiple organ involvement. Exercise intolerance is a common but often an overlooked hallmark of mitochondrial myopathies. The muscle consequences of ETC dysfunction include increased reliance on anaerobic metabolism (lactate generation, phosphocreatine degradation), enhanced free radical production, reduced oxygen extraction and electron flux through ETC, and mitochondrial proliferation or biogenesis (see article by Hood in current issue). Treatments have included antioxidants (vitamin E, alpha lipoic acid), electron donors and acceptors (coenzyme Q10, riboflavin), alternative energy sources (creatine monohydrate), lactate reduction strategies (dichloroacetate) and exercise training. Exercise is a particularly important modality in diagnosis as well as therapy (see article by Taivassalo in current issue). Increased awareness of these disorders by exercise physiologists and sports medicine practitioners should lead to more accurate and more rapid diagnosis and the opportunity for therapy and genetic counseling.

Emerging therapeutic approaches to mitochondrial diseases. Wenz T, Williams SL, Bacman SR, Moraes CT. Developmental Disabilities Research Reviews. 2010 Jun;16(2):219-29.

Abstract

Mitochondrial diseases are very heterogeneous and can affect different tissues and organs. Moreover, they can be caused by genetic defects in either nuclear or mitochondrial DNA as well as by environmental factors. All of these factors have made the development of therapies difficult. In this review article, we will discuss emerging approaches to the therapy of mitochondrial disorders, some of which are targeted to specific conditions whereas others may be applicable to a more diverse group of patients.

Books

American Psychiatric Association. (2000). Pervasive developmental disorders. In Diagnostic and statistical manual of mental disorders (Fourth edition—text revision (DSM-IV-TR). Washington, DC: American Psychiatric Association, 69-70.

DiMauro, Salvatore. Mitochondrial Medicine. Abington, Oxon: Informa Healthcare, 2006.

Websites

Mitochondrial Disease: Symptoms, Physiology, Treatment

- Center for Disease Control and Prevention (CDC), "ASD and Mitochondrial Disease."
  www.cdc.gov

- Columbia University 21stC newsletter, "DNA Unraveled." The other DNA: Research on mitochondrial diseases. Eric Schon and Salvatore DiMauro.
  http://www.columbia.edu/cu/21stC/issue-1.3/dna-mitoch.html

- Facebook Group "You Know you have Mito When…"
  www.facebook.com

- Genetic Health, Genetics 101.
  www.genetichealth.com

- MitoAction Blog archives, podcasts of guest speakers.
  www.mitoaction.org/blog

- MitoAction Clinician's Symptom Management Guide. Mark Korson, MD and Margaret Klehm, RN.
  www.MitoAction.org/guide

- Muscular Dystrophy Association (MDA), MDA Publications (Quest).
  www.mdausa.org/publications/quest

- Online Mendelian Inheritance in Man. OMIM (r), Johns Hopkins University.
  www.omim.org

- Wikipedia, "Oxidative Phosphorylation."
  http://en.wikipedia.org/wiki/Oxidative_phosphorylation

■ Wiley Publishing, Interactive concepts in Biochemistry: "Oxidative Phosphorylation"
http://www.wiley.com/legacy/college/boyer/0470003790/animations/electron_transport/electron_transport.htm

Special Education

■ IFSP web, "Individualized Family Service Plan."
www.ifspweb.org

■ National Dissemination Center for Children with Disabilities.
http://nichcy.org/

■ Special Education Advisor, "Special Education."
www.specialeducationadvisor.com

■ Wrights Law, "IDEA and Special Education."
www.wrightslaw.com

Index

About the Author

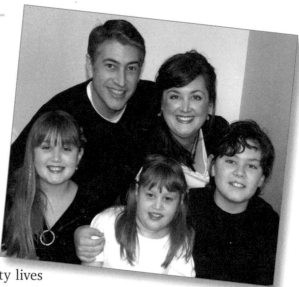

Cristy Balcells RN MSN is a nurse, mother of a child with mitochondrial disease, and tireless advocate for the patient community. She is executive director of MitoAction.org, a national organization that provides quality of life initiatives focused on support, education, and advocacy. Cristy has a Master's in Nursing and Community Public Health from the University of Virginia, and has won awards for her innovative maternal-child health program, "BabySense". Cristy lives with her husband and three children in Boston, MA.